ADVANCES IN ANIMAL WELFARE SCIENCE
1985

ADVANCES IN ANIMAL WELFARE SCIENCE 1985

edited by

Michael W. Fox, D.Sc., Ph.D., B.Vet.Med., MRCVS

Director, The Institute for the Study of Animal Problems
Washington, DC 20037, USA

and

Linda D. Mickley B.S.

Research Associate, The Institute for the Study of Animal Problems
Washington DC 20037, USA

1986 **MARTINUS NIJHOFF PUBLISHERS**
a member of the KLUWER ACADEMIC PUBLISHERS GROUP
BOSTON / DORDRECHT / LANCASTER

Distributors

for the United States and Canada: Kluwer Academic Publishers, 190 Old Derby Street, Hingham, MA 02043, USA
for the UK and Ireland: Kluwer Academic Publishers, MTP Press Limited, Falcon House, Queen Square, Lancaster LA1 1RN, UK
for all other countries: Kluwer Academic Publishers Group, Distribution Center, P.O. Box 322, 3300 AH Dordrecht, The Netherlands

Library of Congress Cataloging in Publication Data

ISBN 0-89838-776-0

PRINTED IN THE NETHERLANDS

IN MEMORIAM

Michael J. McCulloch

His life and work showed us the healing power of concern for animal and human life. We will long remember his pioneering contributions to the study of the human-animal bond.

MANUSCRIPT REVIEW COMMITTEE
ADVANCES IN ANIMAL WELFARE SCIENCE

Ron Kilgour Ministry of Agriculture and Fisheries, Ruakura Animal Research Station, Hamilton, New Zealand

Devra Kleiman National Zoological Park, Smithsonian Institution, Washington, D.C., USA

Elizabeth A. Lawrence Tufts University, School of Veterinary Medicine, Boston, Massachusetts, USA

Michael J. McCulloch Northwest Resource Group of Mental Health, Portland, Oregon, USA

Jenny Remfry Universities Federation for Animal Welfare, Potters Bar, Herts, England

Bernard E. Rollin Department of Philosophy, Colorado State University, Fort Collins, Colorado, USA

Andrew N. Rowan Tufts University, School of Veterinary Medicine, Boston, Massachusetts, USA

Harry C. Rowsell Canadian Council on Animal Care, Ottawa, Ontario, Canada

Joyce S.A. Tischler The Animal Legal Defense Fund, San Francisco, California, USA

G. van Putten Research Institute for Animal Production, "Schoonoord," Zeist, Holland

D.B. Wilkins Royal Society for the Prevention of Cruelty to Animals, The Causeway, Horsham, Sussex, England

Thomas Wolfle National Institutes of Health, Department of Health and Human Services, Bethesda, Maryland, USA

Foreword

This second volume of papers dealing with scientific and ethical aspects of animal welfare covers a variety of topics and areas of investigation. It will be of particular interest to those readers seeking more insight into such subjects as farm animal welfare and humane husbandry systems; animal experimentation, especially in the field of psychology; and pain in animals, notably its recognition and alleviation.

Several of our selections deal with very specific subjects that are germane to animal welfare: the use of T-61 for euthanizing cats and dogs, a new humane method of stunning for livestock and poultry, an innovative alternative to killing animals for rabies diagnosis, alternatives to aversive procedures in teaching experimental psychology, and the need for improved theoretical modeling in animal experimentation and research design.

Following the precedent set in the first volume of *Advances in Animal Welfare Science,* we have included several papers dealing with people's attitudes toward animals. These papers range from a consideration of cultural influences and veterinary ethics to an examination of anthropomorphism, to a discussion of the linkage between the environmental politics and perceptions of the Green Movement and animal welfare and rights.

We wish to express our gratitude to the Manuscript Review Committee for the excellent work they have done and to the twenty contributors to this volume which we believe will do much to advance the science of animal welfare, and the well-being of animals under man's dominion.

M.W. Fox
L.D. Mickley
Washington, D.C.

LIST OF CONTENTS

Part I
Farm Animals

CARDIAC ARREST STUNNING OF LIVESTOCK AND POULTRY

Temple Grandin

University of Illinois
Department of Animal Science
1207 West Gregory Drive
Urbana, Illinois 61201

Introduction

A stunning method that will reliably render an animal insensible to pain and sensation prior to hoisting and bleeding is essential to prevent suffering. Cardiac arrest stunning is more effective than conventional electric stunning. In cardiac arrest stunning, an electric current is passed through both the brain and the heart to produce *permanent* insensibility. Since the animal is killed by the electricity it cannot revive during hoisting, bleeding, or slaughtering procedures. In contrast, conventional electrical stunning induces *reversible* insensibility for a short period of time (Hoenderken 1978a; Grandin 1980a; Warrington 1974; Lambooy and Spanjaard 1982; Blackmore and Newhook 1981).

The advantages of cardiac arrest stunning are outlined below. If the interval between removal of the electric stunner and bleeding (throat cutting) is too long or if the throat is cut incorrectly, an animal may enter the scalding tank or have a limb or skin removed while still conscious. Cardiac arrest stunning practically eliminates this possibility compared to conventional electric stunning. Another advantage of cardiac arrest stunning is if the animal accidentally misses the bleeding station, stopping the heart will probably induce unconsciousness prior to the animal's being transported to the scalding tank or the first leg removal or skinning station. It has been shown that sheep become insensible 28 seconds after the heart stops without bleeding (Gregory and Wotton 1984a) Cardiac arrest stunning is recommended for sheep, pigs, calves, and poultry by many researchers in this area, including Blackmore, and Newhook (1981), Gregory and Wotton (1984d), Lambooy and Spanjaard (1982), Heath (1984a), and the Agricultural and Food Council (1984). A third advantage of cardiac arrest is that its use will help reduce injuries to slaughter plant employees from the animals' kicking during bleeding as the spasms associated with conventional electric stunning are greatly reduced or eliminated (Gilbert 1980; Gilbert et al. 1984.).

Insensibility Times

Table 1 shows the period of insensibility which is induced by conventional electric stunning. It also shows the time required for insensibility to occur due to oxygen deprivation from loss of blood, after both correct and incorrect bleeding methods. For futher information on the assessment of insensibility refer to Lopes da Silva (1983) and Blackmore and Newhook (1983). If the time required to induce unconsciousness from bleeding exceeds the length of the insensibility period induced by the stunner, the animal may feel pain and suffer.

Incorrect bleeding methods may greatly extend the time required for unconsciousness to occur from loss of blood. For example, loss of sensibility may be delayed by cutting the blood vessels on only one side of the neck. Blackmore and Petersen (1981) reported that failure to cut the blood vessels on both sides of the neck of sheep occurred 4 to 47 percent of the time, depending on the skills of the individual slaughter worker. Bleeding by an unskilled person may delay the onset of insensibility in pigs to over 60 seconds (Hoenderken 1978b). In poultry, failure to sever the carotids with an automatic neck cutter lengthened the time required for the bird to die (Agricultural and Food Research Council 1984).

Pigs and sheep lose consiousness relatively quickly after bleeding compared to calves (table 1). Studies by different researchers on pigs and sheep have similar results. Sheep lose consciousness quickly after bleeding because the entire brain is supplied by blood from the carotid arteries (Baldwin 1971; Blackmore 1985, personal communication). In calves, however, the brain is supplied by both the carotid and the vertebral arteries (Baldwin 1971). While the carotids are severed during bleeding, the vertebral arteries are not. After the throat is cut, calves may still receive blood to the brain via the vertebral arteries (Newhook and Blackmore 1982; Blackmore 1985, personal communication). Newhook and Blackmore (1982) report that young calves remain sensible for 65 to 85 seconds after the throat is cut with a possible resurgence of sensibility up to 123 to 323 seconds later. In older calves, 31 to 42 days of age, the onset of unconsciousness was 28 to 168 seconds after bleeding (Blackmore et al. 1983). The results of these two studies are in conflict with the findings of Nangeroni and Kennett (1963), Schultze et al. (1978), and Gregory and Wotton (1984b) (table 1). Blackmore et al. (1983) is unable to explain why their results differed from those of Schultze et al. (1978) and Nangeroni and Kennett (1963).

Gregory and Wotton (1984a) state that calves became insensible within 17 seconds. After the throat cut, responsiveness of the brain was measured utilizing electrocortigrams while a light was flashed in the calf's eyes.

The retina of the eye fails very quickly when it is deprived of oxygen or blood (U.S. Navy 1968; Fraser 1973). Vision is lost almost instantly when acceleration in a centrifuge forces blood out of the retinal blood vessels (Duane 1954; Newsom et al. 1968). Severance of the carotid arteries during slaughter would cut off the major blood supply to the eye in both calves and sheep thereby causing loss of vision (Blackmore 1985, personal communication).

Vision will fail prior to the onset of unconsciousness (Fraser 1973; U.S. Navy 1968; Vecchio 1977; Chambers 1963), but the auditory system is much more resistant to lack of oxygen (Heath and Williams 1977). There is some evidence that hearing may still be functional during the early stages of unconsciousness (Chambers 1963). New research indicates that visually evoked responses and somatosensory evoked responses disappear at approximately the same time after the throat is cut (N.G. Gregory, 1985, personal communication). After bleeding, visually evoked responses persist in poultry for at least one minute after spontaneous cortical activity has stopped (Daly 1985). At the present time, there is no good explanation for the apparent conflict between Gregory and Wotton (1984a), and Blackmore et al. (1983), and Newhook and Blackmore (1982).

Further studies by Blackmore (1984) indicate a large difference in the reactions of sheep and calves after the carotid arteries and jugular veins were cut. Sheep and lambs ceased coordinated attempts to rise after 8 to 11 seconds, and 1 to 7 day old calves stopped attempting to rise at an average of 39 seconds. If one carotid becomes occluded, the time was extended to 385 seconds. The time for an adult bull was 20 seconds.

A stunning method which produces either permanent or prolonged insensibility is essential for humane stunning of calves (Lambooy and Spanjaard 1982; Newhook and Blackmore 1982). I have observed calves reviving during bleeding in slaughter plants when conventional electric stunning was used. Calves may revive even if they are bled immediately after conventional electric stunning. In sheep and pigs, bleeding should take place within 10 to 17 seconds after conventional stunning to insure that the animals do not return to sensibility (Lambooy 1982; Blackmore and Newhook 1981; Leach 1978). In pigs, the absolute maximum allowable interval is 30 seconds (Hoenderken 1978a). Too long an interval between conventional electric stunning and bleeding is, unfortunately, a common occurrence in some slaughter plants (Gregory and Wotton 1984c).

Table 1. Insensibility times.

	Conventional Electric Stunning	Correct Bleeding Method	Incorrect Bleeding Method
Species	Insensibility period	Onset of insensibility due to hypoxia anoxia from bleeding	Onset of insensibility due to hypoxia anoxia from bleeding
Sheep	18–42 sec. (Blackmore & Newhook 1982)	2–7 sec. (Newhook & Blackmore 1982)	29 sec. (Newhook & Blackmore 1982)
	22 minumum sec. X = 43 (Lambooy 1982)	14 sec. Visual evoked potential (Gregory & Wotton 1984)	70–298 sec. (Gregory & Wotton 1984)
		3.3–6.2 sec. (Nangeroni & Kennett 1963)	
		4–6 sec. (Schulze et al. 1978)	
		8–11 sec. Stops attempts to stand (Blackmore 1984)	
Pigs	32 minimum sec. X = 66 (Hoenderken 1978)	12–20 sec. (Hoenderken 1978b)	12–62 + sec. (Hoenderken 1978b)
	34.8 sec. ± 12.45 (Swatland et al. 1984)	25 sec. (Blackmore & Newhook 1981)	

Calves & Cattle			
1 week old		39 sec. Stops attempt to stand (Blackmore 1984) 65–85 sec. up to 123–323 onset Resurgence of possible sensibility (Blackmore et al. 1983b) 17 sec. Visual evoked potential (Gregory & Wotton 1984b)	385 sec. Stops attempts to stand. (Blackmore 1984)
4½ to 8 weeks old	36–61 sec. (Blackmore & Newhook 1982)	4.4–6.9 sec. (Nangeroni & Kennett 1983) 28–168 sec. (Blackmore et al. 1983)	
6 months to adults	21–41 sec. (Lambooy & Spanjaard 1982)	10 sec. (Levinger 1979) 20 sec. Stops attempts to stand (Blackmore 1984)	60 + sec. Walking around (Grandin 1980
Chickens	30–60 sec. (Richards & Sykes 1967) 60 sec. maximum (Kuenzel & Walther 1978)	60 sec. (Gregory & Wotton 1985)	122 sec. (Gregory & Wotton 1985)

Note: All studies electroencephalographic or electrocorticograms unless noted.

Cardiac Arrest Stunning

To reliably induce instantaneous insensibility, an electric current must pass through the brain (Grandin 1980a; Croft 1952; Hoenderken 1978a; Roberts 1954). Enough voltage must be applied to force a sufficient current (amperage) through the brain. Only a small portion of the total applied current actually goes through the brain (Swatland et al. 1984); the rest of the current remains on the surface.

Cardiac arrest stunning can be done three different ways: head-to-back; head-to-leg, -brisket, or -groin; and sequential stun (Gilbert 1980; Lambooy and Spanjaard 1982; Blackmore and Petersen 1981). The electrode which is placed on the head is similar to the electrodes used for conventional electric stunning. The head electrode may be placed on the forehead, on the sides or top of the head, or immediately behind the ears (Grandin 1980a; Hoenderken 1978a; Croft and Hume 1956; Gregory and Wotton 1984d). The head electrode must never be placed on the neck. It is possible to induce cardiac arrest with a head-only stunner, but very high voltages and amperages must be used. A high voltage head-only stunner will not reliably stop the heart in all the animals. When cardiac arrest stunning methods fail to produce cardiac arrest, the animals will be rendered temporarily insensible in the same manner as conventional stunning.

Differences in Sensitivity and Variability

There are large differences in the sensitivity to electricity of different species, and in animals from different regions as well. A stunner setting which will reliably induce cardiac arrest in pigs in one slaughter plant may not reliably induce it in another. Practical experience and research data indicate that an animal's sensitivity to electricity can be affected by factors such as weight, fat thickness, access to drinking water prior to stunning, wetness of the skin, mineral content or salt content in the water which is on the skin, wool or hair coat length, skin thickness and age (Croft 1952; Hoenderken 1978a). A dry pig has twice as much resistance compared to a wet pig, and pigs with thick backfat had a higher resistance (Solis Cortes 1984, personal communication). Old laying hens with scaly legs have a higher electrical resistance than young broilers (Schutt-Abraham et al. 1983). Pigs which have had continuous access to water are easier to stun (Croft 1952). Calves have a lower resistance than pigs (Lambooy and Spanjaard 1982). Another factor which may influence the amount of voltage to induce cardiac arrest is animal contact with electrical grounds (Grandin 1980a). A portion of the electric current may pass through the restrainer or floor instead of between the electrodes. The restrainer should be insulated to isolate the animal from electrical grounds (Grandin 1980a). This is especially important for pigs and calves because they are not covered with insulating wool. The animal should not contact bolts or metal structures which are grounded during stunning. The restrainer should also be examined to make sure that dripping water is not creating electrical grounds. Cardiac arrest stunning can be applied either manually or by an automatic stunner. Three advantages of an automatic system are: safety for employees; consistency because it will not become tired, careless, or sadistic; and labor reduction. Automatic stunners should be rugged, simple, and reliable. Proper maintenance and adjustment is essential to insure that instantaneous unconsciousness is reliably produced.

Electrical Characteristics

The use of a power supply that maintains a constant current (amperage) is recommended. Constant current power sources are used in New Zealand, which is a leader in cardiac arrest stunning technology (Blackmore and Petersen 1981). A constant current power source maintains the amperage setting, and voltage fluctuates depending on the resistance of the animal. It is the *current* which induces unconsciousness (Hoenderken 1978a) and stops the heart. The voltage is the pressure which pushes the current through the animal. Less sophisticated stunners have a constant voltage power source and the current level fluctuates with animal resistance. Thus, the use of a constant voltage power supply is likely to produce erratic results.

The frequency and waveform of the stunning current can affect its ability to induce unconsciousness. Most stunners in the United States and Europe operate on 50 to 60 Hz alternating current (AC). This is the standard frequency supplied by the power company. High frequencies are less likely to induce unconsciousness compared with 50 to 60 Hz. Croft reported that frequencies between 50 to 200 Hz are suitable for stunning; frequencies under 25 Hz or over 500 Hz do not induce unconsciousness (Croft 1952). Hoenderken (1978a) reports that unconsciousness can be more effectively induced at 50 Hz compared to 1800 Hz. High frequencies, it was noted by Van der Wal (1978), seemed to cause pain but these frequencies provide meat quality advantages (Marple 1977; Warrington 1974). High frequencies are less capable of inducing unconsciousness because they stay on the surface of the animal (Horst 1984, personal communication) and stunners with such frequencies that cause pain or fail to produce instant unconsciousness would not be acceptable from an animal welfare viewpoint. Changing the waveform may produce meat quality improvements without compromising animal welfare. The use of 150 Hz square waves on humans reliably induced a seizure and unconsciousness with a 50 percent reduction in energy (Weaver et al. 1977).

Cardiac Arrest Stunning State of the Art

Sheep

Cardiac arrest stunning has been used successfully in New Zealand for many years. For all cardiac arrest stunning methods, the sheep are held in a conveyor restrainer or a restraining chute. As sheep have insulating wool, the electrodes must be designed so as to insure good contact. Manual head-to-back cardiac arrest stunners in New Zealand have a 3⅛ in x 3⅛ in (8 cm x 8 cm) saddle-shaped electrode which is placed on the back over the heart and two pegs which are placed on the head. Water jets in the pegs and in the saddle electrode provide good electrical contact through the wool (Frazerhurst 1975). This method is superior to sharp pin electrodes. The electrodes are spaced 16 in (40 cm) apart (Gilbert and Devine 1982). Some slaughter plants space electrodes 10 in (26 cm) to 13½ in (34.5 cm). The two pegs on the head are spaced 1¼ in (3 cm) apart. The electric current passes from the head electrodes to the back electrodes (Gilbert and Devine 1982).

In head-to-leg stunning, the electric current passes from the head electrodes to a leg electrode which is mounted on the bottom of the conveyor restrainer. To make contact through the wool, water jets wet the legs. Best results are obtained when the leg electrode makes good contact with the front feet. Automatic head-to-leg stunners have been developed in New Zealand.

Blackmore and Petersen (1981) report that 3 seconds' stunning at 0.8 amps at 400 volts and 50 Hz induced cardiac arrest 89.3 percent of the time using head-to-rear legs contacts and 96.8 percent using head-to-forelegs. Due to the wool covering, sheep are the most difficult animal on which to achieve a good electrical contact. Typical New Zealand sheep stunning equipment has a maximum output of 400 volts and is adjustable from 0.5 to 2 amps (Blackmore and Petersen 1981). Settings used to induce cardiac arrest and unconsciousness in sheep varied from 0.7 to 2 amps for 3 to 4 seconds (Gilbert 1980). The voltage varies from 100 to 400 volts depending on the sheep's resistance. Settings of 1 amp, at 300 to 400 volts, 50 Hz for 3 seconds produced unconsciousness and cardiac arrest in 100 percent of adult sheep and lambs (Gregory and Wotton 1984d). A head-to-back stunner with a 15 in (38 cm) electrode spacing was used. Unconsciousness was determined by an epileptiform response on an EEG.

Another cardiac arrest stunning method is split current or sequential stunning. A high current and voltage is used for the initial head stun to induce insensibility, followed by a lower current used to induce cardiac arrest (Gregory and Wotton 1984d; Gilbert et al. 1984). Gregory et al. (1984) used tongs to head stun sheep for 3 seconds at 300 volts 50 Hz, 50 volts were then applied across the chest. Gilbert et al. (1984)

applied 0.75 to 1 amp 50 Hz to the head for 4 seconds with two electrodes spaced 8 cm apart. The heart was stopped two seconds later with a second 0.3 amp current which passed from one foreleg to the other for 4 seconds. To prevent kicking, a third 0.9 amp current was passed from the head to the groin after a delay of 1 to 20 seconds. It was found that 100 volts was the minimum to stop the heart after the head stun. During these experiments, the researchers restrained the sheep by placing them astride a 10 cm (4 in) wide padded bar. This type of restrainer is similar to the one described by Giger et al. (1977).

Gilbert et al. (1984) also experimented with different frequencies to stop the heart. Square waves at 14.3 to 40 Hz and 1000 Hz at 400 volts failed to stop the heart, as did square waves (alternating current) at 14.3 Hz at 400 volts. Alternating current of 50 Hz was found to be the most effective.

Pigs

There has been relatively little formal research on cardiac arrest stunning of pigs. Hoenderken (1978a, 1983) found that 1.25 amps 50 Hz at 300 volts for 1 second was the minimum required for reliable induction of instantaneous unconsciousness in pigs. Practical experience in the United States and Canada indicates that cardiac arrest can be induced with a head-to-back stunner with a wide, blunt, flat electrode or two non-penetrating peg electrodes on the forehead, or immediately behind the ears, and a wide saddle-shaped electrode placed on the back. The wide surface area reduces electrical resistance. The electrodes are spaced 12 (30 cm) to 18 in (36 to 41 cm) apart. Fourteen to 16 inches (35.5 to 46 cm) is the most common spacing. Pigs must be wetted before the stunner is applied (Hoenderken 1978a). Water sprays should be located in the chute where the pigs wait in line to enter the stunning restrainer. Care must be taken that the animals are not dripping wet, as excessive water dripping off the pigs may create undesirable electrical grounds.

Preliminary tests with head-to-foreleg stunning indicated that 300 volts, at 1.5 amps for 1 to 2 seconds induced cardiac arrest in pigs (Swilley 1985, personal communication). Some slaughter plants that did not have constant amperage power units had difficulty inducing cardiac arrest with a head-to-back stunner even when the voltage was considerably higher than 300 volts. Due to the insulating layer of backfat on pigs, head-to-leg may be the preferred cardiac arrest method for pigs.

Many small plants stun pigs on the floor without a restrainer. In England, some plants used standard stunning tongs to stop the heart in pigs. The 90 volt, 50 Hz tongs are first applied to the head in the conventional manner for 15 seconds. After head stunning, the tongs are clamped on the pig's body for 5 seconds (Warriss and Wotton 1981). It is essential that the tongs are placed on the head first. This method must be monitored carefully by slaughter plant management to avoid abuses. This two-phase stunning is a practical solution to the problem of long stunning-to-bleeding intervals in small plants that have slow hoists. Many small locker type plants exceed the 30 second maximum allowable stunning-to-bleeding interval.

An automatic head-to-foreleg stunner has been developed in the United States by Wilson Swilley, Omeco Boss, and the author. The pig rides in a conveyor restrainer which was invented by Regensburger (1940) and is described by Grandin (1980c). Contact is made by the pig's head with a metal flap which is hinged at the top. The forelegs are contacted with two spring-loaded bars. The current is activated when the forward motion of the conveyor causes the pig's head to push the flap up to a 45 degree angle. The current passes from the flap contacting the head to the leg electrode. After stunning, the pig pushes the flap up to a horizontal position and is ejected from the conveyor. Here again, it is essential that pigs be wetted before they are admitted to the stunner. In smaller plants, pigs can be admitted individually into the restrainer with a gate to maintain a separation between animals. In larger plants, a second restrainer must be used to automatically maintain separation between the animals.

An automatic stunning system developed in Holland by Nijhuis will induce cardiac arrest in approximately 70 percent of the animals at a setting of 700 volts for two seconds (Spanjaard 1981). To induce cardiac arrest, the voltages and amperages required are higher than those required for head-to-back, or head-to-leg stunning. While this system by Nijhuis is not a true cardiac arrest stunner because the electrodes are applied to the head, it is an excellent conventional stunner and is used in many plants.

Calves

A stunning method that produces prolonged or permanent insensibility is absolutely essential for humane stunning of calves. Blackmore and Petersen (1981) report that a head-to-leg stunner set at 2 amps for 5 seconds produced 100 percent cardiac arrest. These researchers also report that 1 amp applied for 5 seconds with a head-to-back stunner induced cardiac arrest in 248 out of 250 baby calves while a head-to-back stunner set at 0.8 amps produced cardiac arrest in only half the calves. Present research findings indicate that 1.25 amps for 5 seconds would be the minimum setting for young calves. A constant current power unit is recommended. Head-to-back, and head-to-leg stunning equipment for calves is similar to the equipment for sheep. If the calves are wetted prior to stunning, water jets in the electrodes would not be needed. Sharp penetrating electrodes should not be used.

Lambooy and Spanjaard (1982) tested cardiac arrest stunning on large, 441 lb. (200 kg), six-month-old veal calves. The stunner had two flat metal prongs applied to the head and a saddle-shaped electrode over the back. Setting the stunner at 600 volts and applying it for 1 to 2 seconds killed wet calves immediately.

Cardiac arrest stunning can probably be used on adult cattle. Large versions of the small animal systems would probably work, however, large cattle systems must be carefully researched before they are approved for general use.

Poultry

To accomplish cardiac arrest stunning in poultry, the current must pass from the water bath in which the head is submerged and through the metal shackle from which the bird is suspended by its legs. The electrical resistance of poultry increases greatly as the animals age. For example, two-year-old laying hens required double the voltage for conventional stunning compared to six- to eight-week old broilers (Schutt-Abraham et al. 1983). Older hens have higher resistance due to horny scales on their legs. The electrical resistance of the bird's legs can be reduced by wetting the legs with a water spray (Kuenzel n.d.), or by placing the bird's shank in the shackle. Shank shackled hens had 30 to 40 percent lower impedance compared to leg shackled hens (Schutt-Abraham et al. 1983). The installation of needles or barbs in the shackles to decrease resistance is not acceptable for animal welfare reasons, because the birds hang in the shackles from the truck unloading area to the stunner which may involve considerable time or distance. Another variable which affects electrical resistance is the depth to which the birds are immersed in the water bath. Plunging the birds into the water up to their wings improved stunning (Schutt-Abraham et al. 1983).

A minimum of 120 milliamps (mA) is required to reliably induce cardiac arrest in broilers (Muller 1978; Schutt-Abraham et al. 1983). Heath (1984a) explains that the amperage is divided between the number of birds in the water bath; therefore if seven birds are in the water, 840 mA is the minimum amount of current required to kill them. Cardiac arrest can usually be accomplished by setting the stunner at 200 volts (Heath et al. 1983; Schutt-Abraham et al. 1983). Heath, however, warns that the reading on the voltage dial may over-estimate the actual voltage and amperage of the stunner. A setting of 100 to 120 volts killed only 51 to 75 percent of the broilers (Schutt-Abraham et al. 1983). A setting of 75 volts killed 8 percent of the birds and a setting of 95 volts killed 35 percent (Griffiths and Purcell 1984). The use of a constant current power source would probably improve poultry stunning because amperage would not fluctuate when the number of birds in the water bath changed.

Effects on Processing

Stillness

When conventional head-only stunning is used, the animal will kick violently due to the grand mal seizure which is induced by the stunner. A grand mal seizure must occur to make the animal or bird unconscious (Hoenderken 1978a; Warrington 1974; Croft 1952; Croft and Hume 1956). The spasms and contractions associated with the seizure interfere with shackling and bleeding. Animals are more likely to be bled incorrectly if they are rigid or kicking. When conventional head-only stunning is used, employees in slaughter plants will sometimes turn the stunner voltage down to reduce kicking. This practice may prevent the grand mal seizure and the animal may therefore be sensible during shackling and bleeding.

Cardiac arrest stunning greatly reduces or eliminates kicking, because the electricity passing through the spinal cord depolarizes spinal neurons (Gilbert et al. 1984). Practical experience with pigs and sheep indicates that a stunning time of 4 seconds will produce better stillness than will a 2 second stunning time. Good electrode contact is required for effective stillness. The electrode should be placed as close to the spine as possible. Head-to-back stunning produced better stillness in sheep than did head-to-foreleg stunning (Gilbert 1980; Gilbert et al. 1984). The stillness produced by head-to-foreleg stunning is still good. However, Gilbert and Devine (1982) report that higher currents are required to induce stillness in sheep with head-to-foreleg stunning compared to head-to-back stunning. Properly applied head-to-back, or head-to-foreleg cardiac arrest stunning will produce a relaxed carcass which is easy to bleed and process.

In pigs, head-to-foreleg stunning produced good muscle relaxation and stillness in the forequarters. Observations in the United States slaughter plants indicated that replacing a small back electrode with a large saddle-shaped electrode improved stillness and the carcass was more relaxed and easier to bleed. Cardiac arrest induced by a high voltage head-only stunner often produced a stiff carcass which was more difficult to bleed correctly. One advantage of cardiac arrest stunning is that the more relaxed carcass allows for more accurate insertion of the bleeding knife. This higher accuracy will help reduce the incidence of shoulder sticks which damage the meat. A still, relaxed carcass is required in countries where edible blood is collected through a hose.

Ritual Slaughter

Recently, Moslem religious authorities have prohibited the use of cardiac arrest stunning on animals which are slaughtered in New Zealand for shipment to the Middle East. Head-only electric stunning is still permitted. To maintain adequate stillness, a current that does not stop the heart is passed through the animal after conventional head stun. The current is passed from the forelegs to the hindlegs. Stillness can be maintained by either a brief current (spinal discharge) or a continuous current (immobilization). A 200 Hz 80 volt current applied for 5 seconds is most effective in spinal discharge method for sheep (Gilbert et al. 1984). Immobilization is accomplished by 40 volt square waves at 14.28 Hz. A similar system has been developed for Halal (slaughter according to Moslem law) treatment of cattle. A four-second, 1.5 to 2.5 amp head stun is applied in an automatic stunning pen, and kicking is suppressed by immobilizing the animal with a continuous 80-volt peak, 15 Hz, 5 msec duration square wave current (Devine et al. 1985). The Halal cut is made within 10 seconds after the head stun; before the immobilizing current is applied.

Devine et al. (1985) has tested this method in the laboratory with the EEG and determined that the cattle remained unconscious when the immobilizing current is applied. The immobilizing current appears to prolong the period of unconsciousness which is induced by the head stun. When this method was used under commercial conditions in a slaughter plant there were many serious problems (Blackmore 1985, personal communication). Blackmore states that the method can be further developed to be humane under commercial conditions.

For conventional slaughter, cardiac arrest is the most reliable electrical method to induce and maintain insensibility. Cardiac arrest stunners are simple and would probably be less likely to malfunction. If an animal regained consciousness while the immobilizing current was on, it would feel the shock and be paralyzed. However, electro-immobilization should not be used as a standard restraining method as it is aversive to conscious sheep (Grandin et al. 1985). Sheep will avoid entering a place where they have experienced electro-immobilization. Electro-immobilization was found to be more aversive than a mechanical restraining chute that squeezes and tilts the sheep to a horizontal position.

Carcass Bruises

Sheep and cattle, and to a lesser extent pigs, can still be bruised after stunning. Cattle stunned with a captive bolt can be bruised when they are rolled out of the stunning pen (Meischke and Horder 1976). In sheep, the use of cardiac arrest stunning reduced the susceptibility to bruising by 69 percent (Gregory and Wilkins 1984). The use of cardiac arrest stunning would help reduce the bruises caused by the animal's jerking shackles, falling on the floor, or striking sharp corners during the spasms which occur in the interval between conventional stunning and bleeding.

Bleeding

Livestock and poultry only lose 35 to 60 percent of the total circulating blood regardless of stunning or slaughter method (Warris 1984; Kotula and Helbacka 1966). Research indicates that livestock and poultry will bleed adequately after cardiac arrest stunning. Stopping the heart has no effect on shelf life of the meat, blood content in the muscle, blood pigment levels in the muscle and bacteriological levels (Chrystall et al. 1980-81; Griffiths 1983; Warris 1984; Lambooy 1981; Weise et al. 1982). In poultry, there was little correlation between the amount of blood lost during bleeding and appearance of the carcass (Newell and Shaffner 1950). There sometimes arises in poultry the problem of blood trapped in the larger vessels, which presents an unattractive appearance (Davis and Coe 1954; Newell and Shaffner 1950).

Cardiac arrest stunning applied sequentially to the head and chest of pigs with stunning tongs had no effect on the weight of the blood lost, rate of blood loss, or blood retained in the carcass (Warris and Wotton 1981). In one large pork slaughter plant, head-to-back cardiac arrest stunning caused small amounts of blood to be retained, and subsequently released into the scalding tank. There was no effect on meat quality. There was no additional blood contamination of the scalding tank caused by head-to-back cardiac arrest stunning in another plant. This plant had a well-trained person doing the bleeding and a five minute bleeding time. There were no differences in the appearance or quality of the meat compared with pigs stunned with a conventional electric stunner.

In sheep, the rate of bleeding was slower, and more blood was retained in the carcass (Kirton et al. 1980-81; Crystall et al. 1980-81). The retained blood was located in the thoracic cavity, abdominal viscera, heart and lungs (Warris 1984). This blood drains from the carcass during dressing procedures. There were no differences in meat quality between cardiac arrest and conventionally stunned sheep (Crystall et al. 1980-81). Cardiac arrest slowed bleeding of calves (Lambooy 1981).

Cardiac arrest stunning greatly slows the bleeding rate of poultry, but there were no significant differences in the total blood loss after 180 seconds (Weise et al. 1982; Schutt-Abraham et al. 1983). Blood loss at 90 seconds after bleeding was significantly less. Birds which had not been bled at all could not be distinguished from normally bled birds on the dressing line (Heath et al. 1981). Weise et al. (1982) found that a taste panel could detect no difference in the meat of cardiac arrest and conventionally stunned birds, and there was no adverse effect on muscle pH, juice retention, or keeping quality.

Some people believe that a condition called "redskins" (a cherry red color widespread on the carcass) is caused by killing birds with the electric stunner. Heath et al (1983) found that redskins are probably birds which entered the scalding tank alive. Red skin carcasses are produced when live birds enter the scald tank (Griffiths and Purcell 1984). Cardiac arrest stunning would prevent this problem. Veerkamp and de Vries (1983) report that poultry stunned at 200 volts in a brine stunner had significantly more reddened wing tips and tails than birds stunned at 75 volts. These authors did not indicate whether or not the higher setting induced cardiac arrest. Red wing tips are caused by rupture of small blood vessels when the feathers are removed (Heath 1984b). Reddened wing tips and redskins may be caused by different physiological mechanisms.

Accelerating Bleed-out

One possible disadvantage of cardiac arrest stunning is increased BOD (biological oxygen demand) from blood in the scalding tank and losses in total blood collection. Blood has a high organic content (Harris and Carter 1977) and its presence in the plant's waste water would increase sewage treatment costs. Many poultry plants have a 60 second or less bleeding time (Harris and Carter 1977), and doubling the bleeding time would force some plants to make expensive alterations or entail the building of additions to lengthen the bleeding rail. In general, pork slaughter plants will have minimal problems and poultry plants will have the greatest problems in converting to cardiac arrest stunning. Cardiac arrest stunning is used commercially in New Zealand on sheep; the advantages of increased carcass stillness far outweigh the disadvantage of slightly slower bleed-out.

A simple electrical carcass stimulator greatly reduced scald tank contamination in one pork plant. This device shocks the carcass during bleed-out, at 16 to 32 volts at 60 Hz. Dried blood yields in a plant with a stimulator and cardiac arrest stunning were at normal industry levels. An electrical stimulator used to tenderize and condition beef carcasses increased blood losses from the carcass (*National Provisioner* 1979). The use of rhythmic electrical stimulation to speed up bleeding in poultry has been suggested by Muller (1978). Stunning poultry at 480 Hz was found to improve bleed-out (Kuenzel et al. 1978). The use of high frequencies may make a bleed-out stimulator more effective. There is some concern that stimulating the carcass may lower meat quality in pigs by lowering muscle pH (Jensen et al. 1978). This would not be a problem in veal, beef, or lamb, as in these species, electrical stimulation is used to improve meat quality (Cross 1979). There have been many studies to determine the best voltage, waveform, and pulse time for electrical stimulation for tenderizing and conditioning meat (Cross 1979). Reports from the Commonwealth Scientific Industries Research Organization (CSIRO) in Australia contain information on waveform and frequency (CSIRO 1983, 1981). This information could be used as a starting point to develop inexpensive and practical bleeding rate accelerators. If excessive pH drop is a problem in pigs, the use of vibration may help remove the blood faster.

Bloodsplash, Speckle and Hemorrhages

Electric stunning sometimes produces hemorrhages in the muscle, fat, and connective tissue. These hemorrhages cause economic losses as they damage the appearance of the meat. The wholesomeness of the meat is not affected except in severe cases when bloody meat is trimmed. Sometimes the damage is so severe that an entire ham or chicken may be rejected. The European pork industry may suffer greater economic losses due to hemorrhages because their pork is sold with the skin intact. In the United States, however, superficial speckling in the fat can be trimmed away. Countries and meat plants which export have greater losses due to hemorrhages because the importing country will sometimes reject or downgrade blemished meat.

Failure to distinguish between hemorrhage types may account for some conflicting reports in the literature. Bloodsplashes are hemorrhages which occur in the muscle and internal organs (Leet et al. 1977). Splashes range in size from pin heads to half an inch (1.25 cm). Speckle is small "salt and pepper" hemorrhages which occur in the fat and connective tissue around muscles (Thornton et al. 1979; Gilbert 1980; Petersen and Wright 1982). The biological mechanisms which cause bloodsplash and speckle may be different (Petersen and Pauli 1983).

Animal Susceptibility to Hemorrhages

There are many factors which will either increase or decrease an animal's susceptibility to hemorrhages. The stunning method is only one factor. Observations in pork and beef plants in the United States and Canada indicate an increase in the number of animals with hemorrhages in the fall and early winter when temperatures fluctuate. Hemorrhages may increase when the temperature rises after a cold spell. There is evidence that vasodilation increases the amount of speckle (Devine et al. 1983). As the season progresses from fall to winter, the susceptibility to hemorrhages decreases in lambs (Petersen and Wright 1982). Hemorrhages decrease when the temperature becomes uniformly cold. Natural causes of bloodsplash have a larger effect on bloodsplash severity than do different electric stunning methods (Kirton and Frazerhurst 1983). There is also a tendency for lambs slaughtered early in the day to have less speckle. Bloodsplash levels changed on different slaughter days (Kirton and Frazerhurst 1983). A Danish study indicated bloodsplashing levels in pigs were not affected by holding time in the stockyards, sugar feeding, and type of truck used to transport pigs (Nielson 1977). Observations in the United States and Canada indicate that resting animals before slaughter may reduce hemorrhages, as livestock are transported much greater distances in North America.

There are also differences in hemorrhage susceptibility among groups of animals. For example, sheep from some farms had more bloodsplash than sheep from other farms (Pearson et al. 1977), and lambs that ate coumarin (anticoagulant) producing plants had more bloodsplash (Restall 1980-81). There also may be genetic factors to consider as pigs from different regions or countries may be hemorrhage resistant or hemorrhage prone. Large, heavily-muscled pigs have a tendency to have more hemorrhages and fractures. Younger animals may also be more susceptible (Thornton et al. 1979).

Stunning Method Effects

While captive bolt and CO_2 stunning usually produce less hemorrhages compared to electric stunning (Larsen 1983; Blackmore 1983), problems with these systems do exist. For example, concerns about the humaneness of the use of CO_2 for slaughter have been expressed (Hoenderken 1978; Grandin 1980a). Regarding the captive bolt, this method has a detrimental effect on meat quality in pigs, and therefore, electric stunning is the preferred method (Grandin 1980d; Overstreet et al. 1975). In sheep and calves, electric stunning is more economical and the brains (a consumer product) are not contaminated by a penetrating captive bolt. The nonpenetrating captive bolt which does not contaminate the brains, induces insensibility in only 80 to 95 percent of lambs according to Blackmore (1983), and unless this system is improved, it is not to be considered acceptable for lambs or sheep.

Cardiac arrest stunning produces less bloodsplash in the muscle compared to conventional electric stunning (Kirton et al. 1980-81; Gilbert and Devine 1982; Gilbert 1980). Bloodsplash is reduced because heart stoppage prevents a blood pressure rise after the stunning (Kirton et al. 1980-81). It appears, however, that blood pressure changes during stunning do not influence the amount of speckle (Gilbert and Devine 1982). Gilbert and Devine (1982) report that head-to-back stunning has minimal bloodsplash but will produce speckling in lambs. Head-to-foreleg cardiac arrest stunning was found to be the best method as it produced less speckle and bloodsplash than either head-only or head-to-back cardiac arrest in sheep (Gilbert 1980; Gilbert and Devine 1982). Head-to-back leg application of the stunner will produce more speckling than will head-to-foreleg application when the lambs are held in a V-conveyor restrainer (Blackmore and Petersen 1981). Shortening the distance between the electrodes on a head-to-back stunner reduced speckle in lambs; a span of ten inches (26 cm) was found to produce better results than 13.5 inches (34 cm) (Petersen and Wright 1982). The spring-loaded foreleg electrode must remain in firm contact with the legs as making and breaking the contact may increase bloodsplash and speckle.

Effect of Restrainer

The type of restrainer used to hold the animal during stunning can affect the amount of bloodsplash and speckle. A V-conveyor restrainer with a steep angle of 15 degrees from vertical on each side caused greater amounts of speckle than did a restrainer with the conveyors on a 55 degree angle (Thornton et al. 1979). An electrode position and stunner setting which causes speckle in a V-conveyor restrainer may not cause speckle in some other type of restrainer such as the double rail, or stunning without a restrainer.

When sheep were restrained in a hammock, head-to-back cardiac arrest stunning produced no bloodsplash or speckle, and conventional head-only stunning produced lesions in 10 percent of the animals (Gregory and Wotton 1984d). Observations by Mattson (1984, personal communication) of the Swedish Meat Research Institute indicated that pigs stunned on the floor had fewer hemorrhages. However, accurate placement of the stunner is more difficult when the animals are on the floor, and pigs stunned in such a manner are also more likely to have broken shoulders (Van der Wal 1976).

Human activities may also affect carcass quality. For example, observations in a pork slaughter plant indicated that more bone compression fractures occurred after lunch and coffee breaks. This was probably due to the animals being left in the restrainer. Observations with electrically stunned calves indicated that shortening the period of time the animal remains in the restrainer may reduce hemorrhages. It is the author's opinion that the effect of the restrainer on hemorrhages is not caused by adrenalin secretion or psychological stress, as I have observed pigs sleeping in the restrainer during lunch. Injections of adrenalin do not cause speckle (Gilbert 1980). The increase in homorrhages is due to the skin being stretched just before or during stunning when the animal moves against the side of the restrainer (Gilbert and Devine 1982). In a pork plant, bloodsplash and speckle increased when one side of the restrainer conveyor was broken and the animals' rubbing against the immobile conveyor stretched the skin and muscles. Excitement is likely to cause speckle because an excited animal will struggle and fight the restrainer. Mechanical stretching of the skin and muscle and opposing muscle groups interacting with each other during tonic contracture at stunning is believed to be a cause of speckle (Gilbert and Devine 1982).

The V-conveyor restrainer is an excellent system for the humane handling of animals. All livestock except baby calves will enter the restrainer easily and ride in it with a minimum of excitement. Restrainer induced speckle can be greatly reduced by using head-to-foreleg stunning, changing the angle of the conveyors, and removing the animals from the restrainer when the slaughter line is stopped. The use of the double rail restrainer (Giger et al. 1977) and new restrainer designs should be investigated. The use of a squeeze restrainer may help to reduce hemorrhages in smaller plants. This restrainer holds a pig for only a few seconds between two padded panels.. This system requires less space than a V-conveyor restrainer and it can handle up to 300 pigs per hour.

Stunning Time, Voltage Amperage and Frequency Effects

Shortening the interval between electric stunning and bleeding will help prevent hemorrhages in pigs and sheep (Warrington 1974; Burson et al. 1983; Calkins et al. 1980; Van der Wal 1978). L. Davey, Meat Research Institute of New Zealand, stated that bleeding sheep within 8 seconds after removal of the stunner greatly reduced hemorrhages. Practical experience indicates that when a voltage regulated stunner is used, the number of compression fractures and severe hemorrhaging in the hams of pigs is increased when the voltage was raised. In lambs, long stunning times and higher currents produced more speckle in the leg muscles with a head-to-back cardiac arrest stunner than did short stunning times and lower currents (Devine et al. 1983). In pigs longer stunning times of 12 seconds with 320 volt 50 Hz head-only stunning produced more hemorrhages and broken bones than did a 2 second time (Braathen and Johansen 1984). The use of constant current stunners would help prevent hemorrhages because high current surges would be eliminated. A Danish study on pigs indicated that 700 volt head-only stunning in an automatic system greatly reduced shoulder hemorrhages compared to a 300 volt manual head-only stunning (Larsen 1983). The 700 volt system induced cardiac arrest in many of the pigs. Stunning times were not given but the 700 volt automatic system usually has a shorter stunning time than does a 300 volt manual. The incidence of fractures in both systems was approximately 1 percent.

Increasing the voltage in a poultry stunner greatly increases the number of birds damaged by hemorrhages in the wing joints and broken bones according to R. Lewis Wesley, Virginia State University (personal communication, 1984). Stephen Pretanik, Director of Science and Technology, National Broiler Council (personal communication, 1985) also states that "When electric stunners are set at a level sufficient to kill the bird, considerable internal damage is caused to the bird." Some examples of the damage are broken bones, and bloody areas in the meat and joints. Turkeys have severe contusions of the breast muscles and bloodsplash if the amperage is too high (Howard Hunter 1984, personal communication). Wesley (personal communication, 1984) states that damage can be prevented by conventional stunning at less than 40 volts at high frequency for 7 seconds. Kuenzel and Walther (1978) recommend 480 Hz. There is a need for research to verify that this method of conventional stunning induces unconsciousness. According to Kuenzel and Walther (1978) a peak voltage of 100 volts, average voltage of 30 volts at 480 Hz is required.

Electric Prods

The use of electric prods to drive animals may increase bloodsplash and speckle. Calkins et al. (1980) found that pigs driven with an electric prod had almost twice as many hemorrhages compared with pigs driven with a leather strap. The exact specifications of the prods was not known, but they were either connected to a transformer which stepped down the voltage from 120 volts AC 60 Hz, or they had a small light bulb wired in series to serve as a resistor. Although it is illegal to connect prods directly to the house current without a transformer, some plants still engage in this practice. Observations in Europe indicated that it was difficult to induce hemorrhages by prodding pigs in the leadup chute with a battery operated electric prod (Lambooy 1984, personal communication). A prod wired to a transformer has only a single contact and the electricity flows through the animal to the ground. This causes muscles to tense up. A battery prod has two contacts and the electric shock is localized. Pork plants with electric prods wired through a transformer found they could reduce hemorrhages and broken aitch (hip) bones by lowering prod voltage to 14-16 volts.

Shackle Jerking and Leg Movement

Jerking the leg of a stunned animal by the shackle chain can cause blood vessels to break in the ham. Sometimes hemorrhage problems caused by the jerking of shackle chains are blamed on the stunning method. Systems for conveying the stunned pig should be designed to lift it up smoothly without jerking the shackled leg. The animal's legs must be able to move freely during the spasm which occurs during stunning, otherwise, broken aitch bones and hemorrhages will result if the animal's feet hit an obstruction under the restrainer. Beveling the edges of the restrainer slats at the point where the legs contact may enable the legs to slide more freely during the spasm.

PSE and Electric Stunning

Stunning and slaughter methods can affect the incidence of PSE (pale soft exudative) meat in pigs (Grandin 1980d); Athen et al. 1977;

Larsen 1983). This condition lowers meat quality in pork (Grandin 1980d; Van der Wal 1978), but rarely causes meat quality problems in lambs, calves, or cattle. Shortening the stunner application time from 12 seconds to 2 seconds reduced PSE (Braathen and Johansen 1984; Marple 1977; Van der Wal 1978), because shorter application times have less of an effect on muscle pH (Devine et al. 1984). In sheep, head-only stunning produced a smaller drop in muscle pH than head-to-back-cardiac arrest stunning (Devine et al. 1984; Petersen and Blackmore 1982). In pigs, a lower muscle pH is usually related to increased PSE.

A Danish study in pigs indicated that 700 volt head-only automatic stunning caused slightly less PSE than 300 volt head-only manual stunning (Larsen 1983). The 700 volt stunner induced cardiac arrest in many pigs. A Dutch study by Van der Wal et al. (1983) with similar equipment showed a tendency for the 700 volt stunned pigs to have a lower pH and higher carcass temperature. The conflicting results are probably due to differences in the methods for measuring PSE or confounding of the Dutch trial by carcass grade. PSE measurements with an optical probe and pH sometimes give different results (Larsen 1983).

Swatland (personal communication, 1984), and Van der Wal (1978) state that kicking and muscular contractions after stunning increases PSE. Pigs kick violently after conventional stunning. The use of cardiac arrest stunning with a short application time may help reduce PSE because damaging heat buildup in the muscles caused by kicking would not occur. Pigs kick more violently after conventional stunning than do sheep, and heat buildup may occur more quickly due to the heavy layer of insulating fat. Practical experience in large North American slaughter plants indicates that shortening the interval between stunning and bleeding helped reduce PSE.

Other PSE Factors

There are many causes of PSE which have a greater influence on its incidence than do differences in electrical stunning methods. PSE is a complex condition which is caused by the interaction of many different factors (Grandin 1984; Canadian Meat Council 1980; Eikelenboom 1984). One of the most important factors is genetic stress susceptibility or PSS (porcine stress syndrome) as evidenced by the fact that different pig breeds and strains within a breed or crossbreed have different levels of PSS (Tarrant et al. 1979; Eikelenboom 1984).

Other factors may affect PSE incidence as well. Fluctuating temperatures and unstable weather conditions may double the incidence of PSE. Handling at the slaughter plant is very important also. Well-designed chutes are essential, as is the proper human handling (Grandin 1982, 1985). If they become excited in the chute leading to the stunner, normally stress-resistant pigs will have more PSE and lower meat quality (Barton-Gade 1984). Observations in packing plants indicate that gentle handling in the stunning chute reduces PSE. Showering pigs in the stockyards helped reduce PSE mainly by lowering body temperature (Smulders et al. 1983). In another study, showering had no effect on PSE incidence during cold weather (Mattson 1984, personal communication). These findings illustrate the importance of keeping pigs cool and avoiding overheating. A short, four-hour rest period after arrival at the slaughter plant is beneficial for meat quality (Malmfors 1982). Observations in North American slaughter plants indicate that slaughtering pigs immediately after arrival at the plant is detrimental to meat quality.

A basic principle is that a long-term stress tends to make meat darker and drier than normal and a short-term stress tends to increase PSE (Nielson 1977; Grandin 1980d). Pigs which have been on a long truck ride often have a lower incidence of PSE (Grandin 1980d). Long-haul pigs have less PSE because glycogen (muscle fuel) is exhausted.

There are unknown factors which determine the incidence of PSE. There are some exceptions to the short-term and long-term stress principle. Breeds or strains of pigs that are more excitable may have high levels of PSE after a long truck ride. Fatigued cattle sometimes have a PSE-like condition after electrical stimulation of the carcass (Fjelkner-Modig and Ruderus 1983). A similar condition may exist in electrically stunned fatigued pigs. Some of the confliciting data is due to the possibility that there are different kinds of PSE with different physiological mechanisms (Monin and Sellier 1985; Grandin 1984). Monin and Sellier (1985) found that normal stress-resistant pigs of the Hampshire breed often have inferior meat quality. This breed of pig has higher levels of glycogen. Different measuring methods might provide different readings in genetically stress-susceptible and normal pigs (Barton 1984, personal communication).

Conclusions

Cardiac arrest stunning is definitely recommended for the humane stunning of hogs, sheep, and calves. To induce instantaneous unconsciousness, the electric current must pass through the brain. Humane cardiac arrest stunning can be accomplished by placing the positive electrode on the animal's head and the ground electrode may contact the back, forelegs, hindlegs, brisket, or groin. Another cardiac arrest stunning method is to pass a current through the head first. A second current is then passed through the heart.

Sufficient amperage must be applied to cause unconsciousness. Minimum amperage settings for wet animals with good electrode contact are: market hogs, 1.25; calves, 1.25; shorn lambs, 0.75. Higher settings may be needed to induce unconsciousness if animals are old, dehydrated, have long hair or wool, heavy backfat, or dry hair or wool. There are many variables which will change amperage requirements. Amperage settings higher than these minimums will be required in many slaughter plants.

Author's Addendum

Is Electro-Immobilization Humane? A Review of Recent Studies

There have been concerns about the humaneness of electro-immobilization of livestock. Battery-operated electro-immobilizers have been developed to restrain cattle for veterinary procedures such as dehorning, and sheep for shearing. The devices immobilize the animals by passing a small electrical current through their bodies. The animal is held rigid by contractions of its muscles. The manufacturers of these devices claim that immobilization relieves pain and is less stressful than are conventional mechanical restraints such as squeeze chutes.

Two different research laboratories have found that electro-immobilization does *not* block the sensation of pain. Animals will react to painful stimuli while they are immobilized (Lambooy and van Voorst 1983; Lambooy 1985). Amend (1983) states that there is no reliable evidence that electro-immobilization is a pain reliever. Studies with the EEG in calves and sheep indicate that electro-immobilization does *not* induce electro-anesthesia or electro-sleep (Lambooy and van Vorst 1983). The animals remain sensible during electro-immobilization.

Research conducted by Grandin, Curtis, Widoski and Thurmon (1985) indicates that electro-immobilization is more aversive (disliked) than is restraint in a squeeze tilt table. In a choice test, sheep preferred to be restrained in the squeeze tilt table. The choice tests were conducted in a specially designed sheep handling facility. It had a Y-chute which led to either an electro-immobilizer or to a squeeze tilt table which tilted the sheep to a horizontal position. Each animal was given several choice tests. Ewes which made a choice were rewarded with grain after they were immobilized or restrained in the squeeze tilt table. Ewes that refused to make a choice within five minutes were released. They were not given a grain reward.

Three different commercially available electro-immobilizers were tested. The sheep's choices in three different trials were: electro-immobilizer 13 percent, 13 percent, and 8 percent respectively; squeeze tilt table 79 percent, 57 percent, and 71 percent; and no choice 8 percent, 30 percent, and 21 percent. Ninety-four percent of the sheep chose the squeeze tilt table again after experiencing it once, but 56 percent of the sheep never chose the electro-immobilizer again after experiencing it once.

The sheep became less willing to enter the handling facility after they had experienced both the electro-immobilizer and the squeeze tilt table. Some sheep had to be grabbed and forced into the chute. Electro-immobilization also reduced the sheeps' acceptance of a feed reward. All of the sheep which chose the squeeze tilt table accepted the grain reward, but many of the sheep that were electro-immobilized either refused the reward or only took one bite.

The day after the choice tests were conducted, many of the sheep were still reluctant to enter the handling facility. Gradually the sheep were coaxed into the chute with a bucket of grain and put in the squeeze tilt table. As experience with the tilt table only increased, the sheep became progressively more willing to enter the table for the grain reward. Some animals entered the squeeze tilt table repeatedly and were willing to be squeezed and tilted for the grain reward.

A study by Pascoe and McDonnel (1985) also indicated that electro-immobilization was aversive. They trained Holstein cows to enter a set of stocks. The cows were subjected to four different treatments in the stocks. The treatments were: control (held in the stocks only), saline injection, immobilizer low setting, and immobilizer high setting. These treatments were repeated ten times. Cattle which had been immobilized became more reluctant to enter the stocks. They had higher heart rates upon entering than the controls or the cows which received the saline injection. The immobilized cows also showed a more pronounced emotional reaction before they received the shock. The authors concluded that electro-immobilization was painful.

Carter et al. (1983) reports that one-third of the cattle bellowed when the immobilizer current was turned on. I tried putting all three commercially available immobilizers on my own forearm. The sensation felt like getting a shock, and it was very disagreeable. The sensation was similar at both high and low settings. Different people have reported different reactions to placing the immobilizers on themselves, from a thudding sensation to a very painful one. It is likely that different people and animals may react differently. In sheep and calves, there are large individual differences in the amount of current required to maintain immobilization (Lambooy and van Voorst 1983). Some animals required almost twice as much current.

Carter et al. (1983) measured cortisol (stress hormone) levels in cattle after they were dehorned. There were three different groups: immobilized during dehorning, no immobilization during dehorning, and local anesthetic prior to dehorning. There were no significant differences in the cortisol levels between the three groups. The local anesthetic group may have failed to have lower cortisol levels because they had been handled four times. The other two groups were handled only twice. It is likely that dehorning is such a painful experience that the cortisol levels reached maximum levels in both the immobilized and non-immobilized cattle. More recent research by Lambooy (1985) indicated that electro-immobilization is stressful. The pulse rate and plasma cortisol level increased greatly during current administration in calves, sheep, and pigs. Lambooy (1985) concludes, "Because of the dubious effects on the animal's welfare, the use of such an apparatus (Feenix Stockstill™) cannot be recommended."

For animal welfare reasons, I do not recommend electro-immobilization for routine husbandry procedures such as shearing, dehorning, or castration. A good sturdy squeeze chute is recommended for cattle. Electro-immobilization must never be used as a substitute for anesthetics during major surgery (Pascoe, personal communication).

References

Agricultural and Food Research Council. 1984. A practical guide to neck cutting in poultry. *MRI Memorandum No. 54*. Meat Research Institute. Langford, Bristol, England.

Amend, J.F. 1983. Preliminary verdict for electro-immobilization. *Int. J. Study of Anim. Probs*. 4:11-13

Athen, T.G., Ono, K. and Topel, D.G. 1944. Effect of stress susceptibility or stunning method on catecholamine levels in swine. *Journal of Animal Science*. 44:985-9

Baldwin, B.A. 1971. Anatomical and physiological factors involved in slaughter by carotid section, In: *Humane Killing and Slaughterhouse Techniques*. Universities Federation for Animal Welfare. Potters Bar, Hert, England. pp. 34-43.

Barton-Gade, P. 1984. Influence of halothane genotype on meat quality in pigs and subjected to various pre-slaughter treatments. *30th European Meeting of Meat Research Workers Proceedings*. Bristol, England. 1:3 pp. 8-9.

Blackmore, D.K. 1983. Problems associated with percussion stunning in sheep. In: *Stunning of Animals for Slaughter*. Eikelenboom, G., ed. Boston: Martinus Nijhoff. pp. 146-53.

Blackmore, D.K. 1984. Differences in behaviour between sheep and cattle during slaughter. *Res. Vet. Sci*. 37:223-6.

Blackmore, D.K. and Newhook, J.C. 1981. Insensibility during slaughter of pigs in comparison to other domestic stock. *New Zealand Vet. J*. 29:219-2.

Blackmore, D.K. and Petersen, G.V. 1981. Stunning and slaughter of sheep and calves in New Zealand. *New Zealand Vet. J*. 29:99-102.

Blackmore, D.K. and Newhook, J.C. 1983. The assessment of insensibility in sheep, calves and pigs during slaughter. In: *Stunning of Animals for Slaughter*. Eikelenboom, G. ed. Boston: Martinus Nijhoff. pp. 13-25.

Blackmore, D.K., Newhook, J.C. and Grandin, T. 1983. Time of onset of insensibility in four- to six-week old calves during slaughter. *Meat Sci*. 9:145-9.

Braathen, O.S. and Johansen, J. 1984. The effects of short or long electrical stunning times on pork quality. *30th European Meeting of Meat Research Workers Proceedings*. Bristol, England. pp. 22-23.

Burson, D.E., Hunt, M.C., Schafer, D.E., Beckwith, D. and Garrison, J.R. 1983. Effects of stunning method and time interval from stunning to exsanguination on blood splashing in pork. *J. Anim. Sci*. 57:918-21.

Calkins, C.R., Davis, G.W., Cole, A.B. and Hutsell, D.A. 1980. Incidence of blood splashed hams from hogs subjected to certain antemortem handling methods. *J. Anim. Sci*. 50:15 Supplement A (Abstract).

Canadian Meat Council. 1980. *Guide to PSE Pork*. Canadian Meat Council, Islington, Ontario, Canada.

Carter, P.D., Johnston, N.E., Corner, L.A. and Jarrett, R.G. 1983. Observations on the effect of electro-immobilization on the dehorning of cattle. *Austral. Vet. J*. 60:17-19.

Chambers, R.M. 1963. Operator performance in acceleration environments. In: *Unusual Environments and Human Behavior*. Burns, N.M., Chambers, R.M. and Hendler, E. eds. London: Free Press of Glencoe.

Chrystall, B.B., Devine, C.E. and Newton, K.G. 1980-81. Residual blood in lamb muscles. *Meat Sci*. 5:339-45.

Croft, P.S. 1952. Problems of electrical stunning. *Vet. Rec*. 64:255-8.

Croft, P.G. and Hume, C.W. 1956. Electric stunning of sheep. *Vet. Rec*. May 26. pp. 318-21.

Cross, H.R. 1979. Effect of electrical stimulation on meat tissues and muscle properties: A review. *J. Food Sci*. 44:509-23.

CSIRO. 1981. Effective electrical stimulation of beef carcasses and sides. No. 81/5. 1981. CSIRO Division of Food Research. Brisbane, Australia.

CSIRO. 1983. Effective extra low voltage electrical stimulation of beef—What you need to know. *Meat Research Newsletter*. Vol. 5 (September 26). CSIRO Div. of Food Research. Brisbane, Australia.

Daly, C.C. 1985. Visually evoked responses during slaughter. *Vet. Rec.* (Letters to the Editor). May 25, 1985. pp. 574-5.

Davis, L.L. and Coe, M.E. 1954. Bleeding of chickens during killing operations. *Poultry Sci.* 33:616-9.

Devine, C.E., Gilbert, K.V. and Ellery, S. 1983. Electrical stunning of lambs: The effect of stunning parameters and drugs affecting blood flow and behavior on petechial hemorrhage incidence. *Meat Sci.* 9:247-56.

Devine, C.E., Ellery, S., Wade, L. and Chrystall, B.B. 1984. Differential effects of electrical stunning on the early post-mortem glycolysis in sheep. *Meat Sci.* 11:301-9.

Devine, C.E., Gilbert, K.V., Tavener, A. and Day, A. 1985. The use of electrical stunning followed by electro-immobilization for the humane slaughter of cattle. *New Zealand Veterinary Journal.* 33:47.

Duane, T.D. 1954. Observations on the fundus oculi during blackout. *AMA Archives of Opthalmology* 51:343-55.

Eikelenboom, G. 1984. An overview of PSE in Europe. *Proceedings 64th Annual Conference.* Canadian Meat Council, Islington, Ontario. Paper 9-1.

Fjelkner-Modig, S. and Ruderus, H. 1983. The influence of exhaustion and electrical stimulation on the meat quality of young bulls: Part I—Post mortem pH and temperature. *Meat Sci.* 8:185-201.

Fraser, T.M. 1973. Sustained linear acceleration. Parker, J.F. and West, V.R. eds. *Bioastronautics Data Book.* 2nd edition. Scientific and Technical Information Office, NASA. Washington, D.C.

Frazerhurst, L.F. 1975. Interim report on current developments in electrical stunning of sheep and lambs. Meat Research Institute of New Zealand, *MIRINZ.* 442:1-9.

Giger, W., Prince, R.P., Westervelt, R.G. and Kinsman, D.M. 1977. Equipment for low-stress animal slaughter. *Transactions of ASAE.* 20:571-8.

Gilbert, K.V. 1980. Developments in stunning and slaughter. 21st Meat Industry Conference. *MIRINZ.* Hamilton, New Zealand. pp. 18-25.

Gilbert, K.V. and Devine, C.E. 1982. Effect of electrical stunning method on petechial hemorrhages and on the blood pressure of lambs. *Meat Sci.* 7:197-207.

Gilbert, K.V., Devine, C.E., Hand, R. and Ellery, S. 1984. Electrical stunning and stillness of lambs. *Meat Sci.* 11:45-58.

Grandin, T. 1980a. Mechanical, electrical and anesthetic stunning methods for livestock. *Int. J. Study Anim. Probs.* 1:242-63.

Grandin, T. 1980b. Is your hog stunner insulated? *Meat Processing.* February: 69.

Grandin, T. 1980c. Designs and specifications for livestock handling equipment in slaughter plants. *Int. J. Study Anim.* Probs. 1:178-200.

Grandin, T. 1980d. The effect of stress on livestock and meat quality prior to and during slaughter. *Int. J. Study Anim. Probs.* 1:313-37.

Grandin, T. 1980e. Problems with kosher slaughter. *Int. J. Study Anim. Probs.* 16:375-90.

Grandin, T. 1982. Pig behavior studies applied to slaughter plant design. *Applied Anim. Ethol.* 9:141-51.

Grandin, T. 1984. Reducing PSE losses. *Meat Processing.* 23(3):53,56.

Grandin, T. 1985. How to design hog chutes. *Meat Processing.* May.

Grandin, T., Curtis, S.E., Widowski, T. and Thurmon, J.C. 1985. Aversiveness of restraint by electro-immobilization or in squeeze tilt table. *Journal of Anim. Sci. Suppl.* (Abstract). 61:213-14.

Gregory, N.G. and Wilkins, L.J. 1984. Effect of cardiac arrest on susceptibility to carcass bruising in sheep. *J. Sci. Food Agric.* 35:671-6.

Gregory, N.G. and Wotton, S.B. 1984a. Sheep slaughtering procedures. II. Time to loss of brain responsiveness after exsanguination or cardiac arrest. *British Vet. J.* 140:354-60.

Gregory, N.G. and Wotton, S.B. 1984b. Time of loss of brain responsiveness following exsanguination in calves. *Res. in Vet. Sci.* 37:141-3.

Gregory, N.G. and Wotton, S.B., 1984c. Sheep slaughtering procedures. I. Survey of abattoir practice. *British Vet. J.* 140:281-6.

Gregory, N.G. and Wotton, S.B. 1984d. Sheep slaughtering procedures. III. Head-to-back electrical stunning. *British Vet. J.* 140:570-5.

Gregory, N.G. and Wotton, S.B. 1985. Poultry slaughtering procedures. Paper #2-18. European Meeting of Meat Research Workers. Albena, Bulgaria. pp. 87-91.

Gregory, N.G., Wotton, S.B. and Wilkins, L.J. 1984. The effects of inducing cardiac arrest at stunning on brain function, bleeding efficiency and susceptibility to bruising in sheep. Paper 1:13, *Proceedings 30th European Meeting of Meat Research Workers.* Bristol, England. pp. 25-26.

Griffiths, G.L. 1983. *Proceedings of Technical Sessions World's Poultry Science Assn.* Adelaide, Australia.

Griffiths, G.L. and Purcell, D.A. 1984. A survey of slaughter procedures used in chicken processing plants. *Aust. Vet. J.* 61:399-401.

Harris, C.E. and Carter, T.A. 1977. Broiler blood losses with manual and mechanical killers. *Poultry Sci.* 56:1827-31.

Heath, D. and Williams, D.R. 1977. *Man at High Altitude.* London: Churchill Livingstone.

Heath, G.B.S. 1984a. Slaughter of broilers. *Vet. Rec.* 115:98-100.

Heath, G.B.S. 1984b. The slaughter of broiler chickens. *World's Poultry Sci. J.* 40:151-9.

Heath, G.B.S., Watt, D.J., Waite, P.R. and Ormond, J.M. 1981. Observations of poultry slaughter. *Vet. Rec. J.* 108:97-99.

Heath, G.B.S., Watt, D.J., Waite, P.R. and Meakings, P.A. 1983. Further observations on the slaughter of poultry. *British Vet. J.* 139:285-90.

Hoenderken, R. 1978a. Electrical stunning of pigs for slaughter. Why? *Hearing on Preslaughter Stunning.* Kavlinge, Sweden. May 19, 1978.

Hoenderken, R. 1978b. Electrical stunning of slaughter pigs. Thesis, State University. Utrecht, The Netherlands.

Hoenderken, R. 1983. Electrical and carbon dioxide stunning of pigs for slaughter. In: Eikelenboom, G. ed. *Stunning of Animals for Slaughter.* Boston: Martinus Nijhoff. pp. 59-63.

Jensen, J.H., Jul, M. and Zirck, O. 1978. Electrical stimulation of pig carcasses. *International Congress of Food Science and Technology Abstracts.* p. 124.

Kirton, A.H. and Frazerhurst, L.F. 1983. Effects of normal, light normal or double stunning on the incidence and severity of bloodsplash in lambs. *Meat Sci.* 9:1-6.

Kirton, A.H., Frazerhust, L.F., Woods, E.G. and Chrystall, B.B. 1980-81. Effect of electrical stunning method and cardiac arrest on bleeding efficiency, residual blood and bloodsplash in lambs. *Meat Sci.* 5:347-53.

Kotula, A.W. and Helbacka, N.V. 1966. Blood volume of live chickens and the influence of slaughter technique on blood loss. *Poultry Sci.* 45:684-8.

Kuenzel, W.J., Ingling, A.L., Denbow, M.D., Walther, J.H. and Schaeffer, M.M. 1978. Variable frequency stunning and the comparison of two bleed-out time intervals for maximizing blood release in processed poultry. *Poultry Sci.* 57:449-54.

Kuenzel, W.J. and Walther, J.H. 1978. Heart beat, blood pressure, respiration and brain waves of broilers as affected by electrical stunning and bleed-out. *Poultry Sci.* 57:655-9.

Kuenzel, W.J. (no date) Stunning, killing and bleeding: Specifications, carcass quality and welfare concerns. pp. 63-66.

Lambooy, E. 1981. Electrical stunning and meat quality of veal calves. *27th European Meeting of Meat Research Workers, Proceedings.* Vienna, Austria, August 24-28, pp. 196-7.

Lambooy, E. 1982. Electrical stunning of sheep. *Meat Sci.* 6:123-35.

Lambooy, E. and Spanjaard, W. 1982. Electrical stunning of veal calves. *Meat Sci.* 6:15-25.

Lambooy, E. 1985. Electro-anesthesia or electroimmobilization of calves, sheep, and pigs by the Feenix Stockstill. *The Vet. Quart.* 7:120-6.

Lambooy, E. and Van Voorst, N. 1985. Electro-anesthesia of calves and sheep. In: Eikelenboom, G. ed. *Stunning of Animals for Slaughter.* Boston: Martinus Nijhoff. pp. 117-23.

Larsen, K.H. 1983. Comparison of 300 volt manual stunning, 700 volt automatic stunning and CO_2 compact stunning with respect to quality parameters, blood splashing, fractures and meat quality, In: Eikelenboom, G. ed. *Stunning of Animals for Slaughter.* Boston: Martinus Nijhoff. pp. 73-81.

Leach, T.M. 1978. Pre-slaughter stunning in the E.C. In: Fabiansson, ed. *Hearing on Pre-slaughter Stunning.* Kavlinge, Sweden: Swedish Meat Research Centre.

Leet, N.G., Devine, C.E. and Gavey, A.B. 1977. The histology of blood splash in lamb. *Meat Sci.* 1:229-34.

Levinger, I.M. 1979. Jewish method of slaughtering animals for food and its influence on blood supply to the brain and on the normal functioning of the nervous system. *Animal Reg. Studies.* 2:111-26.

Lopes da Silva, F.H. 1983. The assessment of unconsciousness: General and practical aspects. In: Eikelenboom, G. ed. *Stunning of Animals for Slaughter.* Boston: Martinus Nijhoff: pp. 3-12.

Malmfors, G. 1982. Studies on some factors affecting pig meat quality. *28th European Meeting of Meat Research Workers Proceedings.* Madrid, Spain. pp. 21-23.

Marple, D.M. 1977. The effect of slaughter and stunning methods on meat quality. *Proceedings of the Meat Industry Research Conference.* Auburn University, Auburn, Alabama. pp. 141-6.

Meischke, H.R.C. and Horder, J.C. 1976. A knocking box effect on bruising cattle. *Food Tech. Australia.* 18:369-71.

Monin, G. and Sellier, P. 1985. Pork of low technological quality with a normal rate of muscle pH fall in the immediate post-mortem period: The case of the Hampshire breed. *Meat Sci.* 13:49-63.

Muller, A. 1978. Stunning fowl. *Hearing on Pre-slaughter Stunning.* Kavlinge, Sweden. May 19th.

Nangeroni, L.I. and Kennet, P.D. 1963. An electroencephalographic study of the effects of Sechita slaughter on cortical function in ruminants. *Report.* Ithaca University, Ithaca, New York.

National Provisioner. 1979. Texas firm announces commercial electro-stimulation tenderizing. January 6, 1979. pp. 8-34.

Neilson, N.J. 1977. The influence of pre-slaughter treatment on meat quality of pigs. *NJF Symposium, Muscle Function and Porcine Meat Quality.* Hindsgavl, Denmark. Aug. 28th.

Newell, G.W. and Shaffner, C.S. 1950. Blood loss by chickens during killing. *Poultry Sci.* 29:271-5.

Newhook, J.C. and Blackmore, D.K. 1982. Electroencephalographic studies of stunning and slaughter of sheep and calves: Part 1—The onset of permanent insensibility in sheep during slaughter. *Meat Sci.* 6:295-300.

Overstreet, J.W., Marple, D.N., Huffman, D.L. and Nachreiner, R.F. 1975. Effect of stunning methods on porcine muscle glycolosis. *J. Anim. Sci.* 41:1014-20.

Pascoe, P.J. and McDonnell, W.N. 1985. Aversive conditioning used to test the humaneness of a commercial electro-immobilization unit in cattle. *Vet. Surg.* 14:75-76.

Pearson, A.M., Kilgour, R., de Langen, M. and Payne, E. 1977. Hormonal responses of lambs to trucking, handling and electric stunning proceedings. *New Zealand Soc. Animal Production.* 37:243-8.

Petersen, G.V. and Wright, D.R. 1982. Observations of subcutaneous hemorrhagic speckling in lambs. *New Zealand Vet. J.* 27:166-8.

Petersen, G.V. and Blackmore, D.K. 1982. The effect of different slaughter methods on the postmortem glycolysis of muscle in lambs. *New Zealand Vet. J.* 30:195-8.

Petersen, G.V. and Pauli, J.V. 1983. One stage prothrombin times and subcutaneous hemorrhagic speckling in lambs. *New Zealand Vet. J.* 31:4-6

Regensburger, R.W. 1940. Hog Stunning Pen. U.S. Patent No. 2,185,949, Washington, D.C.

Restall, D.J. 1980-81. Blood splash in lambs—A preliminary study using the one stage prothrombin time test. *Meat Sci.* 5:125-9.

Richards, S.A. and Sykes, A.H., 1967. Physiological effects of electrical stunning and venesection in the fowl. *Res. Vet. Sci.* 8:361-8.

Roberts, T.D.M. 1954. Cortical activity in electrocuted dogs. *Vet. Rec.* 66:561-7.

Schulze, W., Schulze-Petzold, H., Hazem, A.S. and Gross, R. 1978. *Deutche Tierarztliche Wochenschrift.* 85:41-76.

Schutt-Abraham, I., Wormuth, H.J. and Fessel, J. 1983. Electrical stunning of poultry in view of animal welfare and meat production. In: Eikelenboom, G. ed. *Stunning of Animals for Slaughter.* Boston: Martinus Nijhoff. pp. 187-96.

Smulders, F.J.M., Romme, A.M.C.S., Woolthuis, C.H.J., de Kruijf, J.M., Eikelenboom, G. and Corstiaensen, G.P. 1983. Pre-stunning treatment during lairage and pork quality. In: Eikelenboom, G. ed. *Stunning of Animals for Slaughter.* Boston: Martinus Nijhoff. pp. 90-95.

Spanjaard, W. 1981. Automatishce bedwelming/elektrocutic. G.J. Nijhuis b.v., Winterswijk, Holland.

Swatland, H.J., Brogna, R.J. and Lutte, G.H. 1984. Electrical activity in the cerebral hemispheres of electrically stunned pigs. *J. Animal Sci.* 58:68-74.

Tarrant, P.V., Gallwey, W.J. and McGloughlin, P. 1979. Carcass pH values in Irish Landrace and Large White pigs. *Irish J. Agric. Res.* 18:167-72.

Thornton, R.N., Blackmore, D.K., Jolly, R.D., Harris, R.E. and Marsden, N.A. 1979. Petechial hemorrhages in carcass fat of slaughtered lambs. *New Zealand Vet. J.* 27:181-4,189.

U.S. Navy. 1968. *U.S. Naval Flight Surgeon's Manual.* Bio-Technology Inc., Arlington, Virginia.

Van der Wal, P.G., Eikelenboom, G. and Lambooy, E. 1983. The effect of electrical stunning on meat quality. In: Eikelenboom, G. ed. *Stunning Animals for Slaughter.* Boston: Martinus Nijhoff. pp. 83-89.

Van der Wal, P.G. 1976. Bone fractures in pigs as a consequence of electrical stunning. *European Meeting of Meat Research Workers, Proceedings,* Vol. 1. (C3:1, C3:4).

Van der Wal, P.G. 1978. Chemical and physiological aspects of pig stunning in relation to meat quality—A review. *Meat Sci.* 2:19-30.

Vecchio, R.J. 1977. *Physiological Aspects of Flight.* New York: Dowling College Press.

Veercamp, C.H. and de Vries, A.W. 1983. Influence of electrical stunning on quality aspects of broilers. In: Eikelenboom, G. ed. *Stunning of Animals for Slaughter.* Boston: Martinus Nijhoff. pp. 197-207.

Warrington, P.D. 1974. Electrical stunning: A Review of the literature. *Vet. Bulletin.* 44:617-33.

Warriss, P.D. 1984. Exsanguination of animals at slaughter and the residual blood content of meat. *Vet. Rec.* 115:202-205.

Warriss, P.D. and Wotton, S.B. 1981. Effect of cardiac arrest on exsanguination in pigs. *Research Vet. Sci.* 31:82-86.

Weaver, L.A., Ives, J.O., Williams, R. and Nies, A. 1977. A comparison of standard alternating current and low energy brief-pulse electrotherapy. *Biol. Psych.* 12:525-43.

Weise, V.E., Schutt, I. and Levetzow, R. 1982. Effects of stunning broilers by means of alternating current on meat quality. *Berl. Munch Tieraztle.* 95:241-7.

THE DEFINITION, CURRENT KNOWLEDGE AND IMPLEMENTATION OF WELFARE FOR FARM ANIMALS—A PERSONAL VIEW*

Ron Kilgour

Ruakura Animal Research Station
Private Bag, Hamilton
New Zealand

Overview

Being humane to farm animals (welfare) must include (1) having a sound knowledge of their normal and anomalous behavior responses in a farm context and heeding this in a practical way and (2) adopting handling procedures which elicit minimal distress in the species concerned. Building up an ethogram of predictable responses and recording the patterns of behavior during key events, mating, birth, and care of the young are essential. There are still gaps in the recorded ethograms of farm animals. Objective measurements of distress, including an index of its seriousness, are also a priority.

The results from animal preference tests can provide some answers on which to base practical husbandry in the areas of housing design, optimal temperatures, the need for companions, factors which elicit aggression, acceptable feeds, and species' sensory capacities. Handling preference tests could also be undertaken. Overcoming inertia is a problem for both the owners and the animals if changes are to be made within established systems of production.

Gross cruelty can be countered by legislation, but the motivation for ongoing good welfare of farmed animals must come from within the workers/owners on the site. Trying to force it by legislation may be counter-productive. A five-point program for promoting practical animal welfare is outlined.

---

*Original prepared for CENSHARE seminar on "Behaviour and Welfare of Farm Animals," Minnesota, 1983.

Introduction

At times in history, the question of man's use, or exploitation of animals, has been raised for general consideration and this decade appears to be one of these times. It could be beneficial both for husbandry and for animals in farming systems; or it could lead to claim and counter-claim, such that the only loser will be the powerless one in the system, viz. the domestic animal. Since man emerged from hunting, and domesticated plants and animals, some exploitation of both has been practiced to the benefit of civilization. The wide gene pool for some of the basic food plants on which man depends has been whittled away in recent decades. This is also true of farm animal breeds, though a recent renewed interest in rare breeds has in some degree reversed this trend.

The current debate, on welfare matters, involves a reexamination of the "domestic contract" between man and farm animals, pets, fur producers, meat producers, traction animals, and those used for entertainment. The task of this paper is to set some of the guidelines, define some of the terms, so the debate can be creative and lead to some further clarity on the nature, present status, and responsibilities held by each party to the contract: welfarist, husbandman, consumer, scientist, and animal.

Definitions

Domestication

Spurway (1955) stated clearly that a domestic animal is "one which as a dead or alive object is accepted as having an economic function as a source of raw material and/or labor for man." The "social function" of pets and animals used for entertainment or sport should be added to this definition. Such animals will have their slaughter, castration, reproduction, feed, and working tasks organized to some degree by humans. The space in which they live, as well as group size, will be dictated by humans. Sossinka (1982) refers to domestication as the most extensive biological "experiment" ever undertaken by human beings, covering many centuries and still in process. A clear distinction is drawn between "domestication"—a process and a "domesticated animal"—the result or state. Martin (1973) provides an alternative definition of domestication as "adaptation to captivity via population genetic mechanisms in which natural selection is largely replaced by artificial selection." Whatever the definition adopted, mankind has invested in a domestic farm animal for some return (Kilgour 1980).

Questions about welfare come after the acceptance that domestication is permissible and will continue—that domestic animals have a place in current society. Challenging the right of humans to domesticate a plant or animal is quite another issue.

Humane care

Mankind exerts control, therefore, mankind must exercise responsible stewardship over domestic animals. Whereas the domesticated jungle fowl or village pig still had a remote chance of escape and return to the "wild" life-style, modern intensively-housed animals have lost this opportunity completely. They must either adapt, show ill thrift as they try to cope, or die. As the degree of control on animals continues to intensify, so we are challenged with the question, "are we being responsible and just in the way we husband and handle animals?"

A number of definitions of animal welfare have been proposed. For example, Hughes (1976) suggested that "welfare is a state of complete mental and physical health in which an animal is in harmony with its environment." He proposed that an animal should be studied in an environment assumed to be ideal, for comparison with animals in their present intensive farming habitat.

If an attempt is made to apply such a definition to people, few would agree in practice on what constitutes "complete" mental health. Many people who regard their welfare as quite adequate may live with ailments, injuries, or physical disabilities brought on by age, which would be at considerable variance with "complete" physical health. Talking to farmers about "complete" mental health in animals is not very helpful. Even welfare as a term has a paternalistic overtone. The term "humane" is more appropriate.

In being "humane" to animals (Kilgour 1978), we must care for and handle them in a manner which causes them the least amount of distress. This can only be done when we fully understand the behavior of the species and their species-specific requirements. This operational definition of welfare links two fundamental areas of study, stress and behavior (Kilgour 1983). The objective assessment of an animal's behavioral repertoire and some key species' requirements is possible though often we lack the will and resources to systematically document their ethograms fully. Modern assays and sampling devices allow some estimates to be made of the distress of an animal during housing or handling, either by monitoring heart or breathing rates, or hormone levels in the blood.

To assist farmers directly involved with domestic animals, we need to frame up more practical questions like: Are the animals behaving normally? Are they producing normally? Are they free from injury and disease? Are the animals housed and handled without undue distress and in accordance with their species' responses and requirements? If the farming systems met these criteria, it is likely that minimum welfare would be satisfied, though the systems might still be improved. If minimum welfare is not met, then is the system able to be changed to satisfy the criteria? Has the system to be abandoned and if so, what are the appropriate and viable alternatives? Hens will have to live in cages until a real alternative is provided for them (Wegner 1983). It is pointless returning to a deep litter system with all its inadequacies for the laying hen.

The "Welfare" Debate

Parties to the current welfare debate

There are five broad viewpoints in the current "welfare debate" (Kilgour 1980).

Welfarists

Some people are mildly opposed while others strongly reject many or all forms of intensive husbandry and housing of animals. Some have made a balanced study of modern farming methods and have constructive comments to offer. Others use highly emotive claims which may well be counter-productive as farm owners reject out of hand all such suggestions whether helpful or ridiculous.

Owners and farmers

These are the people who have elected to gain a livelihood from farming animals. As units became larger, the proportion of the population directly involved in animal industries has declined. Farmers have greatly reduced political influence and may be subjected to strong economic pressures by the rest of society. They can easily get locked into agribusiness.

The public—consumer

In general, interest in welfare is minimal unless the media draws key issues to the public's attention. On occasions the media provides little background on which to make an informed decision, so the general public tend to remain bewildered spectators. At times, there is resistance to paying more for food even though this might arise as a consequence of improved welfare. Public education campaigns have been promoted by both welfare groups and animal producer boards in some countries. School educational packets for teachers are now available.

Research workers

These people are commissioned among other things to explore the behavior patterns of domestic animals, their nutritional requirements, inoculation programs and general health, housing designs, and the external stimuli which lead to certain emergency reactions or panic in the stock. In theory, researchers are a disinterested group but they will have their own views as members of the public.

The animals

While the debate goes on and more data are collected, the animals still have to live within current systems. Their well-being could improve if husbandry and housing systems are designed to suit their needs more accurately. They may be at risk if ill-informed people force change on the farming industry for change's sake, or corners are cut because of costs. Animals can also be tested to gather more information about their preferences and behavior responses (Klopfer et al. 1981; Kilgour et al. 1984).

The motivation for good welfare

In a recent review of livestock behavior, Kilgour and Dalton (1984) summarized the source of motivation and welfare, "good farm animal welfare grows from the concerned and informed farmer's response. Legislation will do little to change human behavior or affect human motives. Laws are needed to cover cases of gross cruelty, but codes of practice are more helpful guidelines to improve and suggest ways in which the welfare of livestock can be improved. The husbandman must finally be responsible for the animals in the system and their management, as the terms of the 'domestic contract' are upheld. Codes will be the guide."

Much of the pressure for welfare today comes from people in the ever-growing urban centers who may have little practical experience with rural problems. The divorce of understanding between town and country is an issue facing many developed countries at this time. As the media and the legislature are largely urban-based, the urban welfare lobby's power will continue to grow. Unless animal farming systems are changed with care, the welfare of the animals at present in the system will be at very great risk. To this end, encouraging a farmer's pride may in the long run attain more responsible actions than constant harping criticism.

Improved welfare (animal housing, etc.) costs money. An individual farmer with a concern for welfare could place him or herself at an economic disadvantage compared with others without such interest. When animal products cross national boundaries, countries with higher cost structures resulting from new welfare laws may undermine any former export market advantage.

The nature of the debate

Lindgren (1976), when discussing the conflict between technical advances and ethics in animal production, attempts to state the nature of the issues largely from the point of view of the farming industry. He summarizes the debate as follows.

Most objections to modern animal production systems focus on several factors:

A. Cruelty. This is stated to be affected by the following:

i. *Confinement* with animal deprived of adequate space, sunlight, pasture, etc.

ii. *Automation* when animals are dealt with by machines and/or may be deprived of companionship, etc.

iii. *Rough handling* during transportation and slaughter or mutilation such as castration, beak trimming, etc.

iv. Excessive *pressures* for high yields.

B. Impairment of quality of the products. Objections are often raised about too much processing, medication in the food, or the use of growth promotants.

C. Impairment of animal health. As production systems change so do the associated disease syndromes. Larger units also present greater risks of disease outbreak.

D. Environmental pollution. This can be at several levels:

i. Micro-level objections as animals increase their resistance to drugs.

ii. Macro-level objections to the pollution of the surrounding areas by smell and wastes, and

iii. human mental pollution which may arise from humans treating animals purely as industrial raw materials.

In the discussion, Lindgren (1976) suggested that the factors related to "cruelty" are probably over-rated, but that genuine objections can be raised on matters of product quality and animal health as long as people keep to facts and not resort to opinions. He classified objectors to large-scale animal production as: (1) *Primary critics* who include sincere people who support the welfare cause and who have sound reasons for their opinions, or (2) *Secondary critics* who use the issue for political, media, or radical objectives. In summary, Lindgren suggests: (a) that criticism must always be heard, (b) that public education must be continued and (c) that some international standards of sound management covering matters such as feed, wastes, and welfare should be established.

What farm animals are at greatest welfare risk?

It is not appropriate to talk abstractly about *"welfare."* The nature of the species which is at the center of attention is vastly more important.

A proper consideration of the welfare of animals in the system will include: (1) the nature of the species, what their normal and abnormal responses are, the unique features of their life-style which need to be provided for and (2) the ways they can be handled such that they are least distressed by each operation.

Each species is unique and its responses have been shaped by changing conditions during its evolutionary past. Kilgour and Dalton (1984) have provided interim behavior definitions for each of the farmed domestic animals, highlighting what they consider to be the unique attributes of each. In this paper two species, the horse and the sheep, will be used to provide examples of the way points (1) and (2) above should be precursors to welfare considerations.

What is a horse? Firstly, a horse is a large animal. It can be dangerous or difficult to handle. The highest number of farm animal injuries to people come from horses (Kilgour and Houston 1979). Once riders have been hurt they may start to fear and even mishandle horses. Despite current knowledge about their size and the associated dangers, small children are still expected to work with horses! Secondly, horses are non-ruminants which have to eat for many hours, especially when pasture is scarce, to meet their requirements. Feral horses inhabit the drier rangelands.

Thirdly, in feral conditions, horses range over large tracts of country. On their daily movement to water they may cover distances of up to sixteen kilometers and their home range areas may reach a thousand hectares. Horses are an energetic species and appear to delight in exercise.

Fourthly, they are social animals and associate in groups, bands, or harems. Most usually this is made up of a stallion with one or more mares and the offspring. The rest of the males remain solitary or associate in bachelor groups. They develop strong social bonds, interact by grooming, or fight using bites or kicks when aggressive. The stallion protects his harem from the approaches of other bands and he may be able to gather up additional members.

Fifthly, to aid their social associations, horses show a range of communication patterns which include: (1) vocal calls. At least seven of these are used for short- and long-range contact and some of them carry over long distances; (2) body postures with movements of ear, tail, mouth, and head which indicate mood or social status at close quarters; (3) odors often attached to dunging rituals which provide information for the traveling bands of horses and mark the trails regularly used. Odors have a function in keeping bands intact and apart from each other.

The sensory capacities of horses are well developed. They have a good sense of touch, smell, hearing, and can see well at distances though they have limited binocular vision immediately in front of the head. They escape predators by flight and should they be attacked, they kick or buck in defense.

Sixthly, as mating is done within a harem structure, the stallions have little problem detecting estrus in the mares. The mares show a wide variety in their expression of estrus with little synchrony among females—a pattern which serves a harem life-style very well, but which is rather difficult to deal with on farms.

Finally, mares tend to foal at night when it is quiet. The bond between dam and offspring is made quite quickly. The young are precocious and on their feet, staying with the traveling mare within a few hours of birth. They suckle several times an hour and generally "follow" the dam. The dam protects the foal from the interference of other horses and teaches it much of her own behavior responses while it is following, including good and bad habits.

Is current farm or stable practice in line with the behavioral responses and needs of horses as presently understood? (a) Their keenness for exercise every day may not always be met. Stalled horses get little chance for movement and some of the "vices" which commonly appear may be related to the need to be active. Regular riding will be welcomed by horses and treadmills or excercise machines are used in some stables to provide for these needs. (b) Regular social interactions with other horses may not be provided, especially for the mares, which would be association with others in a harem group. The difficulty of detecting mares in estrus when isolated and a number of other on-farm problems may relate to the diminished opportunities for social interactions in the farm system. In stalls, a strong focus on the responses of other horses may mean that "vices" will be copied by others. (c) Horses spend many hours grazing. What happens in the idle time which is artificially created when horses, given their rations twice a day, are able to eat them within a short space of time? A major adjustment must be made by the horse and the occurrence of anomalous behavior (vices) often become part of the horses' adjustment. (d) Foaling at night. As stud animals become more and more valuable, people want to be present at the birth. This may inhibit the normally relaxed parturition of the mare. Sometimes horses are required to foal in stalls which are too cramped. In these ways, the husbandry systems imposed may be to the detriment of foaling. (e) Man rides a horse by getting onto its back. Before a horse is trained this can produce a response similar to that when a horse is sprung upon by a predator, e.g., a mountain lion, and much bucking results.

The best modes of handling a horse, and the critical time in a foal's development when training should begin need study. In many farm species, handling begins shortly after birth. I have heard welfare objections to foster rearing in species like calves as it "may deprive them of the mother love they get in nature" (Brownlee 1950). However, if handling is left until later in life, "horse-breaking" procedures may be required. Astute observers and horse handlers like Jeffreys in Australia or Ray Hunt in the USA make use of the knowledge of horse flight distance, and correct species approach patterns, to be able to touch, harness, and ride horses within minutes of contact without the great struggle of "breaking" horses. Regular handling, gentling, a proper approach, adequate rewards during training are all important for "humane" handling without distress.

What is a sheep? Firstly, a sheep (Kilgour 1976) is a relatively defenseless animal. They gain safety in numbers. Modern day sheep are polled and apart from turning to face or charge a canine predator, and stamping their feet, they have little protection against them. Sheep flock. In fact, most typical species' responses will only be found in groups of three to four sheep or more. Tests of dogs at trials for their ability to work sheep, use three sheep as they tend to split up and make herding a most difficult task for the dog. My rule of thumb is simple, "Four sheep make a sheep." Sheep are also very vigilant and have good vision. They keep in visual contact with other sheep in their group and can flock together quickly should the need arise.

Sheep can be caught by using the blind spot behind the body when they have their heads up, but while they are grazing they can see all about.

Sheep tend to run up hill where they can see their surroundings and they camp at nights on more elevated points.

Sheep grow wool and though this insulates and protects them in cool habitats, it also makes them rather unaware of the cold at key times like lambing. There is little evidence that sheep seek shelter for lambing and under adverse conditions lamb mortality can be high. Pre-lamb shearing however will assist a sheep in making the best use of shelter, and as a result lamb mortality can be reduced where shelter is provided (Lynch et al. 1980). Sheep are open area grazers. They do not reach up and browse like goats nor push through undergrowth as their wool could get tangled. They graze in bouts preferring to take their requirements in less than ten hours a day. They are ruminants. Much of their water is gained from the dew on leaves of plants, though lactating ewes will need extra water. In semi-arid conditions, particularly where the vegetation has a high salt content, the distances sheep walk while grazing will relate to their need to return to watering points (Squires 1981).

Sheep are seasonal breeders in temperate regions, breeding in the autumn or fall. When the rams move into the ewe flocks, they appear to trigger the onset of estrus and help synchronize the ewes. A waxy material in the fleece of the ram is responsible for this "ram effect" (Knight and Lynch 1980). As rams move among the ewes sniff-hunting to find the ones in estrus, they need to be healthy and fit when required to mate a large number of ewes. Dominant rams do much of the mating in peak estrus while subordinate males check out ewes early and late in estrus.

Lambing occurs when a ewe has moved away from the flock. This allows exclusive attention to be given to the offspring and a good bond to be established. When ewe densities are high, lamb stealing or ewe interference can become common. This activity from other ewes usually occurs an hour or so before they lamb. This interference can have a disruptive effect on the lambing ewe and lead to increased lamb mortality especially in ewes with multiples. If the site set up for lambing is steep, lambs can slip and be lost. They may wander after other passing ewes (Kilgour et al. 1983a). A ewe should be undisturbed on the lambing site for four hours for good bonding onto single lambs and longer for twins or triplets (Alexander et al. 1983).

Eventually, sheep move away from the lambing site with their lambs following. Lambs suckle about once an hour and in association with the ewe learn much about the environment, the tracks, and good grazing areas. The whole tendency to flock arises from the early "following" patterns shown by lambs to ewes. Training "leader" sheep can assist the work on farms as sheep "follow" after leaders (Bremner et al. 1980). These are some of the essential and unique attributes of sheep as a species.

Some extrapolations to sheep welfare can be made: (a) Sheep should not be kept in isolation when they travel, are handled, or are slaughtered. A sheep without other companions has a raised heart rate and elevated blood stress hormone levels. It would take them several weeks to adjust to isolated conditions; (b) Shepherding at lambing may be a mixed blessing, especially if it interrupts the establishment of ewe-lamb bonds within a few hours of birth. Some of the benefits of "easy-care" lambing arise from the decrease in disruptive human interventions at lambing time; (c) It is legitimate to adopt husbandry practices which mimic the "ram effect" in the interests of good results at mating.

As a number of studies have been carried out on handling sheep and the measures of distress, it is helpful to focus on this aspect of the welfare of sheep. Kilgour and de Langen (1970) tied sheep up or monitored them as they went through various on-farm handling activities like dipping and shearing, and used blood plasma cortisols to assess their distress. Although the assay used was not a sophisticated one, later studies have borne out their contentions that sheep kept in groups are less distressed by handling than sheep in isolation. Later, Pearson et al. (1977) took serial blood samples from sheep leaving the farm and moving to slaughter to assess catecholamine and cortisol levels over the thirty-six hour period. Again, apart from lengthy water bath washing required by consumer hygiene requirements, the sheep were not unduly stressed until the actual time of stunning. With electrical stunning of the cortex, every physiological emergency process the animal has is switched on full, the catecholamines rise dramatically, reaching levels not shown in any other handling situations and cortisols also rise. But who can argue that "rendering an animal unconscious by the use of electric stunning before its blood is let" is, in fact, not in the animals' best welfare interests? What happens to a sheep in the hours after leaving the farm appears to me to be more important for its welfare then the precise mode of its final slaughter. Slaughter by whatever method takes no more than a minute at the end of a long process in which the transported sheep is washed, dried, and handled over a period of 24-36 hours. Each new hygiene regulation lengthens this stressful pre-slaughter process.

When considering methods of handling sheep without causing them undue distress, the excellent studies at the University of Melbourne (Hutson 1983) tested the principles of sheep handling first recorded by Mr. Hopkins.

Overall, fourteen handling principles have been investigated. Although more work was urgently required in this field, funding for this program was stopped, a tragic loss to sheep welfare studies.

Other Australian studies (Truscott and Wroth 1976) have examined the preparation of sheep for live export to the Persian Gulf ports. When troughs with pelleted feeds were offered to large flocks of sheep, some adjusted very quickly while a small group of "shy" feeders refused to feed. Once the new feed was accepted, most sheep adjusted very readily to shipboard environment although good ventilation is vital. Air extraction systems have been found to be the best. Feed and water containers which prevent spillage during rough seas have now been designed and are now in use.

Apart from the predator harrassment of sheep and the pain and suffering which results, there are few issues which relate to sheep welfare if they are run outdoors. Occasional droughts, or snowfalls can make proper care difficult. More information needs to be gathered by researchers about sheep reactions to housing, what the ideal site for lambing would be like, in what ways the best mating management can be practiced, what are the advantages and the disadvantages of high stocking rates with rotational grazing methods of management, and the relative pressures on twin and triplet lambs when raised by a ewe with only two teats.

A Multi-Faceted Approach to Welfare

Farmers can be given a short list of questions to help them assess the day by day animal welfare on their farms. However, farmers alone are not responsible for the changes in the humane treatment of animals which may need to occur. This is a total community responsibility, devolving especially on groups which decide welfare priorities and have a genuine concern for animals in our society. Five broad approaches to "welfare" issues have been suggested (Kilgour 1983).

1. We must use our knowledge of species' behavior and the distress associated with handling to identify areas of concern and change.

A much greater research effort needs to go into applied ethology or the scientific study of farm animal behavior. What is the current research effort in this field? Are groups which state they have an interest in farm animal welfare willing to fund research in this field to show their genuine interest? More complete ethograms or behavior inventories are needed for each of the farm species. Further studies of animal stress during the normal on-farm routines such as handling, milking, shearing, drenching, weighing, and transport are required. The most reliable indices of distress need further refinement so that there is some unanimity on this matter.

Once the behavior repertoire is documented to act as a baseline for husbandry decisions, there remains the problem of ranking the behavioral needs in sensible order. The need to eat sufficient food is rarely under debate except in decisions relating to backfat thickness in pigs or obesity in domestic dogs. Starving hens as a method of precipitating forced molt arouses a greater debate. Does the fact that pigs and deer wallow in outdoor mudholes make it a behavioral need to wallow? If wallowing is to regulate an animal's temperature, avoid flies, mark territory, or distribute pheromones, there might be no need for such behavior in a domesticated or intensively-housed deer or pig.

2. More care should be taken to pre-condition stock to the farming conditions, housing, transport, handling, etc., which they will experience.

There are a number of studies indicating that tender, gentle care (TGC) has an important place in enabling animals to adjust to farming conditions. Gross and Siegel (1983) have examined aspects of socialization of chickens in groups which are gentled, ignored, or hassled and indicated a relationship with feed conversion and their response to challenges from *E. Coli* infection and RBC antigens. Hemsworth et al. (1981) have assessed the reaction of sows to humans and shown a positive relationship with house productivity as measured by the number of piglets born. Seabrook (1972) has indicated the influence of milker/manager on dairy cow production. Overall, this field is little explored though the advantages of bonding during sensitive periods for pups (Scott et al. 1974) to humans has been utilized by some dog trainers. More knowledge is required of how early shaping and pre-conditioning will enable animals to fit their farming environments.

3. Modifying aspects of the house, cage, feed or drinking unit to better suit the needs of the animals.

In 1969, McBride advised New Zealand poultry men to "fit their farms to fowl." In later research (McBride 1975), the floor area of a large deep-litter unit was restructured to see what changes in behavior would follow. Changes did occur and it was considered that the best quarters ended up like a rather poorly-designed tree. McBride (1976) concluded that a space could be cruel, comfortable, or boring and that attempting to define "cruelty" in terms of measurements of living quarters is not helpful. Tauson (1978) has taken "fitting farms to fowl" seriously. Some of his suggested changes for cages make them better quarters for laying hens.

While the search for more appropriate systems for laying hens continues, it seems wise and appropriate that the existing quarters be remodeled to fit the hen as best as is possible. There have been many reports of studies of cattle in stalls with a view to fitting stalls to cattle, but much more work needs to be undertaken in this area. Which research group has the responsibility of testing proposed engineering designs for new animal quarters or feeding dispensers to see if they in fact suit the animals for which they were designed?

4. Search for strains or breeds better suited to current farming or intensive conditions.

Heart rate studies of light and medium hybrid hens at the Poultry Research Centre in Edinburgh, Scotland, indicated that on presenting a standard "scaring object," the light hybrid, which appeared from behavior to be greatly stressed, in fact, had a rapid return of heart rate to normal. On the other hand, the medium hybrid, while appearing less concerned took much longer to adjust and maintained a high heart rate for much longer. Similarly, we have found in recent field observations on farmed red and fallow deer, that after handling, red deer take time to recover once they are returned to pasture. They appeared not unduly upset while being handled. The fallow get excited and disturbed during the handling process and injure themselves and their handlers, yet settle very quickly when returned to pasture.

Adequate objective criteria are needed together with appropriate tests to measure specific animal responses before any selection procedures can be carried out. The precise definition of the basic traits needed in the indoor or outdoor farm animals of the future is hard to clarify or forecast. In New Zealand, the move to select ewes which always produce twins has resulted in an increased proportion of triplets of lower birth weights and consequently high mortality rates.

If selection is to continue, all the available breed genetical materials must be retained. This is an important priority. The establishment of rare breed survival trusts is an encouraging sign and essential to future genetic programs of selection.

5. Preventing disease and accidents

Disease is considered by the Brambell Report (1965) to be the major source of animal pain and suffering. Programs of preventive health care are an essential requirement for the "humane care" of farm species. This is self-evident and prudent for the large intensive owner. Strict fire precautions, stand-by electricity plants, and early warning indicators of impending dangers such as increasing humidity or a buildup of ammonia are fundamental, and legislation and enforcement of such precautions are legitimate.

Automation, considered by some to be detrimental to the welfare of animals in intensive units, may not necessarily be so. The time saved together with reduced drudgery could free people for more man-animal interactions allowing better care. Many minor faults could be corrected before major breakdowns occur. Tender Gentle Care programs might become feasible with more automation. Automation could free more time to be given to training new stockpersons, take the pressure off existing workers, which in turn might reduce accidents and injury to humans and provide humane care for those who live and work with stock in large intensive farm units.

With this sort of multi-faceted approach, farmers, welfarists, and scientists could work together on the broad field of farm animal welfare for the ultimate benefit for the animals in the system. My concern is that this should be so.

Acknowledgements

I appreciate the constructive comments made by Drs. L.R. Matthews and D.C. Dalton after reading the original manuscript.

References

Alexander, G., Stevens, D., Kilgour, R., de Langen, H., Mottershead, B.E. and Lynch, J.J. 1983. Separation of ewes from twin lambs: Incidence in several sheep breeds. *Appl. Anim. Ethol.* 10:301-17.

Brambell, F.W.R. 1965. Chairman. Report of the technical committee to inquire into the welfare of animals kept under intensive livestock husbandry systems. Command paper No. 2836 (HMSO: London) 96 pp.

Bremner, K.J., Braggins, J.B. and Kilgour, R. 1980. Training sheep as "leaders" in abattoirs and farm sheepyards. *Proc. N.Z. Soc. Anim. Prod.* 40:111-16.

Brownlee, A. 1950. Studies in the behaviour of domestic cows in Britain. *Bull. Anim. Behav.* 1(8):11-20.

Council for Agricultural Science Technology (CAST). 1981. Scientific aspects of the welfare of food animals. Report No. 91:1-54.

Gross, W.B. and Siegel, P.B. 1982. Socialization as a factor in resistance to infection, feed efficiency, and response to antigen in chickens. *Amer. J. Vet. Res.* 43(II):2010-12.

Hemsworth, P.H., Brand, A. and Willems, P. 1981. The behavioural response of sows to the presence of human beings and its relation to productivity. *Livest. Prod. Sci.* 8:67-74.

Hughes, B.O. 1976. Behaviour as an index of welfare. *Proc. 5th European Poultry Conf.* W.S.P.A. Malta. pp. 1005-18.

Hutson, G.D. 1983. Sheep behaviour project: A final report to the Australian Wool Corporation. University of Melbourne. 194 pp.

Kilgour, R. 1976. Sheep behaviour: its importance in farming systems, handling, transport and pre-slaughter treatment. In: Truscott, G.M.C. and Wroth, R.H. eds. *Sheep Assembly and Transport Workshop.* W. Aust. Dept. Agric. Publ. pp. 64-84.

Kilgour, R. 1978. The application of animal behavior and the humane care of farm animals. *J. Anim. Sci.* 46:1478-86.

Kilgour, R. 1980. Animal Welfare—the conflicting viewpoints. In: Wodzicka-Tomaszewska, M., Edey, T.N. and Lynch, J.J. eds. *Behaviour in Relation to Reproduction, Management and Welfare of Farm Animals. Rev. in Rural Sci. IV.* Armidale, N.S.W.: Univ. N.E. Press. pp. 175-82.

Kilgour, R. 1983. Stress and behaviour: an operational approach to animal welfare. In: Baxter, S.H., Baxter, M.R., and MacCormack, J.A.D., eds. *Farm Animal Housing and Welfare.* The Hague: C.E.C. Martinus Nijhoff Publ. pp. 36-44.

Kilgour, R. and Dalton, D.C. 1984. *Livestock Behaviour—A Practical Guide.* London: Collins Professional and Technical Books. 320 pp.

Kilgour, R. and de Langen, H. 1970. Stress in sheep resulting from management practices. *Proc. N.Z. Soc. Anim. Prod.* 30:65-76.

Kilgour, R. and Houston, J.B. 1979. Handling animals safely. *N.Z. Fmr.* 100(18):157-8.

Kilgour, R., Alexander, G. and Stevens, D. 1983. A field study of factors interrupting bonding of ewes and twins. In: Mantell, C.D. ed. *Proc. 2nd Asia-Oceania Cong. Perinatology.* pp. 118-23.

Kilgour, R., Matthews, L.R., Temple, W. and Foster, M. 1984. Using operant tests results for decisions on cattle welfare. In: Hall, W.F. ed. *The Behavior and Welfare of Farm Animals.* CENSHARE: Minnesota Uni. pp. 205-17.

Klopfer, F.D., Kilgour, R. and Matthews, L.R. 1981. Paired comparison analysis of palatabilities of twenty foods to dairy cows. *Proc. N.Z. Soc. Anim. Prod.* 41:242-47.

Knight, T.W. and Lynch, P.R. 1980. Source of ram pheromones that stimulate ovulation in the ewe. *Anim. Reprod. Sci.* 3(3):133-6.

Lindgren, N.O. 1976. The conflict between technical advances and ethics in animal production. *Wld. Poult. Sci. J.* 32:243-8.

Lynch, J.J., Mottershead, B.E. and Alexander, G. 1980. Sheltering behaviour and lamb mortality amongst shorn Merino ewes lambing in paddocks with restricted areas of shelter or no shelter. *Appl. Anim. Ethol.* 6:163-74.

Martin, J.T. 1973. The role of the hypothalamic-pituitary-adrenal system in the development of imprinting and fear behaviour in wild and domesticated ducks. Thesis, Univ. Munchen, Germany.

McBride, G. 1969. Fitting farms to fowl. *Proc. 4th Ann. Poult. Conv.* Massey Uni., N.Z. pp. 1-9.

McBride, G. 1975. Behaviour and the design of the animal-husbandry interface. *Proc. 3rd Comb. Conf. Aust. Chicken Meat Fed. Aust. Stockfd. Manufact. Assoc.* Adelaide. pp. 91-95.

McBride, G. 1976. Improving the welfare of livestock. *Proc. 53rd Ann. Conf. Aust. Vet. Assoc.* pp. 7-9.

Pearson, A.J., Kilgour, R., de Langen, H. and Payne, E. 1977. Hormonal responses of lambs to trucking, handling and electric stunning. *Proc. N.Z. Soc. Anim. Prod.* 37:243-8.

Scott, J.P., Stewart, J.M. and De Ghett, V.J. 1974. Critical periods in the organization of systems. *Devlop. Psychobiol.* 7:489-513.

Seabrook, M.F. 1972. A study to determine the influence of the herdsman's personality on milk yields. *J. Agric. Labour Sci.* 1:45-59.

Sossinka, R. 1982. Domestication in birds. In: Farmer, D.S., King, J.R. and Parkes, K.C. eds. *Avian Biology, VA.* London: Academic Press. pp. 383-404.

Spurway, H. 1955. The causes of domestication: An attempt to integrate some ideas of Konrad Lorenz with evolution theory. *J. Genet.* 53:325-62.

Squires, V.R. 1981. *Livestock Management in the Arid Zone.* Melbourne: Inkata Press. 271 pp.

Tauson, R. 1978. Cage design and welfare. *Proc. 1st Danish Sem. Poult. Welfare in Egg-laying cages. pp. 63-77.*

Truscott, G.M.C. and Wroth, F.H. 1976. Proc. Sheep Assembly and Transport Workshop. W. Aust. Dept. of Agric., Perth. 196 pp.

Wegner, R.M. 1983. Production performance in laying hens kept under different housing conditions. In: Smidt, D. ed. *Indicators Relevant to Farm Animal Welfare.* The Hague: Martinus Nijhoff. pp. 189-96.

THE ATTAINMENT OF HUMANE HOUSING FOR FARM LIVESTOCK

D.G.M. Wood-Gush

The School of Agriculture
The University of Edinburgh
West Mains Road
Edinburgh, Scotland EH9 3JG

In discussing animal welfare it is very easy for the discussion to become bogged down by misunderstandings. Commonly the first misunderstanding arises over the definition of animal welfare. In the content of this article we will take it for granted that any definition includes the physical well-being of the animal as well as ensuring that the animal can fulfill much of its genetically controlled behavioral repertoire. The second misunderstanding arises when the political and scientific assessments of the subject are meshed together. In a scientific assessment, the aim should be to examine welfare problems strictly from what we know about the physiology and behavior of the species under consideration. In relation to the humane housing of farm animals, it should aim at informing the public of the pros and cons of different housing systems with respect to the animals' physiology and behavior. From this knowledge the politicians and their electorate can choose which level of welfare they can adopt while protecting their farmers, for example, from cheap imports from countries where the standards of animal welfare are lower. In this article we shall discuss from the ethological viewpoint how the various ways by which housing systems for farm animals can be assessed with respect to the animals' welfare, and how an ethologically suitable system can be attained.

Many people would advocate the use of production records as a means of assessing the standard of welfare of animals in a particular housing system. The general argument is that only contented animals could perform as well as those found in the average modern intensive system. However, closer consideration shows that production records are inadequate for the assessment of welfare. For example, it is possible for animals that are lame or otherwise injured from their housing to give an adequately profitable return. Furthermore, if production records are to be used legally as a guideline, there is the difficulty of choosing the correct standard. For example, is it to be milk production or milk quality? In addition, it is likely that today's standard may be at variance with the standard required of a certain class of livestock in ten years time. Finally, there is the fact that many animals do not achieve their full potential, for in many enterprises we cater for the average animal.

In order to improve housing systems, it has been advocated that the animal should be allowed to choose its own environment. A number of research workers have investigated this approach. Baldwin and his colleagues (Baldwin and Meese 1977; Baldwin 1974) have carried out experiments in which a pig is allowed to choose its own degree of illumination or to select its own environmental temperature. While such experiments yield some very interesting results, they have certain short-comings. An animal alone in an experiment may behave rather differently from one in a social group. Furthermore, environments have many facets and the desired mixture of these by an animal may differ from the picture obtained by allowing it to choose one at a time rather than in a total combination. In addition, animals may choose a particular environment because it resembles what they are used to (Dawkins 1977; Hughes and Black 1973). Strict interpretation is also difficult. Does the observation that animals choose one environment, or part of it, for a small part of their time, indicate a preference for the other environment or a real need of short duration for the former? Conversely, the choice of one environment over another by the animal may not indicate that the preferred environment is the optimal one. Dr. Marion Dawkins (personal communication), for example, has recently produced data which she interprets as indicating that the hen may not perceive herself as suffering in the battery cage. However, should stronger evidence support this, it does not mean that the battery cage is the best environment for the hen. Several equally objective studies have shown that the hen does find it unsatisfactory in certain respects (Wood-Gush 1972; Vestergaard 1978). Furthermore, when an animal alters the degree of illumination in its environment, is it doing so because it really wants to change the degree of light or because in a dull environment it wants some sort of change? In the wild, animals show a great deal of exploratory behavior for it is advantageous for them to know about their environments and of any changes in them. It is highly likely that this type of behavior is still present in our farm livestock species as studies have shown that they retain many of the behavior patterns of their ancestors (Desforges and Wood-Gush 1975). This tendency to explore the environment and to remain alert to changes in it suggests that the torpidity seen in many animals is likely to be a learnt response to a boring environment, rather than an indication of their true innate behavior.

The assessment of stress by physiological methods is potentially a very useful guide, and a number of endocrine studies have been carried out (Arnone and Dantzer 1980; Barnett et al. 1981), but there are a number of technical snags and more studies are needed on animals under conditions of chronic, as opposed to acute, stress.

When under frustration or when thwarted, animals show particular types of behavioral responses and the use of some of these behavior patterns for the assessment of well-being is promising. However, at present, their use is limited for we have no idea of their levels of occurrence under apparently optimal conditions. Nor have they been systemically studied in all species of farm livestock with the result that we cannot be certain of them in those species.

In some cases the relationship between overt behavior and concurrent physiological measurements are sometimes at variance with expectation. Baldwin and Stephens (1975), for example, reported that in pigs, emotional behavior such as vocalization did not correlate well with the discharge of adrenocortical hormones. In the case of the domestic fowl, a similar finding was made by Duncan and Filshie (1980) using heart rate as the physiological measurement. However, the performance of stereotypies does seem to be useful indicator of an unsuitable environment. These are short sequences of behavior or a single behavior pattern that are repeated over without any apparent objective. In the tethered sow, bar-biting and head-weaving are two examples of this. Experimentally they can be produced by severe frustration in which the animal is presented with an insoluble problem (Duncan and Wood-Gush 1972), but they are also extremely common in animals living in dull environments. Sometimes the behavior can be abolished by the addition of features to the environment. Fraser (1975), for example, found that the provision of a little straw to tethered sows reduced the incidence of stereotypies significantly. More recently, the occurrence of stereotypies in tethered sows has been correlated with release of endorphins (Wiepkema et al. 1984). While the performance of stereotypies may help the animal to cope with a dull, bare environment, the evidence certainly seems to point to the fact that this type of behavior is a good indicator of an unsatisfactory environment. Dull environments can have other effects on the behavior of the animals. Stolba and Wood-Gush (1980, 1981) found that fattening pigs from bare environments react significantly more strongly to a novel stimulus than those from "richer" environments. On the other hand, the barer environments may lead to the piglets being less reactive to environmental changes, such as temperature changes (Wood-Gush and Beilharz 1982). Thus, the absence of stereotypies and mere inactivity cannot be taken to mean that all is well with the pigs' environment.

Another approach is to list the animal's physiological requirements and its behavioral "drives" or motivational systems and to test the present or hypothetical environment against the list by asking whether the environment permits the behavior or not. This approach, however, has many snags on the behavioral side. Quite frankly, we do not know enough about the behavior of our domestic animals and how the various motivational systems are controlled. For example, do animals have behavioral needs or can one, by supplying the animal with the goal, obviate the animal's desire to perform the behavior that usually leads to that goal, or is the performance of the behavior in some cases more, or as important as the goal itself? No categorical answers can be given to these questions at present, although it does seem likely that the provision of a goal will not suppress the behavior. It is known, for example, that if a dog, which eats X grams a day, is given X grams of food directly into the stomach, the dog continues to show signs of hunger. The intragastric meal has to be much larger than a normal meal in order to satisfy the dog. Finally, there is the question of whether certain motivational systems can be considered to be expendable.

Until we know a great deal more about motivation and the behavior of farm livestock, the most valuable approach seems to be to study the behavior of the species under consideration under a variety of environments, including ones that are enriched by a diversity of ecological features and by a social mixture of animals of different ages and both sexes. The study of behavior under such conditions will allow one to see a fuller, if not the full, repertoire of behavior of the animals and furthermore, it will give insight into the motivation and control of behavior. It is important to realize that animal behavior is controlled not only by internal physiological factors but that it is also guided and often elicited by external key stimuli. Investigations have shown that often these are of surprising simplicity. While to us, an animal may appear to be reacting to an entire object or set of objects, it is in fact responding to only some elements of the configuration in a certain context rather as we do when we recognize a politician from a few strokes in a caricature. While the detailed observations on the behavior of animals in an enriched environment will not by themselves allow one to know which part of the object is the actual key stimulus, it will allow one to see which objects are important, and it will usually allow the animals to complete chains of behavior that are seen as enigmatic behavior patterns in intensive conditions. Furthermore, from such studies, once the repertoire of behavior is known together with the important environmental features, then it is possible to make a reasonable assessment of different housing systems (Wood-Gush 1973).

Observations have been carried out on pigs in a semi-natural enclosure at the Edinburgh School of Agriculture over a six-year period. The enclosure, which is about 1.2 hectares, contains woodland, a marsh, a stream, bushes, and grassland. The study population consisted of several groups containing four to five sows, their current litters, an adult boar, a young gilt and a sub-adult boar. This structure and size of population is a compromise between repeating the population structure of the European Wild Boar, in which basically a few females and their current offspring live together while the boars seem to live independently, and the moving of a boar to and from the study enclosure with its attendant management problems. Other populations including mono-caste populations in conventional fattening pens, were studied in environments in some of which the environmental complexity was systematically reduced. In all, thirteen groups were studied in outdoor enclosures, twelve groups in paddocks and yards, and ten groups in conventional fattening pens (Stolba 1982b).

From this process of systematically reducing the environmental complexity, it became apparent that the pigs' behavior is guided by a number of specific features. These were found to be consistently present when certain behavior patterns were performed. For example, in the farrowing sow, nesting material is collected and deposited at the base of vertical structures such a tree or upright brush. In the adults, defecation was found to be statistically more frequent on wide paths where these ran between bushes, rather than anywhere else. Studies on the social behavior revealed that under these conditions of stability in which only the young were removed at bacon weight, close relationships were found between the adults (Stolba 1982b) as well as between the juveniles before weaning (Hutton et al. 1981). The intensity of these relationships is shown by an example cited by Stolba (1982b) in which two new sub-adults were introduced. For over a month they were not permitted to sleep in the communal nest. In another case involving sows, even after 190 days in the enclosure the strong initial social bonds were still evident, for the two sub-groups involved slept significantly more with members of the their own sub-group than with members of the other. In general there are very strong dam-daughter bonds while the boar remains relatively independent. The juveniles tend to form sub-groups at a few weeks of age and later consort a great deal with the sub-adult animals.

Summarizing the results from the studies on the populations in the different environments, Stolba (1982b) concluded that several features, some of which were only in the semi-natural enclosure, were important in guiding the pigs' behavior and that these could be reproduced in the design of a housing environment of enriched pens. They include the following:

A roofed and an open part of the pen to recreate a forest-border habitat where much of the behavior of the pigs in the semi-natural enclosure occurs.

The main feeding area placed away from the resting area.

A sheltered nest site with an open view out of the pen facing the front.

The preferred farrowing nest position against two bushes, recreated by pen walls and farrowing walls.

Space for a nest of 2-3 m in diameter as found outside.

A site for defecating in the morning 4.5-11 m away from the nest site.

A corridor for defecating during the day resembling the paths between bushes.

Peat or bark in a rooting area with a log for the pigs to lever.

A rack for gathering straw sheaves and a post for rubbing against and for marking behavior.

Head partitions between small feeding stalls to ensure sufficient individual space while feeding and to also decrease aggression.

Removable partition walls that allow pigs to hide and thus lower social tensions.

From the studies of social behavior it was concluded that the basic social unit should be small and stable and that the juveniles should remain in the group until the point of sale. Indeed, as will be seen, the system eradicates the practice of the mixing of strange pigs and also does away with the specialist types of housing found in modern piggeries. This basic unit designed by Stolba is reproduced in the *Family Pen System* and consists of four sows, a sub-adult male and a gilt (in case a replacement is needed). Each sow can have her own pen, but the four are linked by a permanently open corridor which is the main defecation site, resembling the paths used for defecation in the semi-natural enclosure. Two of the pens are shown in figure 1. Each pen consists of a peat-bedded rooting area, a straw-covered activity area which contains the feeding stalls, the marking post, the drinking site, and the straw sheaves in a rack. At the back is a straw-bedded nesting area which can be closed off and in which farrowing rails can be placed together with a lamp to form a creep area for very young piglets. Each pen can be closed off with its three components from others but the object is to allow freedom of movement from one pen to another. In the semi-natural enclosure, synchrony of estrus and conception during lactation is a common feature and this has been also found in this new Family Pen system. The boar is introduced on day 20 after farrowing and stays until the lactating sows have been mated and is then moved to another group of four pens if needed. The detailed management has been described elsewhere (Stolba 1982a, 1982b), as has the construction (Stolba 1982a).

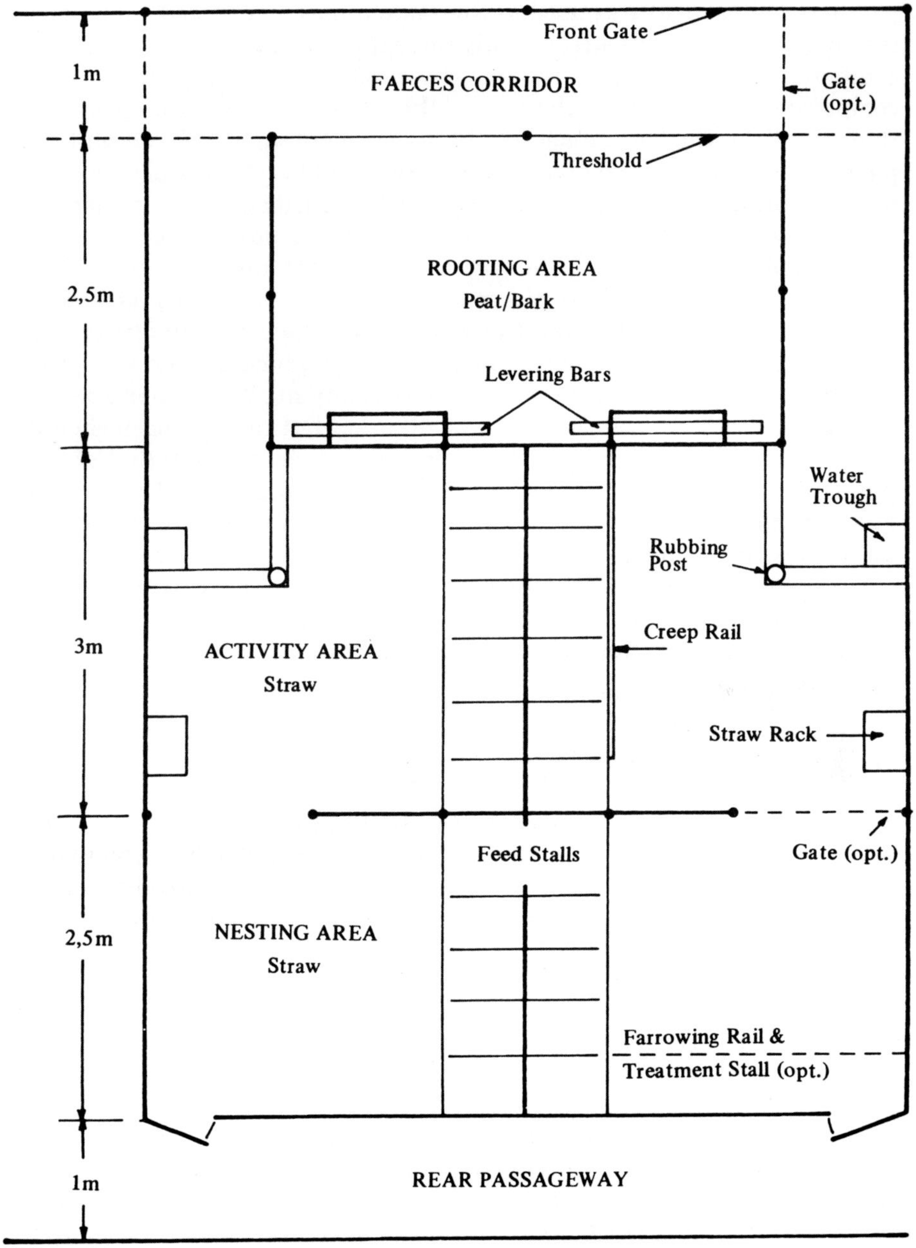

Figure 1. A plan view of two adjacent pens in a unit of four interleading pens in the family pen system. The other two pens are to the left and are linked by the feces corridor.

Many of the features used in the system have been used before but the combination allows a reasonably full expression of the pigs' behavior compared with the pig park and the production records have been comparable with those of the rest of the pig unit. It is with optimism that we enter the next stage of the experiment in which we will be paying more attention to production, as opposed to ethological measurements in order to bring the system to a level where it can be a commercial option, given a political commitment to animal welfare by society which would enable the change from very intensive systems.

The example from the pig study shows the possibility of how a housing system can be be built around the animals' requirements and yet still allow a fairly intensive housing system which also provides the operator with an agreeable working environment. With other species of farm livestock the solutions may be different but the approach should be the same: to study their behavior in habitats resembling that of the putative ancestor, to consider the role of environmental features in guiding their behavior, and to study their social structure under these conditions. While flexibility in social organization or structure is fairly common in wild species it does not always lead to a structure that is fully advantageous (Lott 1984) and therefore all variations should be critically examined from the ethological points of view so that the optimum can be selected.

Acknowledgements

This research on the pigs in the semi-natural enclosure and the Family Pen system was financed by the Royal Society, The Swiss National Science Foundation, Die Stiftung zur Forderung tiergerechter Haltungsformen von Nutztieren and The Farm Animal Care Trust.

References

Arnone, M. and Dantzer, R. 1980. Does frustration induce aggression in pigs? *Appl. Anim. Ethol.* 6:351-62.

Baldwin, B.A. 1974. Behavioural thermoregulation. In: Monteith, J.L. and Mount, L.E. eds. *Heat Loss from Animals and Man.* London: Butterworths. pp. 97-117.

Baldwin, B.A. and Stephens, D.B. 1973. The effects of conditioned behaviour and environmental factors on plasma corticosteroid levels in pigs. *Physiol. Behav.* 10:267-74.

Baldwin, B.A. and Meese, G.B. 1977. Sensory reinforcement and illumination preference in the domesticated pig. *Anim. Behav.* 25:497-507.

Barnett, J.L., Cronin, G.M. and Winfield, C.G. 1981. The effects of individual and group penning of pigs on total and free plasma corticosteroids and maximum corticosteroid binding capacity. *Gen. Comp. Endocrinol.* 44:219-25.

Dawkins, M. 1977. Do hens suffer in battery cages? Environmental preferences and welfare. *Anim. Behav.* 25:1034-46.

Desforges, M.F. and Wood-Gush, D.G.M. 1975. Behavioural differences between Aylesbury and wild Mallard ducks: A study in domestication. *Vet. Rec.* 96:509.

Duncan, I.J.H. and Wood-Gush, D.G.M. 1972. Thwarting of feeding behaviour in the domestic fowl. *Anim. Behav.* 20:444-51.

Duncan, I.J.H. and Filshie, J.H. 1980. The use of radio-telemetry devices to measure temperature and heart rate in the domestic fowl. In: Amlaner, C.J. and McDonald, D.W. eds. *A Handbook of Biotelemetry and Radio Tracking.* London: Permagon Press. pp. 579-88.

Fraser, D. 1975. The effect of straw on the behaviour of sows in tether stalls. *Anim. Prod.* 21:59-68.

Hughes, B.O. and Black, A.J. 1973. The preferences of domestic hens for different types of battery cage floor. *Br. Poult. Sci.* 14:615-19.

Hutton, R., Stolba, A. and Wood-Gush, D.G.M. 1980. Social facilitation as a measure of social relations in piglets kept intensively. *Appl. Anim. Ethol.* 6:391.

Lott, D.F. 1984. Intraspecific variation in the social systems of wild vertebrates. *Behaviour.* 88:266-325.

Stolba, A. 1982a. A Family System of pig housing. *Proc. Symp. Alternatives to Intensive Husbandry Systems.* Potters Bar: U.F.A.W. Publication.

Stolba, A. 1982b. Designing pig housing conditions according to patterns of social structure. *Pigs, problems and prospects.* Report on the Scottish Colleges and Meat and Livestock Commission Pig Conference. Edinburgh Scottish Colleges. East of Scotland College of Agriculture. pp. 11-24.

Stolba, A. and Wood-Gush, D.G.M. 1980. Arousal and exploration in growing pigs in different environments. *Appl. Anim. Ethol.* 6:382-3.

Stolba, A. and Wood-Gush, D.G.M. 1981. Verhaltungsgliederung und Reaktion auf Neureize als ethologische kriterien zur Beurteilung von Haltungsbedingungen. In: *Aktuelle Arbeiten zur artgemassen Tierhaltung 1980.* 264 KBTL - Schrift.

Wiepkema, P.R., Cronin, G.M. and van Ree, J.M. 1984. Stereotypies and endorphins: Functional significance of developing stereotypies in tethered sows. *Proc. Internat. Congr. on Applied Ethology in Farm Animals.* Univ. of Kiel. (In press).

Vestergaard, K. 1978. Normal behaviour of egg-laying birds. *1st Danish Seminar on Poultry Welfare in Egg-laying cages.* National Committee for Poultry and Eggs. Copenhagen. pp. 11-17.

Wood-Gush, D.G.M. 1972. Strain differences in response to sub-optimal stimuli in the fowl. *Anim. Behav.* 20:72-76.

Wood-Gush, D.G.M. 1973. Animal welfare in modern agriculture. *Br. Vet. J.* 129:167-74.

Wood-Gush, D.G.M. and Beilharz, R.G. 1982. The enrichment of a bare environment for animals in confined conditions. *Appl. Anim. Ethol.* 10:209-17.

Part II
Laboratory Animals

Animal Pain

RECOGNITION AND ALLEVIATION OF PAIN IN ANIMALS

P.A. Flecknell

University of Newcastle upon Tyne
Comparative Biology Centre
The Medical School
Framlington Place
Newcastle upon Tyne NE2 4HH
United Kingdom

Introduction

The pain and distress which animals experience as a consequence of their use by man figures prominently in discussions of animal welfare. Some improvements have been made in animal housing and husbandry practices and it is likely that further progress will be made in this field. In comparison, relatively little attention has been given to the problem of minimizing the pain and distress caused to animals by the various procedures to which they are subjected. The most publicized of these are the wide range of experimental techniques which are undertaken using laboratory animals, but also includes procedures such as castration of farm animals and neutering operations carried out on pet animals. The prevention or alleviation of the pain associated with such procedures is a complex problem with no single, simple solution. Consideration must be given to the use of analgesic drugs, the provision of high standards of general care, and the use of special nursing techniques. When dealing with post-operative care, the pre-operative management of the animal, the operative procedures and the anesthetic regime must all be evaluated and, when necessary, modified to minimize pain or discomfort.

Pain Perception in Animals

It is generally accepted that animals perceive and react to pain in a manner similar to man, although the conscious experience of pain may well vary in different animal species and man (Melzack and Dennis 1980; Moloney 1985). Our inability to define precisely the nature of the sensation of pain leads to difficulties, both in its assessment and in recommending methods of pain relief. In man, the common assessment of pain is based mostly on the subjective criterion that "pain is what the patient says hurts" (Smith 1984). In animals, a variety of definitions has been proposed, however as yet none of these are entirely satisfactory (Uvarov 1985).

Although pain is more easily detected in man than in animals, the standard of pain relief following surgery in man is generally poor, with some 40-50 percent of patients receiving inadequate analgesia following surgery (Smith 1984). In a recent survey of the incidence of post-operative pain in children, only 25 percent were found to be pain-free immediately following surgery (Mather and Mackie 1983). In seems reasonable to assume that given the additional difficulties of detection of pain, and the generally lower level of nursing care, that an even greater percentage of animals will experience post-operative pain. The failure to provide adequate pain relief in man has been attributed to a number of factors, including a lack of awareness of the problem by the medical staff concerned and a fear of the undesirable side-effects, such as respiratory depression, which are associated with the use of opiates. It seems likely that similar factors are involved in the provision of pain relief in animals.

If the standard of pain relief for animals is to be improved, it is important to ensure that the possibility of pain in animals is acknowledged, that the staff concerned are trained to recognize pain and distress in animals, and that effective methods of pain relief are employed wherever possible.

In addition to the desirability of relieving pain on humane grounds, pain also has other adverse effects, for example, movement is restricted and food and water intake are depressed. Pain has also been shown to cause widespread vasoconstriction and perpetuate the metabolic and hormonal changes induced by surgery (Kehlet 1978).

Recognition of Pain in Animals

The response of animals to pain varies considerably and it is difficult to offer definitive criteria for the assessment of pain in different animal species. There are, however, a range of behavioral changes that are frequently associated with pain and these are often helpful in determining its degree and thus whether analgesics are required.

In general, animals which are in pain are relatively inactive and may remain completely immobile within their cage or pen. When observed undisturbed, alterations in the pattern or rate of respiration may be noted, and on examination the heart rate may be elevated. If the animal moves it will often have an abnormal gait and when approached or handled may be uncharacteristically aggressive. If the painful area is confined to one limb joint or to a surgical wound, then the animal will usually attempt to prevent the area from being handled and may react violently to attempts to manipulate it. When left undisturbed, the animal may position itself to observe the painful area, and may lick or groom the area excessively. Alternatively, normal grooming behavior may be absent, and as a consequence the coat may appear dirty and unkempt.

Pain may cause the adoption of an abnormal posture, for example a "tucked up" appearance produced by tensing the muscles of the abdomen and back. Animals may also become unusually restless, moving about constantly, or continuously getting up and laying down. Very abnormal behavior such as flailing or extensor rigidity of the limbs, writhing or production of self-inflicted bite wounds, indicates severe pain. Similar behavior may, of course, occur in the immediate post-operative period during recovery from anesthesia, before the animal becomes fully conscious. If, however, such behavior persists when the animal has fully recovered from the anesthetic, then it must be assumed to be experiencing severe pain which must be relieved. If such pain cannot be alleviated rapidly, a decision must be taken as to whether the animal should be humanely killed immediately.

Animals in pain frequently reduce their food and water intake, often to the extent that serious dehydration occurs. If pain persists for a prolonged period, the reduction in food and water intake will result in a fall in body weight which may be a useful index for the assessment of chronic pain, and also for monitoring the efficacy of any analgesia.

Abnormal vocalization may occur—dogs may whine or whimper, cats miaow and cry, or occasionally may purr, rats squeak at an unusual pitch, and primates may scream or grunt when moving. It must be appreciated that vocalization may be elicited in response to non-painful stimuli. For example, the squeals of pigs in response to handling, or in anticipation of feeding, might be interpreted as indicative of pain by those unfamiliar with the normal behavior of the species.

All of the criteria above must be considered in conjunction with the nature of any surgical procedure which has been undertaken, or the characteristics of any disease processes which may be present. As mentioned above, it is also important to be aware of the normal behavioral characteristics of the particular animal species. It is especially useful to discuss the appearance of an individual animal with its owner or handler, since many of the changes in demeanor may be extremely subtle, and apparent only to someone who is very familiar with the animal's previous behavior.

The clinical assessment of pain, distress, and discomfort has been described in small mammals (Morton 1985), dogs and cats (Taylor 1985), horses (Silver 1985), ruminants (Edwards 1985), pigs (Oldham 1985), poultry and birds (Gentle 1985), primates (Tribe 1985), and fish (Brown 1985).

A technique for assessing pain by means of a scoring system based on clinical observation has been described by Morton and Griffiths (1985). The assessment system catalogues a range of clinical signs such as reduced food and water intake, altered posture, change in temperament, and altered respiration and pulse rate. Deviations of these signs from normal are scored according to the severity of the deviation. The total score from all of the listed clinical signs provides an overall assessment of the animal, a high score indicating that pain or distress is likely to be present. This proposed scoring system utilizes many clinical signs that could be produced by other, non-painful factors. Despite this drawback, an animal which has a high score is quite obviously abnormal, and should receive careful attention.

When considering chronic pain of gradual onset, many of the behavioral changes may be ascribed to other factors. A pet dog with a tumor may be thought lethargic and depressed as a consequence of natural aging rather than the pain caused by the tumor. Administration of an analgesic to such animals may result in a marked improvement in its "quality of life" (Yoxall 1978).

It is apparent that although the behavior of animals in pain may be dramatic, in some the response may be so slight as to be almost inapparent to all but those most familiar with the behavior patterns both of the animal species involved, and of the individual animal. Such familiarity is difficult to achieve, and in many instances there will be considerable doubt as to whether an animal is in pain. For this reason it is the author's practice to assume that a procedure or injury which is likely to cause pain in man will also cause pain in an animal. Such anthropomorphic views are open to criticism, and ignore the issue of what significance the animal attaches to its pain. It is possible that the apparent tolerance of injuries that would be acutely painful in man may involve a greater suppression of central pain perception in some animal species. Until unequivocal evidence is produced to support such views, it is obviously more humane to assume that pain is present, and to make every attempt to provide effective pain relief.

Pain Relief in Animals

In most instances pain relief will be provided by the use of analgesic drugs. Although the use of such agents will control pain, an animal may still exhibit signs of distress. Semantic difficulties abound in the field of animal welfare, and numerous definitions of stress and distress have been proposed. In this paper the term "distress" is used to describe the state produced by adverse factors which would not usually be considered to cause pain, but are certainly unpleasant and should be avoided. For example, a cold, wet environment, devoid of suitable bedding material is likely to cause distress to some animal species. Similarly, states of physiological imbalance, such as dehydration caused by inadequate fluid therapy, would not be referred to as painful, but would cause distress. It seems reasonable to include methods aimed at reducing distress in the management of pain. It is also assumed by the author that pain and distress can be heightened by fear or apprehension, and any regime of nursing care must include reassurance and calming of the animal, either by personal contact, environmental manipulations, or by pharmacological means. In addition to analgesics, a range of other drugs including tranquilizers, sedatives, and corticosteroids or similar agents with anti-inflammatory activity may all play a role in the management of pain.

Analgesic Drugs

Of the wide variety of analgesics available for use in man, relatively few have been employed in routine veterinary clinical practice. A certain amount of published information concerning the suitability of analgesics for veterinary use is available, and in many instances the original assessment of a drug's properties in experimental animals provides useful data (Flecknell 1984).

Centrally Acting Analgesics

Narcotics: Agonists

This group of drugs includes the best established veterinary analgesics pethidine (meperidine) and morphine. All are potent analgesics but also produce some undesirable effects on the central nervous system, respiratory depression being of the most clinical significance. Most of the side-effects can be reversed by the use of specific antagonists (see below), although this will, of course, reverse any analgesia which has been produced.

Morphine

Morphine has been used in veterinary practice in the United Kingdom for some years (Hall and Clarke 1983), and its efficacy in the dog has been recently confirmed by Taylor and Houlton (1984). It is an effective analgesic in a wide range of species (table 1), but its undesirable side-effects can include severe respiratory depression and overdosage can cause incoordination or excitement in some species (cat, Davis and

Donnelly 1968, Lumb and Jones 1984; mouse, Pearl et al. 1969, Lumb and Jones 1984) or narcosis in others (dog, primate, rabbit, Lumb and Jones 1984).

Pethidine (Meperidine)

This drug is perhaps the most widely used veterinary analgesic and suitable dose rates have been established for a range of species (table 1), although its respiratory depressant effect can limit its use, particularly in the immediate post-operative period. In addition, pethidine has a relatively short duration of action in some species, for example, less than two hours in the cat (Davis and Donnelly 1968).

Methadone

Clinical use of methadone in the dog has been largely restricted to pre-anesthetic medication (1 mg/kg, i/v or s/c*) (Lumb and Jones 1984). In the horse, in combination with acepromazine (50 mg methadone and 50 mg acepromazine total dose/1000 lb horse), it has been reported to provide effective sedation (Schauffler 1969). The analgesic action of the drug in horses appears variable, although some beneficial effect could be demonstrated (Pippi and Lumb 1979).

D-Propoxyphene

D-Propoxyphene is structurally related to methadone, but has considerably less analgesic potency. It has been recommended for the relief of mild to moderate pain in the dog at a suggested dose of 16.25 mg b.i.d. per os** for small dogs, up to 32 mg/kg t.i.d.† for larger breeds (Yoxall 1978). In the author's experience it is useful at these dose rates for the relief of musculoskeletal pain in this species.

Codeine and dihydrocodeine

These two morphine derivatives have been used to a limited extent in small animals. Oral preparations of codeine may be of use for the control of mild pain in the dog at a dose of 2 mg/kg (Taylor 1985).

Fentanyl and etorphine

Fentanyl and etorphine are two extremely potent analgesics which have been widely used as components of neuroleptanalgesics, and their use for this purpose has been reviewed by Green (1979). The short

* i/v—by intravenous injection
s/c—subcutaneous injection

** b.i.d. per os—twice a day by mouth

† t.i.d.—three times a day.

duration of action of fentanyl limits its value as an analgesic when given by intermittent injection, but it is potentially useful for administration by continuous intravenous infusion (see later).

New Opiates

Alfentanil resembles fentanyl in almost all its pharmacological and clinical effects. It differs in having a very short duration of action (about ten minutes in the rat, Niemegeers 1977), making it especially suitable for administration by continuous intravenous infusion.

Lofentanil, a novel, extremely potent narcotic analgesic, has the longest duration of action of any drug of this group so far discovered. It appears unlikely that the drug will be introduced into human clinical practice, but a drug having such a long duration of action might prove extremely useful in providing analgesia in animals.

Carfentanil, another member of the fentanyl group of analgesics, has a potency thirty-two times that of fentanyl (i.e., about 18,000 times as potent as pethidine). It has been used for the immobilization of wild animals where its high potency enables its use in low volumes (<1 ml for most large animals, De Vos 1978). It has also been used in combination with etomidate as an anesthetic in guinea pigs (Neumann et al. 1980).

Narcotics: Partial Agonists

This group of drugs has mixed morphine-like analgesic and antagonist properties. They were developed primarily in an attempt to produce analgesic drugs free from morphine's undesirable side-effects, and in particular to avoid the problem of the development of addiction.

Pentazocine

Pentazocine has been used to a limited extent in veterinary clinical practice. Its use in the dog to control post-operative pain has been reported by Cooper and Organ (1977) and Taylor and Houlton (1984). It is the author's experience that it can be used effectively to relieve acute pain in nonhuman primates (table 1).

Buprenorphine

This potent, long-lasting analgesic appears to offer several advantages compared to many of the agents mentioned above. Although controlled studies in animals are limited to experimental data in rodents (Heel et al. 1979; Cowan et al. 1977a, 1977b) and a clinical trial in the dog (Taylor and Houlton 1984), the drug has been used clinically in both laboratory and companion animals. Its use in the horse has been reported by Hall and Clarke (1983), and it has been used to provide effective pain relief in a wide range of species by the author (table 1).

Buprenorphine's efficacy in producing pain relief following acute trauma or surgery has also been established in small animal practice in the United Kingdom.

This drug has a considerably longer duration action in most species (> 8 hours) than the other agents described above. In addition, it seems to produce fewer and less marked side-effects.

Butorphanol

This drug has similar pharmacological properties to pentazocine (House 1979), but a somewhat greater potency (Heel et al. 1978). Information concerning its effects in animals is limited (Pircio et al. 1976). Its administration to the horse has been described by Robertson et al. (1981), although its analgesic effects were not evaluated.

Nalbuphine

Nalbuphine has proven to be an efffective analgesic in acute and chronic painful conditions in man, with fewer undesirable side-effects than morphine. Its analgesic action has been studied in mice and rats (Blumberg et al. 1968), however, it would appear to be a potentially useful drug in the dog, since in this species the plasma half-life is 8.3 hours (Fahmy 1983), suggesting that the agent may produce long-lasting analgesia.

Other Analgesic Drugs

A range of low to moderate potency compounds such as aspirin, paracetamol (acetaminophen), and phenacetin are widely used in man to control mild pain. Their use in veterinary practice is limited but these compounds are often administered to pet animals by their owners. Such uncontrolled administration can have serious consequences. Aspirin and paracetamol may both be rapidly and fatally toxic to cats (Wilkinson 1984). In dogs, aspirin is extremely irritant to the gastric mucosa (Davison et al. 1966) and it is preferable to use other preparations such as paracetamol and codeine in this species.

Anti-Inflammatory Agents

Corticosteroids are the drugs most widely used in veterinary practice for the reduction of chronic or acute inflammatory responses. By reducing the degree of inflammation, they diminish the pain associated with such a reaction, but have no specific analgesic action. They are useful in treating conditions in which pain is the result of tissue inflammation. However, since the inflammatory response is a prerequisite for successful healing of damaged tissue, they must be used with caution.

A number of non-steroidal anti-inflammatory drugs have been developed, the most widely used in veterinary practice being phenylbutazone. Phenylbutazone has proven particularly useful in the control of musculoskeletal pain in the dog and the horse, however, its numerous undesirable side-effects may limit its use (Yoxall 1978). Other drugs have been introduced into human clinical practice, and some of these have been used in veterinary practice in the United Kingdom (Taylor 1985). Ibruprofen has been recommended for use in the dog, an initial loading dose of 30 mg/kg per os* in divided doses, followed by a maintenance dose of 16 mg/kg being suggested by Yoxall (1978).

Tranquilizers

This group of drugs has no intrinsic analgesic action, and when used alone they may actually increase pain perception. When administered in conjunction with a narcotic analgesic they will potentiate the effects of the latter. The combination of sedation, analgesia, and a reduction in fear and apprehension is extremely useful, particularly immediately following surgery or trauma. The degree of sedation produced varies considerably in different animal species, for example, diazepam, a sedative which can be used to induce hypnosis (sleep) in man, has little sedative action in the dog, but in rodents and rabbits it produces marked sedation.

Clinical Use of Analgesics

As has been indicated above, the use of analgesics in animals is hampered by the lack of information concerning suitable dose rates and by practical problems associated with drug administration. A major problem with most analgesics is their short duration of action (1-4 hours), so that maintenance of adequate analgesia requires repeated administration of the drug, which is often difficult to arrange in practice. Buprenorphine, unlike other narcotic analgesics, has been shown to have a duration of action of at least 10-14 hours in both animals and man. Veterinary clinical use of this agent has shown that it is effective in controlling severe post-operative pain for at least 10-14 hours. Since buprenorphine has some narcotic antagonistic activity, it can be used to reverse the narcosis produced by neuroleptanalgesic combinations (e.g., fentanyl/fluanisone and fentanyl/droperidol) and yet maintain effective post-operative analgesia.

Slow release preparations of analgesics have been developed for experimental use, (Laska and Fennessy 1978; Frederickson and Smiths

---

* per os—by mouth

1973; McGinity and Mehta 1978), and it would seem feasible to adapt such techniques to provide long-term analgesia. A slow-release morphine preparation for oral administration has become available in the United Kingdom (MST Continus; Napp Laboratories Ltd.), and has been shown to provide up to six hours pain relief in man (Fell et al. 1982). A sustained-release morphine preparation for intramuscular or subcutaneous injection is also marketed (Duromorph, LAB Ltd.), however, no information is available concerning the use of either of these products in animals, although they would appear to be potentially useful preparations.

An alternative method of providing effective pain relief is to use a continuous drug delivery system such as a chronically implanted catheter and a suitable swivel apparatus. The use of continuous intravenous infusion of opiates has been evaluated clinically in man (see review by Mather 1983) and shown to be considerably more effective in providing pain relief than intermittent injections. When using the intravenous route, administration of a drug such as alfentanil, with a short duration of action, enables rapid variation in plasma concentrations should undesirable side-effects occur. In most animal applications, however, the technique will be used to provide analgesia for prolonged periods (for example, overnight) in the absence of nursing staff. Under these circumstances, the main factors influencing the choice of drug will be its therapeutic index and the volume of solution required. If the volume of drug required is small, a light-weight portable infusion pump can be used, bandaged directly to the animal. It is also usually more convenient to use the subcutaneous route of administration. Although this does not enable rapid variations in plasma levels to be achieved should undesirable side-effects occur, it is a much easier technique to instigate and maintain.

When calculating the dose rates required, as a general guide, following administration of an initial standard dose, the quantity of drug needed for continuous infusion will be about half that which would be given by intermittent injection. The animal should, of course, be observed carefully to determine that effective analgesia is being acheived and that undesirable effects, such as respiratory depression, are minimal. When pharmacokinetic data are available for the drug and the animal species concerned, more accurate estimation of infusion rates are possible, and these techniques are reviewed by Mather (1983).

Undesirable Effects of Narcotic Analgesics

Excessive doses of narcotic analgesics can cause severe respiratory depression, requiring assisted ventilation or reversal with an antagonist such as naloxone. Opiate antagonists, of course, reverse any analgesia that has been produced as well as reversing the respiratory depression, so that it may be preferable to use a specific respiratory stimulant such as doxapram. Doxapram has a relatively short duration of action (fifteen to twenty minutes), and either repeated doses or a continuous infusion of the drug may be needed to maintain adequate stimulation of respiration. Use of buprenorphine in animals appears to carry little risk of producing respiratory depression. However, if this does occur, doxapram should be used since naloxone is relatively ineffective in reversing the depressant effects of buprenorphine.

Paradoxically, the potent action of narcotics in abolishing pain has been cited as a disadvantage of their use in clinical veterinary practice. Pain, of course, serves a protective function in discouraging movement of a traumatized area, and so tending to minimize further injury. Complete abolition of pain in the post-operative period has been suggested as likely to lead to disruption of sutures by excessive activity. This is rarely, if ever, a problem providing good wound closure techniques have been used. Excessive activity can be controlled, if necessary, by the addition of a tranquilizer to the post-operative drug regime, and use of appropriate bandaging and splinting techniques can provide additional wound support.

It is the author's view that analgesics should never be withheld on such grounds as those described above. Clinical experience has shown that effective use of analgesics, rather than resulting in tissue damage due to excessive activity, will often prevent undue self-trauma of the affected area.

Additional Components of the Management of Pain

The control of pain requires more than simply the administration of an appropriate analgesic. If a surgical procedure is to be undertaken, it may be useful to include an opiate such as pethidine in any preanesthetic medication to provide pain relief in the immediate post-operative period. If surgery is prolonged, however ($>$ 2 hours), the analgesic effects of the drug will no longer be apparent and a period of acute pain may follow emergence from the anesthetic, unless prompt administration of an analgesic is ensured. This may be avoided to some extent by the use of an anesthetic agent such as methoxyflurane which has been shown to have limited analgesic properties in the post-operative period (Vickers et al. 1984). Alternatively, the technique of reversal of a neuroleptanalgesic combination with a partial agonist such as buprenorphine can be used to try to ensure a completely pain-free emergence from anesthesia.

The pain caused by surgical procedures can, of course, be reduced by good technique, particularly that directed at minimizing tissue trauma.

Preventing tension on suture lines, immobilizing fractures and traumatized tissue, and padding and protecting surgical wounds considerably reduces post-operative pain.

Provision of a special area for recovery from anesthesia and for post-operative nursing is of importance. This enables more appropriate environmental conditions to be maintained and encourages individual attention and special nursing—all important factors in minimizing pain and discomfort.

Such an area should be warm (approximately 25-30 degrees Centigrade for adult animals of most species), draught-free, and quiet. Hypothermia is a common problem during post-operative recovery and a heating pad or heating lamp may be required to provide additional warmth. It is also useful to reduce heat losses by insulating the animal by providing additional bedding materials and by use of specialized blankets. Body temperature should be monitored to ensure that the measures employed are effective, and also to avoid overheating and consequent hyperthermia. Fluid intake is frequently reduced post-operatively so that where appropriate oral intake should be encouraged and hand feeding of fluids undertaken whenever necessary. If these simple measures prove inadequate, dehydration must be corrected by parenteral administration of fluids. Food intake should also be monitored carefully, and supplemented by hand feeding if required.

In all species, every effort should be made to keep the animal clean and dry, since this is more comfortable for the animal and encourages closer attention from the nursing staff. There is little point in preventing pain by the use of analgesics if the animal is uncomfortable and distressed by inappropriate or inadequate post-operative care.

If an animal appears apprehensive, reassurance by personal contact will be effective only in animals which are accustomed to such attentions. Even in these species, and certainly in the case of many laboratory species, use of tranquilizers may be considered necessary.

Future Development

In man, a range of new approaches to the management of pain are being developed. Whilst many of these are unlikely to be routinely used in animals, others hold considerable promise. One technique that may prove particularly useful is the administration of opiates by the intrathecal or epidural routes. This technique has been employed clinically in man and extensively investigated in experimental animals (see reviews by Yaksh 1981, 1983). The technique involves implantation of an epidural or intrathecal catheter to allow repeated administration of small quantities of opiates such as morphine. Profound, long-lasting analgesia is produced, for example, 12-16 hours following intrathecal morphine in primates (Yaksh 1981). The areas of the body rendered analgesic depend upon the spinal cord level reached by the opiate. In most instances the technique has been used to produce analgesia of the abdomen and hindquarters, although successful production of analgesia extending to the forelegs in the dog has been reported by Cohen et al. (1982). In man the technique has been used to control pain following a variety of abdominal surgical procedures, lower limb surgery, and thoracotomy (Camporesi and Redick 1983). The analgesia produced by epidural and intrathecal opiates is not associated with any loss of motor function or loss of sensation to touch, unlike the effects produced by local anesthetics administered by the same routes.

The lower doses of drug used cause few of the systemic effects such as sedation, which develop following intramuscular injection of opiates. Although some undesirable side-effects have been noted including pruritis (Hales 1980) and urinary retention, the latter does not appear to be a problem in animals. The most significant side-effect in man has been the development of severe respiratory depression. The incidence of this problem is difficult to assess, but is certainly low ($<$ 0.5 percent, Reiz et al. 1981; Gustafsson et al. 1982) and has not been noted as a serious side-effect in the limited clinical or experimental studies in the dog (Bonath et al. 1984; Cohen et al. 1982). Repeated intrathecal administration of opiates and maintenance of spinal catheters for prolonged periods (4-16 months) in primates resulted in no demonstrable neurological or pathological changes (Yaksh 1981). It is clear that this technique could be employed in a wide range of situations in animals, particularly following experimental surgical procedures. It might also offer a method of producing long-term analgesia for localized disease processes, or chronic inflammatory conditions. The method of catheter implantation has been described in a wide range of species including the rat (Yaksh and Rudy 1976), the rabbit (Yaksh and Rudy 1976), the cat (Yaksh 1978), the dog (Cohen et al. 1982; Bonath et al. 1984) and nonhuman primates (Yaksh 1978; Bahar et al. 1984). In addition, the continuous epidural infusion of opiates using an implanted pump has been described in the dog (Cohen et al. 1982) offering the possibility of prolonged analgesia without the necessity of repeated injections of drug through an exteriorized spinal catheter.

Conclusions

Considerable opportunity exists for the adoption of better methods for the management of pain and distress in animals. Experimental studies in animals and clinical experience in man are likely to continue to offer new approaches that can be applied to veterinary clinical practice. Major problems remain, for example, the control of chronic pain, particularly in laboratory animals where the prolonged use of analgesics may interfere with the experimental protocol.

The solution of these and other problems requires both the development of new techniques and the better application of existing knowledge. A change in priorities by all those concerned in the management of animals is required, with considerably greater emphasis being placed on the well-being of the animal. Improved education at all levels is needed to disseminate available knowledge, and to promote a greater awareness of the needs of the animals given over to our care.

Table 1. Analgesic drugs for use in animals.

	Morphine	Pethidine	Pentazocine	Buprenorphine
Mouse	10mg/kg s/c 2-4 hourly	20mg/kg s/c i/m 2-3 hourly	10mg/kg s/c 3-4 hourly	2.0mg/kg* s/c 12 hourly
Rat	10mg/kg s/c 2-4 hourly	20mg/kg s/c i/m* 2-3 hourly	10mg/kg s/c 4 hourly	0.1-0.5mg/kg* s/c 12 hourly
Rabbit	5mg/kg s/c i/m 2-4 hourly	10mg/kg s/c i/m* 2-3 hourly	10-20mg/kg s/c i/m 4 hourly	0.02-0.05mg/kg* s/c, i/v 8-12 hourly
Guinea Pig	10mg/kg s/c i/m 2-4 hourly	20mg/kg s/c i/m 2-3 hourly	–	0.05mg/kg s/c 8-12 hourly
Cat	0.1mg/kg/ s/c† 4 hourly	10mg/kg s/c i/m* 2 hourly	8mg/kg i/p ? 4 hourly	0.005-0. 01mg/kg* 12 hourly
Dog	0.5-5.0mg/kg† s/c i/m 2-4 hourly	10mg/kg s/c i/m* 2-3 hourly	2.0mg/kg i/m* 4 hourly	0.01-0.02mg/kg* i/m s/c 12 hourly
Primate	1-2mg/kg s/c 4 hourly	2-4mg/kg i/m* 3-4 hourly	2-5.0mg/kg i/m* 4 hourly	0.01mg/kg* i/m i/v 12 hourly
Pigs	Up to 20mg total dose†	2mg/kg i/m* 4 hourly	2.0mg/kg i/m† 4 hourly	0.005-0.01mg/kg* i/m 12 hourly
Sheep	Up to 10mg total dose i/m †	Up to 200mg total dose i/m †	–	0.005mg/kg* i/m 12 hourly

Dose rates suggested from published data.
*Clinical experience at the Clinical Research Center, Harrow.
†Recommended dosages in veterinary literature (Lumb and Jones 1984; Green 1979; Hall and Clark 1983).

References

Bahar, M., Nunn, J.F., Rosen, M. and Flecknell, P. 1984. Differential sensory and motor blockade after spinal cocaine in the rat and marmoset. *Eur. J. Anaes.* 1:31-36.

Blumberg, H., Dayton, H.B. and Wolf, P.S. 1968. Analgesic properties of the narcotic antagonist EN-2234A. *Pharmacologist.* 10:201.

Bonath, K., Gerlach, K. and Gilber, W. 1984. Peridural catheter and its importance for peridural anaesthesia and pain treatment in the dog. Paper presented at the 2nd FELASA symposium, June 1984.

Brown, L.A. In press. The clinical measurement of pain, distress and discomfort in fish. In: *The Detection and Relief of Pain in Animals.* 2nd British Veterinary Association Animal Welfare Foundation Symposium. London: British Veterinary Association Animal Welfare Foundation.

Camporesi, E.M. and Redick, L.F. 1983. Clinical aspects of spinal narcotics: Post-operative managements and obstetrical pain. *Clinical in Anaesthesiology.* 1:57-70.

Cohen, A.M., Wood, W.C., Bambert, B.S., Risaliti, A. and Poletti, C. 1982. Continuous canine epidural morphine analgesic with an implanted drug infusion pump. *J. Surg Res.* 32:32-37.

Cooper, J.E. and Organ, P. 1977. Pentazocine as an analgesic in dogs. *Vet. Rec.* 101:409.

Cowan, A., Doxey, J.C. and Harry, E.J.R. 1977a. The animal pharmacology of buprenorphine, an oripavine analgesic agent. *B.J. Pharm.* 60:547-54.

Cowan, A., Lewis, J.W. and McFarlane, I.R. 1977b. Agonist and antagonist properties of buprenorphine, a new antinociceptive agent. *B.J. Pharm.* 60:537-45.

Davis, L.E. and Donnelly, E.J. 1968. Analgesic drugs in the cat. *JAVMA* 153:1161-7.

Davison, C., Hertig, D.H. and DeVine, R. 1966. Gastric hemorrhage induced by non-narcotic analgetic agents in dogs. *Clin. Pharmacol. Ther.* 7:239.

De Vos, V. 1978. Immobilisation of free-ranging wild animals using a new drug. *Vet. Rec.* 103:64.

Edwards, G.B. In press. Clinical assessment of pain, distress and discomfort in ruminants. In: 2nd British Veterinary Association Animal Welfare Foundation Symposium. *The Detection and Relief of Pain in Animals.* London: British Veterinary Association Animal Welfare Foundation.

Fahmy, N.R. 1983. Nalbuphine hydrochloride. *Clinics in Anaesthesiology.* 1:164-7

Fell, D., Chmielewski, A. and Smith, G. 1982. Post-operative analgesia with controlled-release morphine sulphate: comparison with intramuscular morphine. *Br.M.J.* 285:92-94

Flecknell, P.A. 1984. The relief of pain in laboratory animals. *Laboratory Animals.* 18:147-60.

Frederickson, R.C.A. and Smiths, S.E. 1973. Time course of dependence and tolerance development in rats treated with "slow release" morphine suspensions. *Res. Comm. Chem. Path. Pharmacol.* 5:867-70.

Gentle, M.J. In press. Measurements of pain, distress and discomfort in poultry and other birds. In: 2nd British Veterinary Association Animal Welfare Foundation Symposium. *The Detection and Relief of Pain in Animals.* London: British Veterinary Association Animal Welfare Foundation.

Green, C.J. 1979. *Animal Anaesthesia.* London: Laboratory Animals Ltd.

Gustafsson, L., Schildt, B. and Jacobsen, I. 1982. Adverse effects of extradural and intrathecal opiates: report of a nationwide survey in Sweden. *Br. J. Anaes.* 54:479-85.

Hales, P. 1980. Pruritis after epidural morphine. *Lancet.* ii:204

Hall, L.W. and Clarke, K.W. 1983 *Veterinary Anaesthesia.* London: Balliere Tindall.

Heel, R.C., Brogden, R.N., Speight, T.M. and Avery, G.S. 1978. Butorphanol: a review of its pharmacological properties and therapeutic efficacy. *Drugs.* 16:473-505.

Heel, R.C., Brogden, R.M., Speight, T.M. and Avery, G.S. 1979. Buprenorphine: a review of its pharmacological properties and therapeutic efficacy. *Drugs.* 17:81-110.

House, R.W. 1979. Analgesic effectiveness of the narcotic agonist-antagonists. *B.J. Clin. Pharm.* 7:2975-3085.

Kehlet, H. 1978. Influence of epidural anaesthesia on the endocrine-metabolic response to surgery. *Acta. Anaesth. Scand. (Suppl)* 70:39-42.

Laska, F.J. and Fennessy, M.R. 1978. Induction of physical dependence on cyclazocine and pentazocine in the rat. *Eur. J. Pharmacol.* 48:57-65.

Lumb, W.V. and Jones, E.W. 1984. *Veterinary Anaesthesia.* 2nd Edition, Philadelphia: Lea and Febiger.

McGinity, J.W. and Mehta, C.S. 1978. Preparation and evaluation of a sustained morphine delivery system in rats. *Pharm. Biochem. Behav.* 9:705-8.

Mather, L.G. 1983. Pharmacokinetic and pharmacodynamic factors influencing the choice, dose and route of administration of opiates for acute pain. *Clinics in Anaesthesiology.* 1:17-40.

Mather, L. and Mackie, J. 1983. The incidence of post-operative pain in children. *Pain.* 15:271-82.

Melzack, R. and Dennis, S.G. 1980. Phylogenetic evolution of pain expression in animals. In: Kosterlitz, H.W. and Tererius, L.Y., eds. *Pain and Society.* Holland: Elsevier.

Moloney, V. In press. Procedures painful in man are painful in animals—true or false? In: 2nd British Veterinary Association Animal Welfare Foundation Symposium. *The Detection and Relief of Pain in Animals.* London: British Veterinary Association Animal Welfare Foundation.

Morton, D.B. and Griffiths, P.H.M. 1985. Guidelines on the recognition of pain, distress and discomfort in experimental animals and an hypothesis for assessment. *Vet. Rec.* 116:431-6.

Morton, D.B. In press. The recognition of pain, distress and discomfort in small laboratory mammals and its assessment. In: 2nd British Veterinary Association Animal Welfare Foundation Symposium. *The Detection and Relief of Pain in Animals.* London: British Veterinary Association Animal Welfare Foundation.

Neumann, G., Erhardt, W., Oberhuber, B., Fritsch, R. and Blumel, G. 1980. A new highly potent and short acting analgesic, carfentanil (R33 799), in combination with the hypnotic agent etomidate (R26 490) as a method of anaesthesia in guinea pigs. *Research in Experimental Medicine* (Berlin) 177:135.

Niemegeers, C.J.E. 1977. R39 209, a potent and very short acting morphine-like analgesic. *Research Report N15340.* Janssen Pharmaceutica.

Oldham, J. In press. Clinical measurement of pain, distress and discomfort in pigs. In: 2nd British Veterinary Association Animal Welfare Foundation Symposium. *The Detection and Relief of Pain in Animals.* London: British Veterinary Association Animal Welfare Foundation.

Pearl, J., Stander, H. and McKean, D.B. 1969. Effects of analgesics and other drugs on mice in phenylquinone and rotarod tests. *J. Pharmac. Exper. Ther.* 167:9-13.

Pippi, N.L. and Lumb, W.V. 1979. Objective tests of analgesic drugs in ponies. *Am. J. Vet. Res.* 40:1082-6.

Pircio, A.W., Gylys, J.A., Cavanagh, R.L., Buyniski, J.P. and Bierwagen, M.E. 1976. The pharmacology of butorphanol, a 3, 14-dihydroxymorphinan narcotic antagonist analgesic. *Arch. Int. Pharm.* 220:231-57.

Reiz, S., Ahlin, J. and Ahrenfeldt, B. 1981. Epidural morphine for post-operative pain relief. *Acta. Anaes. Scand.* 25:111-4.

Robertson, J.T., Muir, W.W. and Sams, R. 1981. Cardiopulmonary effects of butorphanol tartarate in horses. *Am. J. Vet. Res.* 42:41-44.

Schauffler, A.F. 1969. Better equine restraint. *Mod. Vet. Pract.* 50:46-49.

Silver, I.A. In press. The clinical measurement of pain, distress and discomfort in horses. In: 2nd British Veterinary Association Animal Welfare Foundation Symposium. *The Detection and Relief of Pain in Animals.* London: British Veterinary Association Animal Welfare Foundation.

Smith, G. 1984. Post-operative Pain. In: Lunn, J.N. ed. *Quality of Care in Anaesthetic Practice.* London: McMillan Press Ltd.

Taylor, P.M. and Houlton, J.E.F. 1984. Post-operative analgesia in the dog: a comparison of morphine, buprenorphine and pentazocine. *J. Small Anim. Pract.* 25:437-51.

Taylor, P.M. 1985. Analgesia in the dog and the cat. *In Practice.* 7:5-13.

Taylor, P.M. In press. Clinical measurement of pain, distress and discomfort in dogs and cats. In: 2nd British Veterinary Association Animal Welfare Foundation Symposium. *The Detection and Relief of Pain in Animals.* London: British Veterinary Association Animal Welfare Foundation.

Tribe, G.W. In press. Clinical measurement of pain, distress and discomfort in Simian Primates. In: 2nd British Veterinary Association Animal Welfare Foundation Symposium. *The Detection and Relief of Pain in Animals.* London: British Veterinary Association Animal Welfare Foundation.

Uvarov, O. In press. Ethical conceptions and the role and the problems of the veterinary profession in the alleviation of pain. In: 2nd British Veterinary Association Animal Welfare Foundation Symposium. *The Detection and Relief of Pain in Animals.* London: British Veterinary Association Animal Welfare Foundation.

Vickers, M.D., Schnieder, H. and Wood-Smith, F.G. 1984. *Drugs in Anaesthetic Practice.* Sevenoaks, England: Butterworths.

Wilkinson, G.T. 1984. Toxicology. In: Wilkinson, G.T. ed. *Diseases of the Cat and Their Management.* London: Blackwell Scientific Pub.

Yaksh, T.L. 1978. Analgetic actions of intrathecal opiates in cat and primate. *Brain Res.* 153:205,210.

Yaksh, T.L. 1981. Spinal opiate analgesia: characteristics and principles of action. *Pain.* 11:293-346.

Yaksh, T.L. 1983. The principle behind the use of spinal narcotics. *Clinics in Anaesthesiology.* 1:219-32.

Yaksh, T.L. and Rudy, T.A. 1976. Chronic catheterisation of the spinal subarachnoid space. *Physiol. Behav.* 17:1031-6.

Yoxall, A.T. 1978. Pain in small animals—its recogniton and control. *J. Small Anim. Pract.* 19:423-38.

T-61 USE IN THE EUTHANASIA OF DOMESTIC ANIMALS: A SURVEY

Andrew N. Rowan

Department of Environmental Studies
Tufts University
School of Veterinary Medicine
203 Harrison Avenue
Boston, MA 02111

Introduction

A variety of techniques have been proposed and employed for the killing of domestic animals but relatively few have survived as suitable agents for euthanasia—namely, the induction of painless, suffering-free death. Some agents, such as strychnine, curariform agents, or potassium salts cause suffering while others have other disadvantages. Today, dogs and cats are commonly euthanatized with sodium pentobarbital or with T-61 which is a mixture of a central nervous system narcotic, a paralytic agent, and a local anesthetic. The use of T-61 was first reported in the United States in 1963 (Quin 1963). The substance gradually became more popular because it was not a DEA-controlled substance and therefore practitioners did not have to deal with the stringent reporting requirements needed for the barbiturates. However, the presence of a paralytic agent in the T-61 mixture, continuing anecdotal reports of bad reactions when using T-61, and the relatively complicated protocol recommended for its administration have resulted in repeated questions being raised about the appropriateness ofT-61 as a euthanasia agent.

History of T-61 Use and Evaluation

The first reported use of T-61 for the killing of dogs and cats came from West Germany where Eikmeier (1961) concluded from experience on 350 dogs and 300 cats that the material was suitable for small animal euthanasia. According to Carding (1977), T-61 use then spread in Europe, in part because it was cheaper than commercial solutions of barbiturate. In America, T-61 use spread more slowly. For example, the 1972 AVMA Panel on Euthanasia did not mention the agent in its report (AVMA 1972), although it was included in the 1978 revision (AVMA 1978).

Although there was some unpublished electroencephalogram data on T-61 effects in the rats—the EEG became isoelectric in four seconds (Carding 1977)—no studies on the dog were reported until 1978 when the relative effectiveness of T-61 and sodium pentobarbital were compared (Lumb et al. 1978). Nine dogs were injected with T-61 and twelve with sodium pentobarbital under carefully controlled conditions including the recording of EEGs and ECGs. The response of the animals to T-61 and sodium pentobarbital was similar except for three dogs receiving barbiturate in which cardiac output resumed. However, as Reilly (1978) noted, the dose of barbiturate used was close to the minimum lethal dose and the sodium pentobarbital solution was one-half to one-third the strength (at 130 mg/ml) of barbiturate solutions commonly sold for animal euthanasia today (Lumb and Moreland 1982).

The Survey

In view of the continuing questions surrounding the use of T-61 for dog and cat euthanasia, it was decided to survey the reported experience of veterinarians with the agent. Four hundred and twenty-three questionnaires were distributed to veterinarians in Massachusetts. Two hundred and thirty-four completed forms were received. This represents a 55.3 percent response rate, which is excellent.

Over 90 percent of the respondents indicated some experience with T-61 but the majority used sodium pentobarbital for routine euthanasia (table 1). Half of the respondents said they did not use T-61, usually because of one or more bad experiences with the drug. Of the rest, 27.8 percent felt the drug was a satisfactory euthanasia agent (several felt it was excellent) while 21.4 percent had no strong opinion either way. Table 2 provides a more detailed breakdown of the opinions.

Table 1. Summary of sample responses.

		Number	% of Total
Routinely use Na Pent		162	69.2
Routinely use T-61		72	30.8
Attitude to T-61	Pro	65	27.8
	Con (cost)	14	6.0
	Con (bad reactions)	103	44.0
	Neutral/No opinion	52	22.2

Table 2. Opinions on T-61 use

	Na Pent Users		T-61 Users		Total	
	No.	%	No.	%	No.	%
No stated opinion	22	13.6	1	1.4	23	9.8
T-61 too expensive	14	8.6	–	–	14	6.0
Neutral on T-61 use	27	16.7	2	2.8	29	12.4
T-61 causes too many bad reactions	99	61.1	4	5.6	103	44.0
Satisfied with or prefer T-61	–	–	65	90.2	65	27.8
TOTALS	162	100	72	100	234	100

There were a number of comments on some of the perceived problems with T-61. Both users and non-users commented that the heart takes a long time to stop beating. Some talked of the heart continuing for as long as five minutes or more after brain death had apparently occurred. One respondent noted that, in 90 percent of cases, the heart continued beating for several minutes. Another feature of T-61 euthanasia that was mentioned by both groups was the presence of muscle tremors and excitation. T-61 users did not make very much of this and indicated that tremors occurred in approximately 10 percent of cases. However, barbiturate users who did not like the drug spoke of excitation, including convulsions, crying and agonal thrashing, in 20 percent or more of cases.

Of those opposed to the use of T-61, one commented that, while the drug does kill the animal, it is not euthanasia. Another argued that T-61's relatively narrow procedural tolerance, relatively high incidence of adverse reactions, and demonstrated severe excitement reactions in large animals make the drug a liability. A third stated that, while the esthetics of barbiturate euthanasia are not always good, they are usually better than those associated with T-61 euthanasia. On the other side, one person commented that, after fifty years of experience, T-61 was by far the best euthanasia agent or method that has been made available. Another noted that T-61 is an effective euthanasia agent although it would be reassuring to know what it is actually doing in the animal.

There were a number of contradictory comments on specific aspects of T-61 use. Several respondents noted that they had no problems with T-61 because they only used the drug for equine or large animal euthanasia. Others said that the drug was definitely *not* satisfactory for equine euthanasia. Some noted that extra-venous injection of T-61 was very painful and ineffective while others said that intracardiac, intrathoracic, or intraperitoneal injections were effective and did not cause pain. Several respondents argued that one had to use double or triple the recommended dose and there was a wide variation on the question of whether or not T-61 should be administered according to the manufacturer's instructions—namely, two-thirds of the dose should be administered slowly (one milliliter/5 seconds) and the remainder injected rapidly. Table 3 indicates the range of opinions on this matter. In one response, it was noted that a double dose of T-61 injected very rapidly was satisfactory while small doses injected slowly were not.

Table 3. Opinions on importance of injecting first two-thirds of T-61 dose slowly.

	T-61 Users		Na Pent Users*		All	
	No.	%	No.	%	No.	%
Very Important	26	36.1	13	46.4	39	39
Moderately Important	20	27.8	9	32.1	29	29
Not Important	26	36.1	6	21.4	32	32
TOTALS	72	100	28	100	100	100

*Many of those (numbering 134 respondents) who were not using T-61 did not complete the section of the questionnaire dealing with the rate of injection.

The questionnaire results also demonstrated a wide range of opinion on the cost issue. T-61 users were evenly divided on whether the agent was more expensive or less expensive to use than other euthanasia products. Barbiturate users who responded on this question indicated that T-61 was more expensive. According to one survey of suppliers, T-61 is considerably more expensive than Fatal-Plus or Euthanasia-6 but about the same price as Beuthanasia-D (Barocio 1983). This is confirmed by Lumb and Moreland (1982) who note that the cost per pound to euthanize an animal with T-61 or Beuthanasia is about three to four times that of the simpler pentobarbital products.

During analysis of the questionnaires, it often seemed as though respondents were reporting on two different drugs, so contradictory were some of the responses and comments. Part of the reason for this may well be due to the fact that T-61 administration does have narrow procedural tolerances and slight differences in technique may produce large differences in reported responses. Some of the reports appear to contradict the published results of Lumb et al. (1978) who noted that the ECG activity lasted longer in the barbiturate-injected dogs than in those receiving T-61. There were a number of reports of the heartbeat continuing for up to a minute or more by respondents who had used T-61 and some uneasiness was expressed over this.

While there are some problems with the survey (self-reporting is not as reliable as recorded observations), and the questionnaire did not identify precisely how much experience individuals had had with T-61 (it is possible that some comments were based on very limited experience), it is possible to draw some conclusions. For example, it is clear that T-61 is not always used in the clinic according to the manufacturer's recommendations. It is also clear that there are many questions about T-61 that still need to be resolved. For example, what is the clinical incidence of muscle tremors and/or convulsions and what causes them? Is the prolonged duration of the heartbeat after the injection a problem that needs to be addressed? What is the reason for contradictory reports of T-61 euthanasia in large animals? This survey cannot answer such questions but merely adds to the anecdotal data indicating that the continuing use of T-61 as a euthanasia agent needs to be subjected to close and critical review.

References

AVMA. 1972. Report of the AVMA Panel on Euthanasia. *J. Am. Vet. Med. Assoc.* 160:761-72

AVMA. 1978. Report of the AVMA Panel on Euthanasia. *J. Am. Vet. Med. Assoc.* 173:59-72

Barocio, L.D. 1983. Review of literature on use of T-61 as a euthanasic agent. *Int. J. Study Animal Problems.* 4:336-42

Carding, T. 1977. Euthanasia of dogs and cats: An analysis of experience and current knowledge with recommendations for research. *Animal Reg. Study.* 1:5-21

Eikmeier, M. 1962. Experiences with a new preparation for painless destruction of small animals (T-61). *Die Blauen Hefte Tierarztl.* 5:22-23

Lumb, W.V. and Moreland, A.F. 1982. Chemical methods for euthanasia. *Lab Animal.* 11(4):29-35

Lumb, W.V., Doshi, K., and Scott, J.R. 1978. A comparative study of T-61 and pentobarbital for euthanasia of dogs. *J. Am. Vet. Med. Assoc.* 172:149-52

Quin, A.H. 1963. Observations on a new euthanasia agent for small animals. *Vet. Med.* 58:494-5

Reilly, L.L. 1978. Euthanasia of dogs. *J. Am. Vet. Med. Assoc.* 172:984

Editor's Commentary

Euthanasia means a humane death. For euthanasia to be humane, therefore, it must induce unconsciousness, not arrest respiration before unconsciousness occurs, and bring about the onset of death swiftly and consistently.

T-61 cannot be regarded as a suitable euthanasia agent because it fails to meet this second criterion, namely, consistency. T-61 does not act consistently: it can cause animals intense pain soon after initial administration, or even a curare-like paralysis of respiration before *the animal is unconscious.*

If T-61 were consistent in its pharmacological effects and caused death swiftly and without pain or distress to animals, then veterinarians would be consistent in their recognition and acceptance of T-61 as a humane compound for euthanasia. But the truth is that there is no unanimous consensus in the veterinary profession to this end as evidenced by Andrew Rowan's survey.

That only 27.8 percent of respondents approved of T-61 and 44 percent experienced bad reactions in animals to this compound is clear evidence that T-61 does not meet the humane euthanasia criterion of consistency or reliability.

Bad reactions reported by veterinarians in Rowan's study included: muscle tremors and excitation, including convulsions, crying, and agonal thrashing; and prolonged heart activity, the heart beating for five minutes or longer after brain death had apparently occurred.

The manufacturers will claim that such undesirable reactions occur because the veterinarians have not followed their printed instructions for proper administration of T-61. But surely so many veterinarians who are opposed to the use of T-61 in Rowan's survey cannot be that illiterate and incompetent as to be incapable of administering T-61 properly.

Furthermore, since the manufacturers clearly admit that improper administration can result in inhumane side-effects on animals, it is self-evident that since competent and experienced veterinarians have had problems with this compound, animal shelter and animal control personnel using T-61 are likely to encounter problems even more frequently.

Thus T-61 should not be approved for use by laypersons in animal shelters and it is for these reasons that The Humane Society of the United States (HSUS) has concluded in a recent publication that "T-61 is an impractical and unacceptable euthanasia drug. It is not a controlled substance, but it is one of the more expensive euthanasia drugs." This publication also emphasizes that T-61 is of limited use because "a major limitation...is that it should be injected only *intravenously and not administered by any other route; an additional limitation is that it should be administered at a precise rate. Not only does the skill of the euthanasia technician vary from person to person, but the reactions of the animals are variable and unpredictable."*

This publication approves of sodium pentobarbital as the best euthanasia method available and endorses the use of FP-3 (sodium pentobarbital plus lidocaine), the added benefit being that this is easier to obtain as a Schedule III drug rather than Schedule II as sodium pentobarbital is classified.

Further evidence in support of T-61 being rejected as being an unsatisfactory and unreliable euthanasia compound comes from the United Kingdom, where T-61 is not accepted by the veterinary profession. British veterinarian Deborah J. Baker, employed by Hoechst Company, manufacturers of T-61 states, in a letter to The HSUS (7 August 1980):

> *"...for the last four years, this product has been unavailable in the U.K. It was withdrawn because although for Euthanasia the mode of action seems good, in practice, I gather that animals euthanized with this tended to have rather distressing, painful convulsions accompanied by howling prior to their demise, this being because the phases, i.e. induction stage, anaesthetic stage and respiratory paralysis do not occur in that order, and one tends to get respiratory paralysis prior to anaesthesia being completed. I, myself, therefore, would not recommend its use for euthanasia purposes."*

A study by Dr. William Lumb comparing T-61 and sodium pentobarbital published in the Journal of the American Veterinary Medical Association *comparing the effects of sodium pentobarbital and T-61 (January 15, 1968) is often cited as showing that T-61 is superior because some of the dogs given sodium pentobarbital did not die. While it might be unfair to suggest that this study, funded by the manufacturers of T-61, was rigged to ensure a favorable outcome for them, it is obvious that the investigator avoided overdosing the dogs with sodium pentobarbital in order to ensure that they would not recover, which is common practice when using this drug for euthanasia. Dr. Lumb used a weaker (anaesthetic-surgery) strength solution of sodium pentobarbital in this study, than is routinely used when this drug is employed for euthanasia. Little wonder therefore that some dogs recovered.*

It is obvious from the above evidence, and in view of the fact that there are more humane alternatives to using T-61 as a euthanasia agent, that T-61 should not be approved for euthanasia purposes in animal shelters. Nor should it be recognized as an acceptable agent of euthanasia.

ETHICAL ASPECTS OF ANIMAL EXPERIMENTATION

Wolfgang Scharmann

Bundesgesundheitsamt
Postfach D-1000
Berlin 33 West Germany

If inquiries are made of people regarding their attitudes towards animal experimentation, there will no doubt be various answers corresponding to the different ethical attitudes today. Three principle points of view are imaginable. The two extremes are: an unrestricted support of all animal experiments; and a radical rejection of any such experiment. These two positions, in all likelihood, are taken by only a minority of the population. The majority will approve of animal experimentation in principle, however, only insofar as it is really necessary to preserve human life. So, the point of controversy arises from the question: When is an animal experiment necessary and indispensable?

The easiest solution, of course, (especially for legislators and authorities responsible for regulations on animal experimentation), would be to provide clearly defined statements as to which animal experiments are really necessary, that is, a catalogue of all experiments that are justifiable on ethical grounds. There cannot, however, be such a classification due to the fact that opinions regarding which animal experiments are necessary are largely divergent among the scientific as well as the lay community. Ethical demands will always be binding only in the individual case. Such demands can serve as a basis for legal regulations only after having become generally recognized.

So, the decision as to whether or not the purpose of an experiment is justifiable in terms of animal suffering would seem to rest with the individual scientist. The investigator will be able to accept this responsibility in a fair manner only if he/she recognizes the animal as a sentient, animated individual capable of suffering and with whom he/she feels connected through a common history of evolution. To many scientists, this demand may seem to be emotionally exaggerated. Their knowledge of the animal has been formed by scientific studies which are almost exclusively limited to morphological description and measurement of physiological parameters which provide the young scientist with a unilateral mechanistic picture of the phenomenon of life. Modern veterinary medicine still adheres considerably to the Cartesian belief that animals are merely automatons, incapable of feeling distress and suffering. Therefore, we have to ask ourselves how to what degree the prevalence and extent of animal experimentation may be associated with the conversion of the animal into an object by the teachings of the natural sciences. Does the downgrading of the animal to the status of a measuring instrument, a live apparatus, reduce the threshold inhibiting humans from manipulating an animal, inflicting pain on it, or killing it? What is the value of compassion when the realization of scientific goals are at stake?

I ask this question, since I personally know very well how powerful the authority of science is, especially to young scientists. The investigations of Milgram (Milgram 1974) and others have revealed that science is regarded as an authority which is not questioned even if the scientific method appears to be doubtful. Although Milgram's studies have often been cited, they shall be described in brief because they may be significant also in regard to animal experimentation.

In his experiment, Milgram designated naive subjects as "teachers" and made them believe they would inflict electric shocks to a test person (the "learner") as part of a scientific study on learning capability. The "learner," however, was an actor who had been informed of the experiment. Guided by a scientist, most "teachers" inflicted the alleged shocks with rising intensity until there was the warning: "Danger—severe shock." Even protests and agonized screams of the "victim" did not cause most of the teachers to discontinue with the experiment when the scientist enjoined in continuing the shocks. They considered themselves as cooperators of an important research program which had to be performed to the benefit of society even if in its course nasty situations and sacrifices could not be avoided. An action which normally appeared evil to the naive subjects acquired a totally different meaning and legitimacy when carried out by the authority of science.

Albert Schweitzer, known for his precept of "reverence for life," deplored a tendency in his contemporaries to give up thinking for themselves and instead to rely on truths spoon-fed by authority. "The man," he said, "who has truly become a thinking being feels a compulsion to give to every will-to-live the same reverence for life that he gives to his own" (Schweitzer 1952). If we nevertheless consciously overrule the will-to-live of animals because we relate more strongly with the suffering fellow human being than with the suffering animal, we inflict guilt upon ourselves. In my opinion, only a human being conscious of becoming guilty and accepting guilt should be able to perform animal experiments.

Thus it will be more important than ever to raise and to strengthen the understanding by scientists, animal caretakers, and all others involved in animal experimentation of the will and the right of the animal to live. Approaches for this goal should be found above all else in the training curricula for scientists. The animals used for experiments should no longer be represented, viewed, and handled as objects, as is too often the case. A system of critical self-control of scientists by means of animal care or ethical committees (which exist in a number of countries already) may contribute to a sensitization of researchers. Conceivably, within this system, when research projects are discussed within ethical committees, the experimenter will be reminded of his/her responsibility to the animals. In the planning stages of experiments, the researcher will be expected to take into account scientific criteria, but show equal consideration for the animals even if this results in additional work and trouble. Such consideration and handling of the animal in the most careful manner possible will not only correspond to ethical concepts, but eventually also result in benefits for research as it is logical that experimental results will be of greater reliability when obtained using animals that are not stressed or in pain.

However, even if voting in favor of animal experimentation (with the reservation that experiments should be carried out only for indispensable purposes), we should ask ourselves whether the oppressingly high number of animal experiments does not exceed by far those justifiably necessary to maintain human life in dignity. In this respect, I refer to the great number of experiments conducted in connection with the control of civilization-associated diseases accounting for the major part of medicaments administered today in the industrialized nations. The major part of these illnesses have been caused by man himself when pursuing a wrong style of life. A comprehensive long-term study over a period of ten years (Schweiker 1982) involving seven thousand American male and female adults has demonstrated that the observance of a few positive health practices, such as not smoking, getting enough sleep and exercise, consuming alcohol only in moderation, maintaining proper weight, and eating breakfast, is of far greater importance for the maintenance of health than all the advances of twentieth century medicine, including those garnered by animal experiments.

I also ask myself whether in order to maintain man's existence, is it in fact necessary to introduce more than one thousand new chemicals annually into the market worldwide (Balls 1983)? Estimation of the associated risk requires experiments of between two thousand and six thousand animals per agent. One segment of these animal experiments is toxicological studies which involve severe suffering. When looking at the victim we must ask ourselves whether the price of economic growth, affluence, and a comfortable life (and animal experiments stand only for a fraction of this price) can still be justified.

Finally, I ask myself whether scientists, who thus far have decided upon the objective of their research mainly under their own responsibility, should not increasingly regard the public as their partner in discussion. The assertion of scientists that research would serve progress and human well-being has lost its credibility for many people. We have to ask whether or not there should be a re-thinking of what should be the essence of progress in the natural sciences. Will scientists alone be able to find a way out of the ecological crisis?

At least one thing has been clarified. We shall have to learn how to handle nature in a less destructive and more careful way. In my opinion, this would also include a higher examination of the will-to-live of animals, irrespective of whether they belong to wildlife or experimental species.

These questions and doubts should not be understood as attribution of guilt to a certain group, but rather as self-criticism and a suggestion to re-think our everyday actions. Such self-evaluation should also include the demand being voiced by so many people to reduce animal experiments, especially the painful ones. Their concerns should not be regarded simply as a nuisance impairing scientific work, although what is said by animal activists may often be exaggerated or even technically wrong. Rather it should also be understood as a call for a humane society in which nature is no longer taken as the object of exploitation but instead as a partner within the overall association of life.

References

Balls, M. 1983. *Veterinary Record.* 113: 398.

Milgram, S. 1974. *Obedience to Authority: An Experimental View.* London: Tavistock

Schweiker, R.S. 1892. *Public Health Reports.* 97:196.

Schweitzer, A. 1952. Aus meinem Leben und Denken. Hamburg: Fischer-Bucherei. (English translation: 1961. *Out of My Life and Thought.* New York: Holt, Rinehart, and Winston.)

ANIMAL PAIN

Bernard E. Rollin

Department of Philosophy
Colorado State University
Fort Collins, Colorado
80523

Introduction

Some time ago, I received a telephone call from an eminent primatologist asking me to give the keynote address at a scientific seminar on animal pain. My first response was to express surprise that they were inviting a philosopher. His reply was remarkable, if only for its rarity among scientists: "The truly interesting and important issues concerning pain in animals are not scientific ones," he said. "They are moral, philosophical, and conceptual ones. And the total failure of science to engage or even acknowledge these issues discredits biomedical science and weakens its conceptual base." I hope to show you that my colleague was indeed correct, and that the scientific community's attitude towards animal pain is muddled, inconsistent, incoherent, and perpetuated by self-serving ideological positions which are rarely subjected to logical scrutiny.

The Dilemma of Pain Research

Perhaps the primary issue which needs to be brought forth is the fundamental ambivalence displayed by the scientific community regarding the reality and knowability of animal pain. As I shall indicate, this is just a special case in a generalized ambivalence endemic among scientists towards matter of animal consciousness and awareness. Simply stated, the ambivalence in the case of pain manifests itself as follows: On the one hand, scientists are loath to speak of animals experiencing pain or pleasure (or any mental state) for such claims are felt to be unverifiable at worst (and hence unscientific), and anthropomorphic at best. On the other hand, scientists often find themselves incapable of doing and describing their own work if they do not presuppose and speak of animal pain (and other mental states). The foregoing dilemma, which puts scientists in a logically incoherent position, is rarely resolved —most often, in fact, it is simply ignored.

This point revealed itself clearly at an American Association of Laboratory Animal Science (AALAS) seminar at which I lectured, held a few years ago on standards of care for domestic farm animals used in research (AALAS 1982). Participants found themselves unable to discuss the welfare of farm animals without talking about the conditions which make these animals happy, but were professionally reluctant to advance claims about animal happiness, claims which were seen as unscientific. Most participants sailed over the difficulty by talking about what conditions make animals "happy"—a move which doubtless made them terminologically more comfortable, but which simply glossed over the issue we are discussing. (What, for example, is the difference between happy and "happy"?)

A moment's reflection will reveal that, on some level, science is absolutely committed to the belief that animals feel pain (and experience other mental states) which are, to a significant degree, analogous to what human beings experience. If animals did not, it would surely be absurd to do pain research on them, and to study dose responses to anesthetics and analgesics. In fact, not only does such research logically presuppose that animals feel pain, it even attempts to provide some quantitative measures of the pain and of its control by analgesics through such tests as the hotplate (writhing) test, the tail-flick test, skin-twitch test, the head-withdrawal test, pressure tests involving tails and digits, and electrical stimulation tests (Lineberry 1981). Further, such tests also presuppose some meaningful analogies between animal and human pain, for they are employed in part to screen substances for potential analgesic effect in humans.

A similar tension, of course, exists in psychology. Psychologists reject allegedly anthropomorphic ascription of human mental states like fear, anxiety, depression, boredom, and hopelessness to animals, as being outside the scope of legitimate scientific claims. However, the unstated presupposition of psychological research is that these states are analogous in humans and animals, and that their study in animals provides valuable insights into their nature in humans. The currently popular work in hopelessness and learned helplessness provides a very clear example of how psychologists who do such animal work must presuppose analogous states in men and beasts. Presupposing such analogies leads to the inevitable and much discussed "psychologists' dilemma" (which is also the "pain physiologists' dilemma"): If these noxious mental states in animals are sufficiently analogous to those of humans to provide adequate models for human experience, what right have we to induce them in animals? And if they are totally disanalogous, what is the value of studying them? Such embarrassing conclusions again lead to a form of learned helplessness among the psychologists—unable to resolve the tension between their professed skepticism about animal consciousness and their implicit reliance upon it, they avoid the issue altogether, and simply wish it out of existence.

Some five years ago, I personally experienced an extraordinary example of the contradiction we have been discussing. I had served on a panel on animal pain with a well-known pain physiologist who spent the better part of an hour trying to show that since the electrochemical activity in the cerebral cortex of a dog differed dramatically from the electrochemical activity in the cerebral cortex of humans, and since the cerebral cortex is the information processing area of the brain, the dog didn't *really* feel pain in any sense that humans do.

The time came for my rebuttal, and although I am usually long-winded, in this case my response was quite brief. I said, "Dr. X, you are justly acclaimed for your work in pain." "Thank you," he said. "You do that work on dogs, do you not?" I queried. "I do," he replied. "You extrapolate the results to people, do you not?" I queried. "That is correct," he said. "In that case," I said, "I have nothing else to say!" In other words, either his paper was false, or his research work was—he could not have it both ways.

Moral Consequences of the Dilemma

If a lack of intellectual coherence in science were the only consequence issuing from the scientific community's ambivalence on animal pain and awareness, that alone would justify a vigorous attempt to resolve the problem. But more is at stake than coherence. Moral issues also suffer. It is, of course, a fundamental principle of logic that from a contradiction anything at all may be deduced, and this is precisely what occurs in this area. For what essentially occurs is that whenever it is pragmatically expedient, one term of the contradiction is simply suppressed and ignored. If it is convenient to study pain mechanisms or analgesia in animals, it is taken for granted that animals feel pain. But when it is convenient or conscience-salving to ignore the painful consequences of one's research or teaching manipulations on animals, out comes the claim that one cannot really know what or even *that* animals experience. This in turn enables researchers to avoid having to deal with the infliction of pain as a moral problem. Almost anyone who has been trained as a veterinarian in this country will at some point have encountered the claim that animals don't really feel pain as we do, or if they do, it is purely momentary and transient. Not too many years ago, I am told by my older veterinary colleagues, this was a mainstream ideology, commonly asserted. A leading veterinary pain expert, Dr. Michael Kaplan, estimated that probably 75 percent of veterinarians still view anesthesia as chemical restraint (personal communciation), and I myself encountered this very dramatically at a veterinary college. I had just finished asserting that veterinarians at least couldn't doubt that animals feel pain or else why would they study anesthesia and analgesia. Up jumped the associate dean, livid with rage. "Anesthesia and analgesia have nothing to do with pain," he declared, "they are methods of chemical restraint." (An Austrailian scientist in the audience responded beautifully: "He's daft," he declared. "What the hell do they need restraint for if they are not in pain?")

The moral cash value or consequence of all this is readily documentable: Little is done in the course of animal research to control even "unnecessary" pain—i.e., pain not essential to the protocol in question. If animal pain is not real, why treat it? This philosophical position goes a long way towards explaining why so few protocols embody provisions for laboratory animal analgesia; and why, incredibly enough, virtually no conferences have been held on laboratory animal analgesia (the seminar I attended was only the second one ever held) (Erickson 1983), and why, indeed, the use of analgesia is so rare in ordinary veterinary practice and so little taught in veterinary schools. It also helps explain why few scientists have, until very recently, addressed the ethical questions arising from inflicting pain on animals.

In fact, many researchers do not even understand that the infliction of pain constitutes an ethical question. I recall one group of researchers telling me that the failure to use anesthesia and analgesia in certain protocols has nothing to do with ethics—it is solely a scientific decision arising out of a desire not to introduce new variables which might skew the data! It also explains why many scientists see the social demand for control of pain as an illegitimate intrusion by non-experts into their freedom of inquiry, rather than as a legitimate moral claim, and thus oppose legislation which would only require control of pain "not essential to the protocol." It is ironic that rodents are the most infrequent recipients of analgesia in the course of research done on them, yet that, jumping to the other side of the contradiction, virtually all analgesics have been tested on rodents, so dose response curves are well known.

To summarize: The philosophical problem built into the ambivalence about animal pain that we have been discussing may be restated as follows: Either animals feel pain or they do not. Science, in its activities, and insofar as its practitioners are people of good common sense, has presupposed that animals do feel pain, and the consequences of current biological theory assert this is surely the case. Conversely, the ideology of science has tended to claim either that animals do not feel pain, or at least that we cannot know if they do, just as we cannot know about any mental state in animals. (The latter two claims tend, of course, to slide into the former.) This in turn circumvents the need for ethical theorizing about when pain-infliction is justifiable.

Mechanization of Pain and Stress

In actual practice, the scientific community has sometimes tended to try to smooth over this paradox. It has done so, in general, by treating pain as a mechanical physiological or neurophysiological occurrence, rather than as a mental state or mode of awareness. In this way, it has tried to avoid "unscientific claims," and has also assuaged common sense and moral reluctance to inflict uncontrolled real pain on animals. On this essentially Cartesian view, pain responses are objectively studiable, physical, mechanical states, rather than states of awareness. Such an approach admits the existence of physiological mechanisms of pain, while ducking the issue of how the animal feels. A good example of this approach may be found in the aforementioned old view of anesthesia as chemical restraint. A more recent example may be found in the American Physiological Society symposium held on animal pain, which deals in exquisite detail with the neurophysiology and neurochemistry and mechanisms and behavior involved in animal pain, while almost never discussing the psychic and morally relevant component, namely, that the animal hurts (Kitchell and Erickson 1983).

A similar conceptually problematic attempt to deny other states of awareness, especially unpleasant ones, by reducing them to mechanical processes rather than mental states may be found in the widespread and notoriously fuzzy use of the concept of stress as a catchall for fear, anxiety, and other sorts of misery. Stress is often felt to be objective and measurable, and is defined primarily in terms of activation of the pituitary-adrenal axis, or in other physicochemical terms. What is rarely, if ever, mentioned in the scientific literature is the psychological-experiential component; the fact that the stressed animal is doubtless having unpleasant sensations at least somewhat analogous to sensations humans have under similar circumstances, which are responsible for the activation of the mechanisms studied. In other words, an animal would surely not show physiological signs of stress under various unpleasant conditions if it did not experience them as unpleasant. (Fully unconscious animals do not react to most stresses.) Some recent work has begun to recognize this point, and argues, as I have done, that the purely physicalistic explanation of stress is senseless without an explicit or implicit reference and appeal to what the animal is experiencing, which experience in turn activates these mechanisms (Archer 1979). In short, much of the literature is guilty of confusing physical signs and effects of stress with stress itself, and with using these physical signs of stress as a catchall for a variety of noxious mental states in its effort to avoid reference to animal thought and feeling.

Some scientists have carried this sort of mechanization of animal experience to incredible lengths. One of my colleagues in zoology recently took me to task for saying that horses prefer the taste of rolled oats with molasses to that of ordinary rolled oats. "You can't scientifically say that," he told me. "At most you can say that there is a mechanical process which leads them to be drawn towards the molasses, much as a thermostat is affected by temperature."

In other words, insofar as many scientists have addressed the dilemma we described, they have done so by eliminating reference to mental states, and reducing such notions as pain and fear to the physical processes associated with them. Why has this occurred? Why have they not gone the other way, and simply assumed, along with common sense and Darwin, that such animal experiences as pain are, *mutatis mutandis,* something like our own?

Philosophy of Science and Animal Consciousness

An answer to this question requires that we make a brief excursus into the history and philosophy of science. In the late nineteenth century, along with the ascendance of Darwinian biology, came a belief that psychological or mental states like pain, fear, anger, grief, and the like were surely as phylogenetically continuous as morphological and physiological traits. Highly respectable scientists like Darwin, Romanes, and H.S. Jennings took for granted the evolutionary continuity of thought and feeling, and their studiability in animals. Darwin himself, of course, wrote of the *Expression of Emotions in Man and Animals,* and studied the problem-solving ability of earthworms. Much interesting research was done under the assumption that animals could think and feel. By 1920, however, this view had been banished. Ironically, its banishment had nothing whatever to do with new empirical scientific discoveries which falsified it, or even with new conceptual analyses which showed it to be logically flawed, as Einstein had done with certain concepts of classical physics. Rather, what occurred was the rise of a new philosophy of science, which promised to set science on the right path, eliminate excess baggage from science, and banish anything that could not be verified factually, and which further introduced new values into science while claiming that science ought to be value-free. This movement peaked in positivism and behaviorism, both of which denied the cogency of talking about mental states in man *or* animal (though much of positivism was phenomenalistic), and in the case of behaviorism, came perilously close to asserting that we don't have thoughts, we only think we do (Rollin 1985). Psychology became the study of behavior, and subjective states of any sort were ordered out of existence in the name of scientific methodology. Most scientists working today continue to pick up some version of this simplistic philosophy of science along with their science in the course of their training, even though it has been largely abandoned by philosophers of science in recent years. So powerful is this ideology that it serves to eclipse common sense, coherence (as represented by evolutionary theory's clear presumption of continuity of mentation), and the acknowledgement of legitimate value questions in science.

The philosophical denial of consciousness and its studiability have certainly shaped the form of twentieth century science, but far more radically with regard to animals than to humans. After all, no scientist, not even the most ardent behaviorist, can ever doubt that he is conscious, or that his co-workers are conscious, or that they are feeling pains when they describe their thoughts and feelings to him in boring detail. On the other hand, in the case of animals, this new philosophy meshed nicely with convenience. If one's research necessitates hurting animals, one's work is made ever so much easier by a philosophy which suggests that animals aren't really feeling pain, they are "exhibiting pain behavior," aren't really crying out, but "vocalizing," aren't really suffering, but only "exhibiting mechanical responses." One need no longer feel morally ambivalent about hurting animals to advance knowledge, or feel compelled to assess that hurt morally and mask it with analgesia which may skew results if animals aren't really hurting, only responding. As we said earlier, this was buttressed by the notion that science was value-free, and that such judgments are scientific, not moral.

Thus the skepticism about animal pain and awareness which dominates twentieth century science has a variety of sources which reinforce one another. In the first place, it was part of a general move to allegedly eliminate the unverifiable from science. In the second place, it was part of a general move to make all science as reductionistic and as close to physics and chemistry as possible for the sake of exactness. In third place, it provided an effective method for closing off moral reservations and ambivalences about invasive animal research—if animals were in essence neurophysiological machines, imputing unpleasant mental states to them was just anthropomorphism, a prescientific bias which need to be guarded against.

What happened in the twentieth century was the same thing that happened with Descartes in the seventeenth—philosophy was invoked in order to overcome common sense. In the seventeenth century, Descartes had said that animals were machines with no souls, minds, or feelings, thereby reconciling in one master stroke the demands of Catholicism that animals not have souls with the demands of a growing science of physiology which forced in its quest for knowledge to do what common sense called atrocious and painful procedures to animals without any way of controlling the pain. No need to control the pain, said Cartesian physiologists, since it is not really experienced pain, it is rather merely mechanical response.

Other Arguments for Ignoring Animal Pain

To the general skepticism about animal consciousness in the early twentieth century were added other palliative arguments designed to teach young scientists and veterinarians that concern for animal pain was largely sentimental anthropomorphism. As many older veterinarians have told me, they were taught that animal pain is merely momentary—with teachers citing as evidence, for example, the fact that a cow will eat immediately after surgery. Such arguments, of course, neglect the fact that it is a selective advantage for a cow to behave that way regardless of how it feels. A cow that didn't eat would be weakened considerably, a cow that didn't graze with the rest of the herd when hurt would be flagged as vulnerable to predators.

In a similar vein, sometimes it was said by philosophers *and* scientists that animal pain, while perhaps momentarily present, was insignificant, for animals lack concepts enabling them to anticipate and remember. For example, the suffering engendered for us by worrying about and anticipating going to a painful situation such as the dentist which often makes the pain ever so much worse, simply does not arise in animals. Aside from the fact that animals clearly do anticipate and remember (for how else could they learn), another point is relevant here. If animals are indeed locked into what is happening at the moment, we are all the more obliged to try to relieve their suffering, since they themselves cannot look forward to or anticipate its cessation. For them there is no *hope*.

Spinoza pointed out that understanding the cause of an unpleasant sensation can diminish its severity, and not understanding its cause can increase its severity (Spinoza 1677). If this is the case, (and Spinoza's conjecture has been borne out by empirical work on humans), then surely we have reason to believe that animals, especially laboratory animals, suffer perhaps more severely than humans since they have no grasp of the causal chain occasioning the pain. At least one leading animal pain psychologist, Professor Kitchell, takes a similar line. He divides pain into a sensory-discriminative dimension and a motivational-affective dimension. The former concerns itself with locating and understanding the source of pain, the latter with escaping from it. Kitchell speculates that since animals are more limited than humans in the first dimension, lacking human intellectual abilities, it is plausible that the second dimension is correlatively stronger. In short, since animals cannot intellectually deal with danger and injury as we do, their motivation to flee must be correlatively stronger than ours—in short, they probably *hurt* more (personal communication).

Perhaps the most ironic and perverse argument against concern with animal pain is related to the two just discussed. It is often said that worrying about animal pain is misplaced anthropomorphism, for given painful circumstances where humans would be screaming and writhing, many animals show very few such signs. Aside from the point made earlier that stoic behavior doubtless confers a selective advantage on animals, we can make a much more ironic point. It is not the people who impute pain to animals who are anthropomorphic—they have good evolutionary, neurophysiological, and behavioral reasons to do so as I shall discuss shortly. It is those who deny pain to animals on the grounds that their behavior is unlike humans who are anthropomorphic—who else but someone guilty of the grossest anthropomorphism would expect a bovine in pain to behave like a human in pain. Animals do show unique pain behavior—it just doesn't happen to be human pain behavior. (People who know horses well in some cases are aware that the tightening of the palpebral (eyelid) muscles can eloquently bespeak great agony.)

It is difficult to believe that many of these beliefs were taken seriously intellectually. They seem, rather, to have been perpetuated by extra-logical factors. So perpetuated, of course, was the general lack of social concern for animals—even though common sense acknowledged the existence of animal pain, such people did not worry very much about it morally. We should also consider the probability that perpetuating the above ideology served as a highly useful defense mechanism for researchers enjoined in invasive work on animals. Researchers are, of course, as decent and reluctant to inflict pain as anyone else, even if they believe that what they are doing is important. Simply denying that animals felt or really felt pain helped forestall guilt and compunctions. If one did not genuinely believe that animals were not hurting, one would be forced to look into an abyss from which it is not easy to return.

Philosophical Bases for Affirming Animal Awareness

Philosphically, the denial of thought awareness and pain to animals on the grounds that we cannot experience them is not cogent. In the first place, as is well known, if we are so positivistic as to claim we cannot know anything we do not directly experience, we can make no claims about anyone's mental states but our own. Therefore, we cannot claim to know that other humans have minds or pains either. For that matter, as Berkeley showed (Berkeley 1710), if we restrict knowledge to our own sensations and perceptions, we can't even know that there is an external, public world existing independently of our perceptions of it! So the same hard line which claims we cannot know animal mental states, if carried to its logical conclusion, would render impossible both science (of an objective world) and interaction with our fellow humans.

In fact, the same sorts of things which count in favor of attributing mind, awareness, and pain to other human beings count in favor of attributing them to animals. Looking at pain, we find in the first place that the *behavioral* evidence which helps license us to attribute pain to other humans is also present in the case of animals. Animals cry out when injured, are tender at point of injury, cringe before blows, avoid electrical shock and heat, etc., etc. True, their behavioral responses are not always the same as ours—compare the horse's wincing rather than crying out when in pain—but, for that matter, human pain responses across different cultures and subcultures are not the same either. Compare, for example, the way in which middle class Jewish children are encouraged to express pain when they fall down as toddlers as contrasted with children raised on western ranches ("Get up, you aren't hurt!"). Compare athletes or runners who glory in pain, with others who think they are masochistic or mad. Much research has been done showing that cultural determinants loom large in shaping the experience, threshold, and expression of pain.

Classical research indicates that sociopsychological factors are major factors in shaping the experience of pain in humans. It has been shown, for example, that Northern Europeans are less susceptible to painful stimuli than are Southern Europeans, and this is explained by cultural rather than biological differences (Wolff and Langley 1975). In Beecher's classic work earlier this century (Beecher 1956), he showed that wounded soldiers required less analgesia than non-military surgical patients, even though the injuries to the soldiers were far more massive. He explained this by the fact that the soldiers were seeing a real benefit in the wound (i.e., no longer having their lives at risk on the battlefield), whereas the surgical patients were just focused on the pain. Such facts have sometimes been used to claim that animal pain is qualitatively different from human pain, because it is untouched by psychological factors. In actual fact, clinical veterinarians dispute this. A wounded animal seems to suffer less pain in the presence of an owner, less when treated at home or in familiar surroundings and when reassured, less when rapport is established with the clinician, less when stroked, etc. (If you doubt this, ask any vet who makes house calls.)

Second, in defending the view that animals feel pain, we may cite neurophysiological analogies between humans and animals, at least through the vertebrates. Ironically, the Cartesianism which made the science of physiology possible led to its own undoing, by an ever increasing demonstration of the identical neurophysiological mechanisms in humans and animals, mechanisms which make it highly implausible that animals are merely machines if we are not. Thus, here as elsewhere, we have scientific grounds for the reappropriation of common sense. Pain and pleasure centers in the brain, analogous to those found in humans, have been reported in birds, mammals, and fish (Walker 1983), and the neural mechanisms responsible for pain behavior are remarkably similar in all vertebrates. Anesthetics and analgesics control what appears to be pain in all vertebrates and, perhaps most dramatically, the biological feedback mechanisms for controlling pain seem to be remarkably similar in all vertebrates, involving serotonin, endorphins and enkephalins, and substance P (Kelly 1984). The very existence of endogenous opiates in animals is powerful evidence that they feel pain. In certain shock experiments, large doses of naloxone have been given to traumatized animals, reversing the effect of endogenous opiates, and it has been shown that the animals so treated will die as a direct result of uncontrolled pain (Fettman 1984).

Third, we may cite evidence from evolutionary theory. The pain mechanisms seem to remain remarkably constant among at least the vertebrates. Here, as elsewhere, there is reason to believe that evolution preserves and perpetuates successful biological systems. If the mechanisms are the same, it would strain credibility to suggest that the experience of pain suddenly emerges at the level of humans. Not only is such a hypothesis *ad hoc*, it is not plausible. We know from cases among human beings that the ability to feel pain is essential to survival; people with a congenital inability to feel pain or with afflictions such as Hansen's disease are unlikely to do well or even survive without extraordinary heroic attention. (The same, of course, is true in animals—witness Dr. Taub's deafferented monkeys.) The *feeling* of pain and its motivational influence are essential to the survival value of the system—to suggest that the system is purely mechanical in animals but not in man is therefore highly implausible. If pain worked well as a purely mechanical system in animals without a subjective dimension, why would it suddenly appear in man? (Unless, of course, as my wife pointed out, one invokes some such theological notion as original sin and pain as divine punishment—hardly a legitimate scientific move!)

Fourth, when scientists express the view that we cannot legitimately make claims about animal pain because we can't directly experience it, they seem to forget that much science in fact presupposes animal pain. More importantly, they seem to forget that the actual practice of science, as opposed to its positivistic ideological rhetoric, has never really taken seriously the injunction that one must only deal with what is directly observable. If science did take this notion seriously, it could hardly concern itself with genes, quarks, and black holes, indeed all theoretical, non-observable entities. Animal subjective experience enjoys a similar status—it is postulated to explain observed behavior and physiological activity. As long as it continues to provide explanatory and predictive power, it seems legitimate and indeed necessary to admit its existence (Rollin 1985).

Conclusions

If what we have been arguing is correct, it is not at all problematic—philosophically or scientifically—to attribute pain and other mental states to animals. Granted that we are always in danger of excessive anthropomorphism when we do so, but it surely doesn't follow that just because an idea can be abused, it shouldn't be used at all. (If we followed that dictum, we'd have no ideas at all!) We have good scientific and philosophical reasons to postulate animal pain and other modes of awareness; indeed we must do so in order to even do such a thing as pain research. Furthermore, this postulation is not mere speculation; it generates all sorts of research which regularly puts the hypothesis to test. In addition, it explains what animals do and how they behave, and is consistent with the evolutionary theoretical approach upon which modern biology rests, as well as with common sense and ordinary practice. (D.O. Hebb (1946) has shown that zookeepers are unable to do their job if they are not allowed to apply mentalistic terms to animals in describing their states and behavior.) How many of us could deal with the family dog if we weren't allowed to say things like "He wants to play"; "He is afraid of sirens"; "He doesn't like the taste of dry dog food"?

Given everything we have said, why has the scientific community, and more particularly, the veterinary community, been so cavalier about animal pain? I say cavalier, for example, because of the rarity in which analgesics are used either in research or in veterinary practice. This point has been made forcefully in the only contribution to the aforementioned American Physiological Society volume on animal pain which displays any concern with the moral and conceptual aspects of such pain. In his paper, Professor Davis (1983) remarks that:

> One of the psychological curiosities of therapeutic decision-making is the withholding of analgesic drugs, because the clinician is not absolutely certain that the animal is experiencing pain. Yet the same individual will administer antibiotics without documenting the presence of a bacterial infection.

The answer has less to do with science than with philosophy. Until recently, little value has been put on concern for animal pain in research and in scientific and veterinary education. Common sense questions of the form "surely that hurts the animal" were countered with ideological pronouncements about animals not feeling pain, animals not really in pain, animals feeling only momentary pain, or our inability even to address this notion. (At a recent scientific meeting, one speaker spoke derisively of the attempt by the Wisconsin Primate Center to develop a scale of invasiveness of procedures using animals—as if it were as scientifically absurd as a scale of holiness.) These teachings were partially a matter of dogma concerning what science could know and more than partially a matter of convenience—it is much easier to do invasive things to animals if one believes they aren't being hurt. I once had some students come to me to tell me that their instructor, a wildlife biologist, has taught them that fish did not feel pain. In response to my query, he told me that of course one couldn't know one way or the other, and that while insofar as one could tell, all evidence indicated that they could feel pain, it made his job infinitely easier if the students didn't *worry* about animal pain.

In general, either out of considerations of ideology, convenience, or emotional self-defense, animal pain and its control are not dealt with a great deal in science. I recall asking a medical researcher why so few federally funded projects wrote in provisions for laboratory animal analgesia, even when such use would not compromise the data. Up jumped a friend of mine, the chief of veterinary surgery at this institution; "Oh," he said, "that's because the use of analgesia isn't standard veterinary prac..." His hand flew to his mouth and he turned pale as he realized what he had said. "Oh my God," he went on, "I've been doing major surgeries like thoracotomies for twenty-five years, and it never dawned on me that these animals surely experience post-surgical pain."

Fundamentally, the basic reason that the scientific community has been so cavalier about animal pain is the fact that animals enjoy no socially sanctioned or legally codified moral status. People—even ordinary people who don't doubt that animals think and feel—are not used to thinking of animals in "the moral tone of voice." (Human pain has at various times and places been similarly ignored in medical research in the case of human groups with no real moral status—women, slaves, blacks, indigents, convicts, political prisoners, etc.) Animals are generally seen as tools, and cheap ones at that, which should be kept in decent repair (i.e., fed and watered), but beyond that, need no great concern. (Ironically, this has compromised a great deal of research by leading to a failure on the part of the researchers to think about, reckon with, and control stress variables which have enormous effects on physiological parameters—witness Gärtner's (1980) work with simply moving rats in a cage a distance of three feet and thereby markedly affecting a variety of plasma variables in a manner indicating microcirculatory shock reactions.)

But science can no longer afford the luxury of ignoring the moral status of animals and not dealing with animal pain. For society as a whole, in the last decade, has begun to change its *gestalt* on animals, and ever-increasingly sees animals as objects of moral concern. Ever-increasing ferment in Britain, Europe, and the U.S. provides evidence for the claim that animal welfare issues may well be "the Vietnam of the 80s." For an ever-increasing number of people, how we treat animals needs to be assessed by moral criteria, not merely by criteria of efficiency and convenience. And, clearly, the very first question which needs to be addressed by anyone looking at animals morally is whether they are suffering any pain at our hands which could be eliminated, avoided, or mitigated.

In today's society, such traditional practices as multiple survival surgery, uncontrolled post-operative pain, and housing which makes no allowance for animals' social and behavioral needs, are no longer considered acceptable. And common sense, tempered with moral concern for animals, will have no patience with the old notion that animals do not feel pain, or that we cannot know that they do. A continued failure on the part of science to address moral issues concerning laboratory animals will not be tolerated. And thus, the inconsistent, self-serving, ideology of science which defines animal pain out of existence can no longer serve as a valuational basis for scientific activity. As anyone who has tried to get research funding knows, the idea that science is value-free is a myth; ignoring one's valuational presuppositions does not mean that they are not there.

The moment has come for science to reassess its valuational presuppositions regarding the moral status of animals, and their use. This is not merely a moral requirement, and a scientific one, but necessary to the very survival of science in the current social milieu. While this is certainly a challenge, it need not be viewed as a threat. If such reassessment is rationally accomplished, everyone concerned will benefit. The public will feel secure that full moral concern has been extended to animals; animals will no longer suffer useless, needless, controllable pain; science will inevitably benefit from greater attention to pain and stress variables, and scientists will no longer have to entertain a double standard; officially denying the reality and significance of animal pain as part of the ideology of science, while presupposing it in their work and acknowledging it in their daily interactions with family pets. As I have argued elsewhere, science is inseparable from value questions, including moral ones, and the question of animal pain is inescapably as much a moral question as a scientific one.

One final note: The day I finished this paper a recent neuroscience textbook crossed my desk. The first sentence of the chapter on pain perhaps betokens a change in scientific attitudes on this issue. The author writes that "pain is a primitive, protective *experience* (not mechanism, emphasis mine,) which we share with all living organisms" (Kelly 1982). I take this as a positive sign that for whatever reason, perhaps the sorts of social concerns we discussed, scientists are beginning to soften their attitudes, both on whether animals experience pain and on whether we can know this, and perhaps the next generation of scientists will take this for granted. It is also noteworthy that there is no argument in this chapter for the quoted claim; perhaps, given the current moral climate on animals, scientists will go from a "Well, we can't really know if animals feel pain, so let's assume that they don't" attitude to "Well, even if we can't know, let's give them the benefit of the doubt" stance, a position I have in fact seen articulated in science journals (cf the *Laboratory Animals* article mentioned earlier and Davis' article). This is unfortunate, for only when good philosophical arguments on this issue have driven out bad ones can we feel confident that science will not slip back to either denying or ignoring the pain of animals.

References

AALAS annual meeting. Seminar on "Standards of care for domestic farm animals used in research." Washington, D.C., October, 1982.

Archer, J. 1979. *Animals Under Stress.* Baltimore: University Park Press.

Beecher, H.K. 1956. Relationship of significance of wound to pain experienced. *J.A.M.A.* 161:1609-13.

Berkeley, A. 1710. *Principles of Human Knowledge.*

Davis, L. 1983. Species differences in drug disposition as factors in alleviation of pain. In: Kitchell, R. and Erickson, H. eds. *Animal Pain: Perception and Alleviation.* Bethesda, MD: American Physiological Society.

Erickson, H. 1983. Preface. In: Kitchell, R. and Erickson, H. eds. *Animal Pain: Perception and Alleviation.* Bethesda, MD: American Physiological Society.

Fettman, M. 1984. Naloxone therapy in awake endotoxemic yucatan minipigs. *Jour. of Surg. Res.* 37:208-25.

Gärtner, D. 1980. Stress response of rats to handling and experimental procedures. *Lab. Animals.* 14:267-74.

Hebb, D.O. 1946. Emotion in man and animal. *Psychology Review.* 53:88-106.

Kelly, D.D. 1982. Central representations of pain and analgesia. In: Kandel, E. and Schwartz, J. eds. *Principles of Neural Science.* New York: Elsevier.

Kitchell, R. and Erickson, H. 1983. *Animal Pain: Perception and Alleviation.* Bethesda, MD: American Physiological Society.

Lineberry, C.W. 1981. Laboratory animals in pain research. In: Gay, W. Ed. *Methods of Animal Experimentation.* VI. New York: Academic Press.

Rollin, B. 1985. Animal consciousness and scientific change. *New Ideas in Psychology:* forthcoming.

Spinoza, B. 1677. *Ethics.* Part V.

Walker, S. 1983. *Animal Thought.* London: Routledge and Kegan Paul.

Wolff, B. and Langley, S. 1975. Cultural factors and the response to pain: a review. In: Weisenberg, M. ed. *Pain: Clinical and Experimental Perspectives.* St. Louis: C.V. Mosby.

Animal Experimentation in the Psychology Setting

THREE BLIND MICE, SEE HOW THEY RUN: A CRITIQUE OF BEHAVIORAL RESEARCH WITH ANIMALS

Michael A. Giannelli

The Fund for Animals
12548 Ventura Blvd.
Suite 141
Studio City, CA
91604

Introduction

Animal research has been a traditionally accepted and respected part of modern psychology from its earliest days. The prevalent view of animals in contemporary psychology has origins far more basic than the scientific method. Its roots are deeply imbedded in Judaeo-Christian culture, a tradition which postulates a wide gulf between humankind and the animal world. The Darwinian revolution and the ethological outlook it fostered, while of immense biological significance, has for the most part been neglected by modern American comparative psychologists in favor of a positivistic-behaviorist orientation with a heavy reliance upon laboratory experimentation.

In recent years, opposition to animal research (some of it rational, some not) has experienced a profound resurgence. Psychologists have received a disproportionate share of the criticism considering the relatively small numbers of animals sacrificed in psychology laboratories. In this paper, I propose to review this development, critically examine the response of orthodox psychology to it, and offer suggestions for improvement.

Animal research in psychology has come under fire from a variety of sources and for a variety of reasons. Mellgren, et al. (1984) described the problem in relatively mild terms:

> Animal psychologists have been undergoing an identity crisis, with increasingly common criticisms of the traditional field revolving around the assumption that laboratory preparations alone will reveal laws of learning having generality. Such criticisms have taken many forms but may be reduced to the criticism that animal psychologists have ignored the biological predispositions of their subjects and by doing so may have distorted the true nature of the subjects' learning capacities, motivational processes, and so on (p. 142).

Rollin (1981) offered a more vociferous critique:

> It is perhaps better to focus upon the field most consistently guilty of mindless activity that results in great suffering. This is the field of experimental, behavioral, comparative, and sometimes physiological psychology. Nowhere are researchers further removed from theory, nowhere are researchers less engaged in trying to develop a picture of some aspect of the world, nowhere are researchers less able to discuss intelligently the significance of their experiments, nowhere are researchers less concerned with the morality of what they do (p. 124).... Besides the potential pernicious consequences for human beings, the lack of theory, the empirical dabblings, and the trial-and-error approach that characterize behavioral and physiological psychology are extremely mischievous from the point of view of animal suffering. Suffering is essential to psychological research in a way that is unparalleled in all other research, except research on anesthetics and analgesics. A basic feature of behavioral psychological research is the use of negative reinforcement (i.e., pain, anxiety, stress, etc.) to condition animal behavior in various ways. It is for this reason that I am so strongly critical of psychological research.... It is extremely revealing and interesting that other scientists who work with animals, even strong defenders of the researcher's right to use animals, have great contempt for behavioral psychology and point out that by far the most cruel and useless experiments are done by psychologists, and that these experiments give *all* researchers a bad name (p. 126).

Regrettably, spokespersons for institutionalized psychology (e.g., King 1984; Miller 1985) have conveyed the impression that their only serious critics are animal rights advocates with little understanding of or appreciation for science. This defense is demonstrably false and misleading as this paper will show. Additionally, specific written assurances have been offered by the American Psychological Association (APA) purporting to describe legal and professional safeguards for the "humane" treatment of laboratory animals. While it is beyond the scope of the present work to comprehensively counter these claims, elsewhere I have discussed the major defects in the relevant laws and professional guidelines (Giannelli 1985). It will suffice to say at this point that the great majority of species used in psychological work (i.e., mice and rats) are *not* covered by Federal regulation, the Animal Welfare Act (1966, 1970, 1976). Further, such laws and guidelines as do exist expressly allow the infliction of pain *without* benefit of anesthesics, analgesics, or tranquilizers.

In an atypical presidential address to the APA, William Bevan (1982) made the following appeal: "We must somehow reconcile our needs for a technology based on science with those for a humanely inspired culture.... We can no longer confidently believe that the effects of science and technology upon the fate of society are always unidirectional and beneficent."

I suspect that the majority of my colleagues in psychology would readily see the reasonableness of Dr. Bevan's point, but would be miffed at the suggestion that *we* psychologists share the blame. The tradition of untrammeled inquiry in the behavioral sciences has been at best a mixed blessing. Animal experimentation in psychology should neither be universally condemned nor universally applauded. However, the orthodox scientific and ethical justifications for much of this work are rightfully being challenged, especially the behaviorist methodology which is the predominant animal research paradigm in psychology.

I became a clinician because I am keenly interested in people. During my undergraduate training at the University of California, Los Angeles (UCLA), I learned about the work of famous animal researchers such as Pavlov, Thorndike, Harlow, Skinner and others. The ethics of such work was not discussed by my professors. This omission struck me as odd, particularly in light of some research we learned about. For example, in *Abnormal Psychology and Modern Life* (Coleman and Broen 1972), the most popular introductory text of its day, one finds a table (p. 149) titled, "Effects of Early Deprivation and Trauma on Adult Behavior of Animals." It mentioned the following early experiences: "raised in darkness or with restricted tactual stimulation," "immobilization of movement in early infancy," "partial starvation in early infancy," "total social isolation for six months or more after birth," "subjected to aversive stimulation such as electroshock or loud noise," "raised in an overcrowded environment," and "trained to fight over food." The book had graphic descriptions of "experimentally induced neuroses":

> Monkeys, in addition to anxiety and phobic reactions, like those shown by the cats, displayed even more profound disturbances. Somatic and motor dysfunctions included diarrhea and gastrointestinal disorders resulting in rickets and severe neuromuscular weakness. In contrast to their previous behavior, some monkeys after experimental treatment spent long periods in stereotyped repetitive activity such as "pacing" back and forth in the experimental cage. Sometimes this behavior alternated with states of tense, apprehensive immobility. Some animals would stare fixedly for hours if left undisturbed. Often thse monkeys would sleep or lie immobile in their home cages until midafternoon. Homosexual and autoerotic activity increased markedly, even in the presence of receptive females. One monkey attempted coitus only once in six months. "Neurotic" animals also lost their former positions of dominance in relation to other animals and were frequently attacked by other members of the colony (p. 258).

All of this might have been rationalized by reference to "essential clinical insights" which benefit people and which could not have otherwise been obtained. But, the qualifier was found elsewhere, "It is risky, of course, to assume that conclusions drawn from animal studies will be found to apply on the human level." No one ever said anything. I said nothing. What could one say?

People are often surprised to hear that in the course of my graduate level clinical studies at UCLA or in my clinical internships, animal research was not formally discussed at all. This, I came to realize, was not an oversight in my training (a program still considered one of the best in the country) but rather it reflected a conspicuous lack of practical importance animal experiments have had in the making of a psychotherapist. Of course, animal research in psychology has generated an enormous amount of sheer *information*. We have learned a great deal about how primates, dogs, cats, pigs, pigeons, and rodents behave in highly artificial (and often stressful) situations. But the practical importance and relevance to people of much of this data is highly questionable. Over the years, I regrettably came to the conclusion that many psychological experiments with animals are a particularly clear illustration of how animal research can and often does become an end-in-itself, a self-perpetuating (and often self-congratulating) industry.

The Black Box Revisited

As the prime research paradigm in psychological animal research, Skinnerian behaviorism merits brief review, if for no other reason than to understand the theoretical and methodological floor the system stands on.

Learning theory has its roots in the work of the Russian physiologist, Ivan Pavlov (1849-1936). While studying the digestive process in dogs, he discovered that if a stimulus (A) which naturally produces salivation is consistently paired with a stimulus (B) which has no natural salivation-eliciting properties, (B) eventually will produce salivation even in the absence of (A). From this base, Pavlov refined the technique to identify factors such as unconditioned stimuli, conditioned stimuli, the effects of contingency (order), higher-order conditioning, extinction, stimulus generalization, etc., in a system which came to be known as classical or respondent conditioning. During the course of studies on stimulus discrimination, Pavlov produced an "experimental neurosis" in a dog required to make increasingly difficult discriminations between a circle and an ellipse.

The term "behaviorism" was coined by the American psychologist, John B. Watson (1850-1907). Dissatisfied with the introspectionist approach of his day, Pavlov's classical conditioning paradigm seemed to Watson to promise a means by which the scientific study of psychology could be accelerated by concerning itself only with observable stimuli and responses. Edward L. Thorndike (1874-1949) expanded upon this approach in his "Law of Effect," which on the basis of animal studies, proclaimed that learning can take place without reason, insight or understanding.

B.F. Skinner (1904-) renamed Thorndike's Law of Effect "the principle of reinforcement" and studied the effects on animals' learning which are determined by the consequences of their behavior, i.e., operant or instrumental conditioning. Utilizing rodents and pigeons, Skinner explored various operant factors such as positive and negative reinforcement, escape conditioning, punishment, avoidance conditioning, shaping of behavior, chaining of behaviors, and the effects of various schedules of reinforcement. Skinnerian behaviorism is a "black box" approach in that the psychologist's task is to describe behavioral input into the organism (stimulation and reinforcement) and the resulting output (responses and behavior). The strict behaviorist, such as Skinner, sees no need to speculate about the inner workings of the organism, preferring instead to carefully record the observable consequences of various experimental conditions. Behaviorists employ the classical methods of experimental psychology to ascertain the concomitant variation among variables, such as the effects of various treatments on subsequent responses, or response-reinforcement relationships.

Segal and Lachman (1972) have noted that the behavioristic paradigm is grounded in the philosophy of Logical Positivism, a movement which emerged from Vienna in the 1920s. In very simplified fashion, this school believed that all sentences could be classified as: (1) analytic (logical; true by definition); (2) synthetic (belonging to science and verifiable by empirical observation); and (3) nonsensical. Radical behaviorists purport to investigate only "synthetic" issues and reject the direct study of subjective experience because it does not meet their criterion of verifiability. Science must be a public phenomenon, they argue, based upon strict observable methods capable of replication.

Another philosophical underpinning of behaviorism was referred to by Skinner (1975), "The issue is, of course, determinism. . . . I suggest that the spontaneous generation of behavior in the guise of ideas and acts of will is now at the stage of the spontaneous generation of life in the form of maggots and microorganisms 100 years ago."

Behavior, asserts Skinner, is no more "free" than digestion or any other physiological process. Behavior is caused by our environment (including environmental reinforcement history) not by alleged "free will." The principles learned about our overt behavior can be extrapolated to explain our covert behavior as well, without unnecessary reference to hypothetical subjective states, cognitions, or metaphysical constructs.

Endler and Magnusson (1976), among others, have referred to the behavioristic approach as "situationism." They note that little attention is given to biological or inherited factors in this model, which prefers rather to focus on social learning processes. Behaviorism is thus biased toward empiricism as opposed to nativism.

Another essential facet to realize about the behaviorist approach is its goal from the scientific inquiry, namely to predict and eventually control behavior (Wertheimer 1972). From this angle, if a behavior cannot be successfully predicted, it has not really been understood. The principle of operant conditioning is intended to help predict behavior by demonstrating how new responses are shaped from simple movements through control of the consequences of those movements, i.e., getting positive or negative reinforcement. Furthermore, principles such as operant conditioning can only be developed from inductive, empirical investigation.

Skinner and his followers came to believe that the complex psychological processes of man could be reduced to principles or subcomponents essentially present in "lower" mammals. The conditions of learning were presumed to be the same across species. This position appeared reasonable at that time and received support from comparative anatomy and the reductionist positions of physiology and biochemistry (Segal and Lachman 1972). A classic illustration of the rampant optimism characteristic of early behaviorists can be seen in the concluding passage of Keller and Schoenfeld's (1950) *Principles of Psychology*, a popular text which appeared around the zenith of American behaviorism, "In a science that takes the whole of behavior as its province, what part of man's activities shall be said to lie out of bounds and exempt from scrutiny? Who can justly deny her the right of passage through any meadow, and on what basis declare that she trespasses?"

The Case for the Opposition

Spokespersons for psychological research with animals have responded to criticism basically by rejecting it. King (1984), Chairman of the APA's Committee on Animal Research and Experimentation (CARE), has flatly stated, "Basic psychological research with animals has led to important achievements in the interest of human welfare."

Rajecki (1983) asks, then answers a key question, "Whether or not one is correct in speaking of animal and human behavior in the same breath, has there been any real impact of animal data on general advances in modern psychology? Actually, there are quite affirmative answers to my rhetorical questions." Rajecki cites four examples, two from child psychology and development (infantile attachment and dominance relations among peers) and two from clinical/experimental psychology (learned taste aversions for the treatment of alcoholism and learned helplessness for the study of depression). We will later return to these and other examples of well-publicized research for more analysis.

Perhaps Miller (1985) has provided the most extensive defense of animal research in psychology. Miller's abstract cites the following list of animal research benefits:

> . . . treatment of human urinary and fecal incontinence; psychotherapy and especially behavior therapy and behavior medicine; rehabilitation of neuromuscular disorders; understanding and alleviating effects of stress and pain; discovery and testing of drugs for treatment of anxiety, psychosis, and Parkinson's disease; new knowledge about mechanisms of drug addiction, relapse, and damage to the fetus; treatment enabling extremely premature infants to gain 47% more weight and save $6000 per child in hospital care; and understanding mechanisms and probable future alleviation of some deficits of memory that occur with aging (p. 423).

Other areas mentioned by Miller include: principles of learning and behavior (classical conditioning, operant conditioning, motivation, reinforcement, drive, etc.), automated training devices, visual learning and biofeedback, effects of noise, effects of early experience, and prevention techniques. With reference to the latter area, Heffernan and Albee (1985) appear to reserve credit, not simply for the past achievements of psychology, but even for *future* ones, "When prevention activities in health and mental health are firmly in place, it will have been psychological expertise that is needed to answer prevention's central question: How do we change behaviors and attitudes?"

Simultaneous with articles such as those cited, the APA's CARE committee has been busy at work producing "exemplars" and explanations of animal research in psychology. Many of these papers were widely distributed at a recent APA convention (Toronto, 1984). One particular brochure entitled, *Behavioral Research With Animals* asked the rhetorical question, "Why is behavioral research with animals so important?" (side 1) to which the following reply is provided:

> Research psychologists are both explorers and verifiers. They reach into the unknown in search of answers which must be tested and verified against real life conditions. Verification is the crucial step that separates truth from error. Humans are the focus of most psychological research experiments. But in seven or eight percent of behavioral investigations, animals are the focus of study. Animals are complex enough and similar enough to us to be informative not only about themselves but about human nature (side 1).

Whether the case for the opposition represents balanced and responsible scholarship or merely "*behavioral bravado*" is the question to be examined in the next two sections.

Theoretical Thin Ice

Before reviewing the empirical track record of behavioral research with animals, it will be wise to dissect its rationale. Ulrich (1985, unpublished paper, "Animal Research and the Utopian Dream;" himself a former animal researcher widely published in the area of aggression), restated the fundamental premise, "The assumption that animals and humans are alike has been the cornerstone upon which scientists have built their rationale for laboratory experimentation." Singer (1975) put forth what has come to be known as "the psychologists' dilemma," "The researcher's central dilemma exists in an especially acute form in psychology; either the animal is not like us, in which case there is no reason for performing the experiment; or else the animal is like us, in which case we ought not to perform an experiment on the animal which would be considered outrageous if performed on one of us."

Rollin (1985) underscored the matter in noting that:

> ...at least some animal research in psychology is predicated upon the assumption that the animal mind or animal behavior is a good model for the human mind or behavior...And if the animals are to be adequate models for research into the effects of pain, pleasure, fear, anxiety, grief, depression, addiction, hopelessness, helplessness, and other mental modalities, or for research into such phenomena as learning, problem-solving, aggression, and mothering, the assumption obviously must be made that these states or behaviors are fairly similar in animals and in humans. If animals do not approximate the humans in their ability to experience such states, why use them? However, if animals are sufficiently similar to humans to be good models, what right do we have to do to them what we would not do to humans? (p. 925).

An immediate paradox comes to light. On the one hand, contemporary psychology implicitly (when not explicitly) accepts the cultural dogma that there are vast qualitative *differences* between humans and other animals. These differences are presumed to be especially great in dimensions traditionally of a psychological nature; e.g., intelligence, rationality, cognition, motivation, etc. On the other hand, the presumption of strong *similarities* between human and animal psychology constitutes the scientific basis for using "animal models" of human experience in the first place. What better illustration might one have of (to use an intentional play on words) "having your animal and eating it too."

In the past twenty-five years, numerous authors have offered reservations and objections to the behavioristic approach. Shapiro (1982) expressed the basic two-part objection to the animal researcher's rationale, "The use of these animal models is 'twice removed' from the phenomenon: First, the subjects are not humans; secondly, the animals are not themselves, i.e., they are themselves reared in artificial environments and subjected to artificial conditions. Any gain in precision and control is likely offset by losses through extrapolation across species and from artificial to natural environments and conditions."

Elsewhere, Shapiro discussed in more detail the problem of extrapolating from animals in laboratory environments to humans in real world settings:

> On the laboratory side, clearly we no longer see other animals as simple organisms that somehow consist of certain states such as hunger or deprivation, states readily controlled, measured, and analyzed in the laboratory setting. When we divorce these or any animals from their natural habitat and from what we now are only beginning to learn of their natural social organizations, their patterned behavior, their communication, and their various adversarial, parasitic, and reciprocal relations with their environment and other species, do we really believe we have any idea of what we have a measure? On the clinical side, in most quarters it is no longer held that human psychopathology...is intelligible as a disease entity, certainly not that group of infectious diseases which partially prompted the animal model research strategy. It is not a matter of infecting another species with a human disease, then to follow and eventually affect its course. Even that limited part of human psychopathology that might be attributable to constitutional or neurological defect does not express itself in physiological symptoms that are straightforward signs of a certain disease. Our disorders are not diseases so much as they are at base peculiarly human phenomena, inseparable from culture and history, from language and meaning...(p. 5).

Mahoney (1977) noted that the key behavioral concepts are notoriously difficult to operationally define beyond the laboratory context; e.g., stimulus, response, reinforcement, behavior, environment, and learning. Fletcher (1984) voiced a similar concern, "In this fashion, Skinner attempts to purge commonsense language of mentalistic terms, purportedly producing a tight scientific discourse. I say 'purportedly' because one of the major criticisms leveled at Skinner concerns the status of these behavioral translations; namely, that although Skinner's concepts, such as reinforcement, are defined in a precise enough way in the laboratory with rats and pigeons, their meaning becomes crass and undifferentiated when applied to human social relations."

Influential critics such as Chomsky (1959, 1968) and the Transformationalist school of linguistics argued that because of man's capacity for rule-following behavior and creative language use, there was a great gap between "lower" animal conditioning and human learning which could not be bridged by generalization. On this theme, Shotter and Gauld (1971) commented, "The total failure of 'empirical' and neobehaviorist theories to handle even concept possession augurs ill for any 'empirical' theory of rule-following behavior....The inability of 'empirical' theory and of traditional empirical methods to cope adequately with our linguistic abilities and performances thus emerges as only a part (but a central part) of their general inability to cope with human rule-following actions."

As one moves along the animal continuum from pigeons to people, reinforcement principles progressively explain less and less about organismic behavior (Smith 1978). It has already been demonstrated (Brewer 1974; Weimer and Palermo 1974) that the principles of conditioning are not equal to the principles of learning. Despite these commonplace objections, Bannister (1981) noted that:

> Strangely, the theoretical assumptions underlying this vast undertaking have rarely been debated. The vast mass of animal work in psychology is published as if its fundamental value were unquestionable and only its detail needed to be examined (p. 307)....If the assumptions underlying animal experimentation in psychology are, at best, highly questionable, then how does it come about that they have not frequently been questioned? It may be due to the fact that the massive stream of published work in the field of animal experimentation is presented in such a way that its assumptions are deeply inferred within it, are so implicit that they neither arouse, nor are they readily accessible to, questioning (pp. 310-311).

Sometimes the theoretical import of animal research to psychological issues is not even available for analysis. Any cursory review of comparative psychology publications reveal a large number of articles which seem more appropriately found in zoological or biological journals. One is not inclined to challenge their relevance to human psychology because they claim none, except by implication by appearing in a psychological journal. Bannister (1981) put it, "Only by crediting the *psychologically* vast and vacuous statement 'man is an animal' can we believe that it will cast light on the psychology of humankind." It would seem that, insofar as Skinnerian behaviorism is concerned, relatively little has changed in nearly ninety years. London (1972), borrowing from Franks (1969) and Lazarus (1971), noted that all of the principles behavior modifiers ever refer to can be reduced down to about "one and one-half principles," namely that learning depends on the connections between what you do and what subsequently happens to you.

The failings of radical behaviorism have been all the worse because of its dogmatic insistence that valid knowledge could only be achieved via this model, thus relegating other approaches to myth, delusion, and superstition (Smith 1978). The attitude toward quantitative analysis is an excellent illustration of the differences between behaviorism and humanism. Wertheimer (1972) wrote, "Quantification, particularly premature quantification, may yield a totally false picture of a person or a phenomenon." Formulas, functions, and frequency distributions are usually abstractions or statistical fictions which may not really characterize anyone or anything. Wertheimer has argued that, in a seemingly counter-intuitive way, it is the strict experimentalist who is *most* subjective in his/her research:

> The phenomenon the experimentalist concocts in his laboratory may be nothing more than some artificial curiosity, some meaningless monstrosity whose relation to real-world events is remote indeed. It is the experimental scientist, says the intuitive clinician, who goes too far in imposing his views in nature, whose methods permit him to see only what he wants to see. The design of a study precludes certain events: the scientist deliberately blinds himself. Rather than permitting nature to speak to him, he presumptuously tells nature what it is he wants her to tell him and what channel she must use, irrespective of whether the channel is appropriate to what nature could tell him if he would only let her. Why impose your conditions on nature? Why not open yourself fully to whatever she is saying, in whatever form the message can come through? (p. 250).

The foregoing theme has been expressed by Gadlin and Ingle (1975) who urged, "We ought to begin with a reversal of the present emphases: psychology should initially address itself to phenomena, not methodology. Rather than selecting for research those phenomena suited to our methods, we ought to shape and develop our methods to fit phenomena." Koch (1969) pointed out that psychology, "was unique in the extent to which its institutionalization preceded its content and its method preceded the problem."

The critique of "method-oriented research" has been undertaken by numerous other authors (e.g., Maslow 1954; Giorgi 1970; Romanyshyn 1971; Bakan 1972; Kvale 1973). Indeed, Baron (1971) argued that the main criterion in past financial support for research was methodological sophistication, sometimes with little regard for the question being researched. In a similar vein, Smith (1973) wrote, "I only deplore the sterility of much ritualistic research that is guided more by fetishism for the trappings of science than by any inner light." Any study purporting to provide insight into human nature which ignores the flux, the flow, the originality and the creativity of personal experience has hopelessly handicapped itself. Even Skinner's rats lever-pressed spontaneously before operant conditioning was introduced.

Another basic theme in the humanist critique of behaviorist methodology is that human research is relational. By ignoring the relationship between the experimental subject and himself, the strict behaviorist violates his own criterion of objectivity. Skinnerians see their subject matter and their methods as independent of one another, but this dichotomy is not only questionable, it encourages the scientist to see his subjects as *objects*. This approach, it is argued, has negative repercussions for both subjects and researchers alike.

Demarest (1983) finds fault with those psychologists who fail to clarify their theoretical assumptions, "Unfortunately, most people in psychology do not explicitly state what their assumptions are when reporting research or formulating hypotheses. This can present problems because many times the implicit assumptions underlying a research program provide the theoretical foundation for interpreting and generalizing the results. Ironically, although most scientists are well aware that their observations of nature are determined in large part by tacit theoretical assumptions, few ever stop to consider what these assumptions are or how they came to hold them."

Although Skinner openly promotes an "atheoretical" orientation, even basic analysis of the operant conditioning paradigm is problematic. For example, the hallmark of an operant or instrumental response (as opposed to a Pavlovian or respondent response) is that it is "freely" emitted. The likelihood of repeating an operant response is said to depend upon its consequences, i.e., rewards or punishments. Clearly, a laboratory animal (in a Skinner a box, for example) cannot truly be said to be "freely" emitting operant responses in any way analogous to human operant behavior. First and most obvious, the animal is confined to the experimental apparatus and would likely escape if given the opportunity. Secondly, in order to motivate action, laboratory animals are typically deprived of some basic necessity (e.g., food, water, etc.) or coerced by aversive stimulation (e.g., shock, noise, etc.). Thirdly, the customary protocol of animal experiments is designed to radically limit the range of available activities and thus elicit highly artifical behaviors which are not part of the animal's natural repertoire. Fourthly, in terms of theoretical impediments, one cannot argue that: a) animals' operant behavior is reflective of "freely" emitted choices; and b) the animals do not possess "free will" and therefore are acting on instinct. One can't have it both ways.

The rapid rise since the 1970s of behavior modification techniques employing cognitive elements, e.g., Beck et al. (1979), is evidence of the limitations inherent in strictly behavioristic approaches to human psychology. In this light, behavioristic aspirations for building an objective scientific psychology without a self-concept and other cognitive dimensions can be seen as a futile mimicking of the physical sciences, or as one wag put it, "physics envy." Psychology, hopefully, is regaining consciousness—as well as conscience.

Social Blessing or Psychology Pie (In the Sky)

> Psychology... is an amalgam of humbug, platitude, piercing intuition, *naiveté*, soaring flight of the imagination, dull dogma, incisive reasoning and sheer drivel. Hence a certain fastidiousness in deciding what to read and what not to read on the subject is not to be despised. A system for protecting the less wary who venture into the swampy zones

> of psychological literature may be commended to Psychological Librarians. Every text on the shelves of the psychological library should have inscribed on it the number of grains of salt to be taken when reading it, and on the library table an ample bowl of salt should be placed and replenished at regular intervals. (Anonymous)

In terms of practical psychological benefits to humanity, how important has animal research been? This is a short and deceptively simple question with no easy answer. Avid proponents and avid opponents alike are frequently inclined toward exaggeration and distortion.

There are a variety of ways to approach this issue. One preliminary might be to get an overview of psychology's contribution as a whole to society, including *both* animal and human research. While I share a general sense of pride in and respect for my profession, it must be acknowledged that by no means has the field achieved consensual acclaim. Pion and Lipsey (1984) noted that, "Many critics have argued that psychology has a less than impressive record in understanding and explaining human behavior, especially social behavior (e.g., Dunnette 1966; Koch 1969; Meehl 1978; Sarason 1981; Smith 1972)."

In summarizing the results of a nationwide survey of graduate students and faculty in psychology, Lipsey (1974) noted, "The issue that generated the most heat was social relevance, the demand that psychology involve itself constructively in the widespread social problems that beset society. A large majority of both students and faculty felt that the discipline should be contributing to the solution of social problems and an equally large majority felt that at present it was making no important contribution."

In a recent article, Kimble (1984) reiterated a familiar theme, "Psychology has an identity problem. After more than a century of official existence, it still lacks a coherent set of values, there is little harmony among groups of us who practice very different professions, and there is even debate over the definition of our subject matter. . . . The disagreements have been around for so long, in such varied contexts, and expressed by so many different individuals with no indication that we are moving toward consensus."

This is not to suggest, of course, that psychology has contributed nothing (as some overzealous critics have contended). The point here is that, if the entire field of psychology (including human-based research) has been of less than dramatic utility, overinflated claims from the animal-based research lobby within the profession must be taken with the proverbial grains of salt referred to previously.

Another measure of the contribution from animal research in psychology is the percentage of publications in the two APA journals which publish such work. The 1983 figures are representative of the past several years. According to the APA Summary Report of Journal

Operations, 1983, the *Journal of Comparative Psychology* and the *Journal of Experimental Psychology: Animal Behavior Processes* have a combined rejection rate of 62 percent. Rejection rates for social science journals tend to be high anyway, but in this area, that cold statistic may amount to a lot of animals which experienced pain and/or death in vain.

Another measure of the contribution of animal research in psychology is the historical trend for specialty fields of new psychology doctorate recipients. According to studies by the National Research Council and the National Science Foundation (Pion and Lipsey 1984), the percentages of newly awarded doctoral degrees in animal research specialty fields (experimental, comparative, physiological) has changed as follows: 30.7 percent (1966); 21.7 percent (1972); 18 percent (1975); 16.1 percent (1977); and 13.7 percent (1979-80). It would be hard to explain these findings, which reflect a steady decline in those psychologists entering animal research fields, in terms of a theory which ascribes monumental importance to animal research results. Indeed, the theory would predict the opposite trend.

Another consideration in this analysis requires a better differentiation of the global term "animal research." While some animal rights advocates have irrationally called for an end to all animal research in psychology, a more representative position of the animal advocate community is opposition to vivisection. Defined in a modern sense (c.f., the *Encyclopedia Americana, International Edition* 1974), the term vivisection is no longer limited to surgical interventions but refers to any traumatic procedure which gives a medical or psychological problem to a previously healthy animal (e.g., inflicting diseases, injuries, deprivation, restraint, fear, stress, etc.). This is an extremely important concept methodologically, ethically, and in terms of the case which needs to be made by either side of the controversy. For example, most animal rightists would not object to properly conducted clinical research with animals done for their own benefit, nor to noninvasive laboratory work which respected the biological and social needs of the animal subjects, nor to ethological research in natural habitats.

Failure to consider this differentiation leads to unnecessary confusion. Consider the work of Rajecki (1983) cited earlier. In discussing the value of comparative research in understanding infantile attachment, Rajecki cites two ethological reports (Bowlby 1969; and Ainsworth 1969) alongside the vivisection studies of Harlow (to be discussed elsewhere). In making the case for animal research in the area of dominance relations among peers, Rajecki cites three ethological works (Tinbergen 1951; McGrew 1972; and Deag 1977) along with an entire table of conclusions based solely on ethological studies (p. 81). This is, so to speak, the academic version of "bait and switch," i.e., making a case for animal vivisection by reference to *non*vivisection research.

Another method for assessing the social relevance of APA published animal research is to sample recent journal articles in light of APA's stated policy that, "Psychological studies are aimed at understanding and alleviating the behavioral and health conditions that are problems for human society and for animals themselves" (*APA Backgrounder* 1984). To test the genuineness of this claim, a review of APA publications was conducted for studies appearing in the first half of 1984. Highlights included:

Journal of Comparative Psychology
March 1984, Volume 98, Number 1

Page	
3 *Subject*:	how mockingbirds respond to recorded spring and fall mockingbird songs during the two seasons
35 *Subject*:	social behavior of young rhesus monkeys raised either with a surrogate "dog mother" or plastic hobbyhorses
45 *Subject*:	differences in the sexual behavior of two different species of male voles (a type of rodent) given access to one, two, three, or four females
66 *Subject*:	differences in aggressive attack behavior of female golden hamsters permitted one vs. multiple "biting attacks" upon a smaller "target" hamster
91 *Subject*:	"maternal" behavior of young male and female rats exposed either to rat pups or pup-sized rubber toys
100 *Subject*:	the effect of reward levels on the learning and loss of learning behaviors of honeybees

Journal of Comparative Psychology
June 1984, Volume 98, Number 2

Page	
119 *Subject*:	learning behavior of blowflies subjected to a heart disturbance and a motor response elicited by an illuminated disk while in a dark room
137 *Subject*:	development of species identification calls in wood ducklings
189 *Subject*:	motion sickness in Japanese quail exposed to rapid body rotation on a 70 RPM turntable and a conditioned aversion to fluid
219 *Subject*:	responses of 200 male and female college students upon exposure to the smell of a male sex hormone from pigs

Journal of Experimental Psychology: Animal Behavior Processes
January 1984, Volume 10, Number 1

Page	
1 *Subject*:	the ability of rats to process two simultaneous events
30 *Subject*:	the ability of rats to learn a string of information by "chunking" the material into sections
90 *Subject*:	the influence of the predictability of a conditioned stimulus (light) to the orienting response ("what-is-it?" reflex) in rats

Journal of Experimental Psychology: Animal Behavior Processes
April 1984, Volume 10, Number 2

Page	
138 *Subject*:	the ability of pigeons to differentiate between complex musical sequences
168 *Subject*:	the role of odor given off by rats exposed to inescapable shock on the escape performance of other rats later exposed to shock in the same setting
182 *Subject*:	social transmission of learned pecking preferences in newborn chicks
221 *Subject*:	The "startle reflex" in rats exposed to loud bursts of sound

Journal of Experimental Psychology: Animal Behavior Processes
July 1984, Volume 10, Number 3

Page	
273 *Subject*:	time discrimination ability of rats exposed to various stimulus conditions
333 *Subject*:	the ability of pigeons to discriminate between events that they cause and those that they don't cause based on time cues

The intent of the survey was not to critique the design or analyses of these specific experiments per se. The sole question in mind was the relevance of this recent work to significant social problems and issues. The survey (complete form available from the author) suggests that typical animal research published in APA's journals, while academically impressive, bear little or no relationship to society's health problems or practical therapeutic techniques. Indeed, it is of more than passing interest to note that such relevance was rarely claimed even by the investigators themselves. It comes as no surprise that animal psychologists have sometimes been suspected of "scientific eccentricity."

In a *New York Times* essay by Nicholas Wade ("Smart Apes, or Dumb?" April 30, 1982), the author reported on a contemporary *Psychology Today* article in which "eleven of the best minds in the field" were surveyed as to their opinions on the most significant work in the field in the previous fifteen years. Wade noted:

> Several contributors mention experiments of their own. Well, if they think that, there is no need for false modesty. But no work is cited by any other Best Mind except for purposes of criticism; each trumpet blower blows his own tune, which makes for a conspicuous absence of harmony. The failure of the 11 psychologists to agree on almost anything evinces a serious problem in their academic discipline. Physicists or biologists asked the same question would not concur on everything but there would be a substantial commonality in their answers. Can psychology be taken seriously as science if even its leading practitioners cannot agree on its recent advances?

To bring the phenomenon closer to home, I compared the reference lists for two recent and extensive papers, referred to earlier, both written for the explicit purpose of demonstrating the value of animal research in psychology: Rajecki's (1983) review chapter entitled, "Successful Comparative Psychology" and Miller's (1985) review article entitled, "The Value of Behavioral Research on Animals." Rajecki listed ninety-four references and seventy-eight authors. Miller listed one hundred and eighteen references and ninety-five authors. Cross-referencing the papers, I found only one common citation and only four common authors (neither Rajecki nor Miller mentioned the other's work).

As the longer and more recent article, I then compared Miller's (1985) reference list with the combined five-volume reference lists of the 1985 Association for Advanced Training in the Behavioral Sciences (AATBS; arguably the best and most comprehensive course for the national licensure exam in psychology). Of Miller's one hundred and eighteen specific citations (hand-picked to demonstrate the critical value of animal research to psychological knowledge), only seven (5.9 percent) could be found in the massed AATBS references. Of Miller's ninety-five authors, only seventeen (17.9 percent) were also noted by AATBS. To an impartial observer, this might lead one to conclude that Miller's reconstruction of the history of psychology placed undue emphasis on the role of animal research.

Perhaps the most convincing empirical evidence that Miller and his colleagues have greatly inflated the importance of animal research to the development of therapeutic psychological techniques comes from recent research by Kelly (1985). Kelly conducted a detailed examination of all reference citations appearing in every article published by the *Journal of Consulting and Clinical Psychology (JCCP)* and *Behavior Therapy* during calendar year 1984. These two journals, both rigorous in their publication standards, were chosen because treatment research topics represented in their 1984 volumes coincide with those areas touted by Miller (1985) as most indebted to laboratory animal research. In 1984 (Volume 52), *JCCP* contained a total of 3,293 reference citations to the work of others. Of these, only ten (or less than one-third of one percent of the total) were citations of laboratory animal studies. Indeed, only nine of the 164 articles published by *JCCP* contained any references at all to animal research. In 1984, *Behavior Therapy* (Volume 15) contained a total of 1,132 reference citations. Of these, only twenty-three (or two percent of the total) were citations of laboratory animal studies. Only six percent of the articles published that year in *Behavior Therapy* contained any references at all to animal research.

Based upon these empirical findings, Kelly concluded:

> Miller argues that treatments for a myriad of clinical disorders in humans depend critically on laboratory animal research. However, clinical researchers who publish in these two high-quality journals rarely cite animal studies. If we assume that researchers reference those previous studies that they deem most critical to their own work, it is evident that Miller's conclusions are inaccurate.... Moreover, as

confirmed by my reference citation study, most current clinical interventions, including behavioral interventions, for the human disorders described by Miller depend far more closely on previous behavioral research with people rather than animals (p. 3).

Before examining specific examples of research cited by Miller (1985) in terms of the level-of-benefit claimed, a fundamental point of clarification is in order. It is not enough for the vivisection proponent to cite clinical techniques which utilized animals at some stage of development; one must also make the case that such use of animals was *indispensible.* I do not establish the "necessity" for a carnivorous life-style merely by showing that animal flesh has been a major source of protein and fat in the human diet. Drewett and Kani (1981) expressed this idea as follows:

> Whether behavioural research on animals is responsible for clear substantial advances in clinical practice that could not be attained without it is something that is more difficult to assess. The rider is important. The critical question, for those who wish to make a serious attempt to reduce the number of animals used in experimental work, is not whether research on animals makes a contribution, but whether it makes an indispensible contribution.... But it would be curious to argue that it would have been *impossible* to carry out the relevant research on human subjects; for how could a therapeutic method for use with human beings be based on principles of learning which could be demonstrated and investigated in dogs and rats, but which could not be demonstrated and investigated in human volunteers? Indeed, one could argue that the development of behaviour therapy might have been more rapid if more of the relevant research had been carried out on human volunteers rather than on animals (for instance, the importance of imagery would probably have been defined earlier) (pp. 196-197).

To cite another analogy, the statement, "Ninety percent of the transportation benefits enjoyed by people in the last century are attributable to the exploitation of fossil fuels," may be a factual historical assertion, but this obviously does not prove that transportation benefits *required* this type of technology. Given the massive exploitation of animals in psychology, the truly surprising observation is that so much basic knowledge and practical advances remain elusive. The point here is that a statement such as, "X and Y necessitated the use of animals," is a decidedly nonscientific claim. Ultimately, the only way to empirically demonstrate such an assertion is to do the impossible, i.e., turn back the clock and proceed along alternative research lines to determine the level of achievement possible. This obviously cannot be done, therefore such claims are not subject to scientific confirmation or refutation. Such assertions must be recognized as politically motivated speculation.

A comprehensive review of the proclaimed benefits of behavioral research with animals is clearly beyond the scope of this paper. In all of the following sections, primarily based on Miller's (1985) report, it must be acknowledged that significant and sometimes substantial advances have been made in all of the areas mentioned. Nevertheless, the following is intended to raise legitimate questions about the level of benefits claimed or implied.

Principles of Learning

There is no debate that the use of animals was instrumental in this area, but there is no convincing evidence that animals were absolutely essential. For example, did Pavlov require the use of dogs to demonstrate the principles of respondent conditioning? This seems implausible given the fact that, "Classically conditioned responses have been established for a variety of other subjects including human beings" (Mancucella 1984). Indeed, classically conditioned responses (which are not under voluntary control) can be established on resistant, drugged or even unconscious subjects. Likewise, there is no clear evidence to suggest that Skinnerian or operant principles of conditioning could not have been explored using human volunteers. As discussed previously, the concept that operants are "freely emitted" breaks down in the case of laboratory animals which are confined, deprived, coerced, and given an artificially restricted range of possible behaviors. Even Skinner (1975) has bemoaned the futility of trying to apply laboratory-derived principles to the human condition, "Why has it been so difficult to be scientific about human behavior? Why have methods that have been so prodigiously successful almost everywhere else failed so ignominiously in this one field?" As Smith (1978; past president of APA) put it, "Behaviorism has had a full and fair chance over more than half a century to show its worth; it has failed."

Treatment of Enuresis

The work of Mowrer and Mowrer (1938) in development of the "bell-and-pad" technique is said to be based on learning principles derived from animal experiments, but again, no compelling evidence is presented to show that the former depended upon the latter. Indeed, Azrin and Thienes (1978) have found that a treatment without a conditioning apparatus which involves training in rapid awakening, correct toileting, and social reinforcement for nonenuretic behavior is even more effective.

Automated Training Devices

The claim is made by Miller (1985) that teaching machines and programmed learning were dependent upon animal research. As before, it strains the imagination to suggest that such approaches necessitated the use of animals, particularly considering the qualitative differences in learning which apply to human subjects. In any event, such devices are hardly a panacea. As Mancucella (1984) noted, "In spite of the fact that programmed instruction has proven to be a useful tool for certain kinds of learning and in certain situations (e.g., in teaching material to large groups of students), it has several drawbacks: Students often dislike working with machines, programmed instruction tends to limit teacher-student and student-student interactions, and, especially in the case of computerized program instruction, costs can be prohibitive."

Behavioral Therapy

The term behavior therapy encompasses a wide variety of therapeutic techniques. A widely accepted definition of the term provided by Yates (1978) was referred to by Becker (1984):

> Note that Yates' definition makes no specific reference to learning theory as the only underlying basis of behavior therapy. Instead, Yates has provided a definition which describes the unique, systematic approach taken by behavior therapists in attempting to understand and treat a variety of behavioral problems (p.7).... One of the first major contributors to the future field of behavior therapy was William James. As early as 1890, James included a chapter on habits in his textbook *Principles of Psychology*. This chapter set forth many of the principles which are still considered essential to the practice of behavior therapy (p.3).

The point here is that behavior therapy as currently defined and practiced can hardly be said to be a direct application of learning theory based on animal research. Indeed, behavior modification techniques currently most in use are increasingly reliant upon cognitive factors which strictly traditional respondent or operant conditioning ignored (e.g., rational-emotive therapy, Ellis 1962; cognitive restructuring, Meichenbaum 1973; anxiety management training, Suinn and Richardson 1971; stress inoculation, Meichenbaum and Cameron 1973, etc.)

Recognition of the limitations of "animal models" of human neuroses, phobias, and obsessions has long been noted. Consider, for example, the observations of Marks (1977), Kubie (1939) and Hunt (1964), respectively:

> A major problem encountered in conditioning experiments on fear acquisition is that clearly traumatic events—a definable US (unconditioned stimulus)—can rarely be pin-pointed at the start of human phobias and obsessions.... Because there is usually no history of a clearly traumatic onset to human phobias or obsessions, we cannot assume that they have been conditioned, only that they have been acquired. Traumatic conditioning is uncommon in humans, and experiments on this issue are understandably rare. In a typical animal experiment, a single CS (conditioned stimulus) and a single US are arranged to produce fear. In contrast, a variety of situations usually trigger a patient's clinical distress, and those are seldom traceable to particular traumatic experiences. No one knows the original US, or if indeed one ever existed. The phobia or obsession simply appears, and search for the equivalent of unconditioned shock is fruitless (p. 204, 207).

> The dream of the scientist in the field of psychiatry is to find an equivalent of Koch's postulates. His despair has been the impossibility of translating the voice and behavior of lower animals into anything

> comparable to the symbolic language of *Homo sapiens*. This has limited the significance of efforts experimentally to produce neuroses in laboratory animals; because language is necessary for the communication of ideas, without which nothing comparable to a human neurosis is conceivable... The experimentally induced disturbances in animals are quasi-neuroses, not in any true sense indentical with human neurosis (p. 541).

> Despite all this promise and appeal, the animal neurosis experiments seem not to have amplified our knowledge about human psychopathology materially. More characteristically, these experiments receive favorable attention because they illustrate, duplicate, or confirm things already known about the human case. While illustration and confirmation are not trivial contributions, we must ask why this comparative sterility? (p. 28).

While behavior modification techniques offer hope in the treatment of human psychopathology, one must always be on guard against excessive claims. Case in point: Miller's (1985) reference to Wolpe's (1976) optimistic report entitled, "How laboratory-derived principles of learning have conquered the neuroses." The writers of the *Diagnostic and Statistical Manual of Mental Disorders III (DSM III,* 1980) found a more expedient solution by dropping the term "neurosis" from its current classification scheme, primarily due to a general lack of consensus among clinicians on the term's definition.

Behavioral Medicine

The extension of psychological treatment into areas traditionally associated with the practice of medicine is a promising new development. Yet, as always, one would do well to consider claims from scientists which may be more politically based than scientifically based. As an antidote to the former, I offer the following commentary by Kaplan (1984b):

> The expected health benefits from behavioral programs may not match the enthusiasm espoused by some health psychologists.... As an enthusiastic supporter of health psychology and behavioral medicine, I am pleased to see the field developing and thriving. Yet, the art should not precede the science. The rationale behind many applications in health psychology depends on a series of as yet unverified assumptions (p.755).... In the following sections, I will argue that these and other assumptions in the clinical practice of health promotion are not uniformly supported by research data. As a result, we are in danger of losing credibility by overenthusiastically announcing the expected benefits of our services (p.757).... My only concern is that we recognize the complexities of the problems and the general absence of definitive evidence on the relationship between behavior interventions and disease prevention. There is no quarrel with health promotion, only with the promotion of health promotion (p. 763).

Biofeedback

The work of Miller (1978, 1980) was highly important in demonstrating that human subjects could alter autonomic responses (salivation, blood pressure, temperature, heart rate, etc.) when given systematic performance feedback on their physiological status and selective reinforcement. This technique, which represents aspects of both classical and operant conditioning, has been applied to a wide variety of physical ailments. Once again, one is frustrated in the search for convincing evidence that this technique depended upon prior animal research. For example, Miller (1985) cites the human subjects research of Basmajian (1963) on the firing of single motor units and work of Kamiya (1969) which examined the voluntary control by human subjects of EEG rhythms. Miller then asserts, "But these two types of human behavioral experiments were dependent on earlier physiological experiments with animals that studied the electrical activity of nerves and that discovered the existence of single motor units." Why, one might reasonably ask, is this the case? It can hardly be argued that human volunteers would have been exposed to excessive risks, nor can it be suggested that the efficacy of biofeedback techniques depends upon the subjects' comprehension of the physiological mechanisms involved. In fact, successful biofeedback subjects typically cannot even articulate how they voluntarily elicit changes in their physiological functions.

On the clinical level, the successful application of biofeedback has been moderate at best and carries practical disadvantages. Becker (1984) took note:

> Initial enthusiasm for biofeedback has, however, diminished somewhat due to mixed research results and practical shortcomings. In terms of research results, one of the initial claims concerning the use of biofeedback was its ability to enhance the production of alpha waves which have been associated with states of euphoria and relaxation. Subsequent research has, however, shown that biofeedback is not necessarily a reliable method for increasing alpha waves (e.g., Plotkin and Cohen 1976). Additionally, it has been found that some individuals have great difficulty learning to regulate physiological responses. Finally, the use of biofeedback not only requires a large monetary investment in equipment, but also extensive technical knowledge to use such equipment (p. 34).

Effects of Stress

After acknowledging that clinical and epidemiological work (and hopefully some common sense) has indicated that stress can exacerbate a wide variety of medical disorders, Miller (1985) discussed a number of animal studies, "in which confounding factors can be rigorously controlled." This is arguably tunnel vision in that he presumes that captive, manipulated animals experience no stress other than that experimentally provided by the investigator. He specifically cites research summarized by Henry and Stephen (1979) on a mouse colony where the animals were forced to compete for food, water, and space. Miller concluded that these experiments provide a good animal model of "psychosocial stress." In my judgment, it is scientifically hollow (not to mention ethically reprehensible) to expose animals to hellish conditions and then analytically observe that they deteriorate into hellish behavior. Even in terms of the applicability of such work to human populations, Gangsei (1983) observed:

> The detrimental effects of overcrowding among animals was demonstrated by Calhoun (1962) who found that increased population density in a population of rats resulted in a variety of pathological behaviors (e.g., reduced fertility rates, increased mortality rates, sexual aberrations and increased aggressive behavior). Several mental health researchers have similarly investigated the effects of increased population density on human behavior. Unfortunately, the results of human research, although suggesting the existence of an important relationship between population size and behavior, have been less consistent than those obtained in animal research (pp. 9-10).

Miller (1985) contends that animal experiments "are demonstrating a point-to-point correspondence between the after-effects of unpredictable, uncontrollable electric shocks and the behaviors characteristic of human depression as described in the latest manual for psychiatric diagnoses, *Diagnostic and Statistical Manual of Mental Disorders (DSM III;* American Psychiatric Association, 1980)." This rather remarkable conclusion is disconfirmed elsewhere in the literature on learned helplessness and uncontrollable stress. Rajecki (1983) observed (sadly):

> Alas, despite their valuable contributions in the past, the place of dogs in future learned helplessness research is doubtful. The original theoretical formulation for helplessness effects was that a lack of contingency between response and outcome led to a reduction in the incentive for operant responding (Miller et al. 1977). By now, this relatively simple hypothesis has been supplanted by a more complicated formulation that incorporates ideas of (for example) universal versus personal helplessness, general or specific helplessness, whether future helplessness will be chronic or acute, and whether it will lower self-esteem or not (Abramson, Seligman and Teasdale 1978). Many features of the newer formulation rest on cognitive and attributional processes that are not usually associated with dog behavior. Indeed, Abramson, et al. (1978) state that: "Investigators of human helplessness . . . have become increasingly disenchanted with the adequacy of theoretical constructs originating in animal helplessness for understanding helplessness in humans. And so have we." (p. 102).

Even more discouraging is the report from Mineka, et al. (1984):

> Over the past 15 years an enormous amount of research has been directed toward understanding the differential behavioral and physiological effects that stem from exposure to controllable as opposed to uncontrollable aversive events. The general conclusion has been that exposure to uncontrollable aversive events is considerably more stressful for the organism than is exposure to controllable aversive events. The greater stress has been indexed by a wide range of behavioral deficits and physiological changes, including impaired ability to learn control in subsequent tasks, passivity, lowered aggressiveness, alterations in levels of certain important neurotransmitters, ulcers,

> analgesia, and many others (p. 307).... Nevertheless, we believe our results are important in highlighting the importance of two issues. First, they raise some question about the validity of the conclusions of the hundreds of experiments conducted over the past 15 years or so that have compared the effects of controllable versus uncontrollable shock on a variety of dependent variables.... The second issue highlighted by our results concerns the importance of examining the dynamics of fear conditioning in more complex contexts than those in which it has traditionally been examined (p. 322).

It is no wonder that Pratt (1976) bemoaned, "On this obsessive study of terrorized small animals the cumulative outlay of public funds has been enormous, even though the research can hardly claim relevance to human problems."

Pain

Miller (1985) illustrates the classic mixed message of the animal research advocate in contending both that, "Considerable progress has been made in controlling pain ... [and] chronic pain is the most costly health problem in America." Unfortunately, it is not difficult to document the low payoff from the massive volume of pain research on animals. A leading expert in the field (Lineberry 1981) soberly observed:

> The control of pain in humans has always been a difficult problem. As a consequence, considerable basic research on pain has been conducted on laboratory animals, but the results have provided few consistently effective weapons for the physician. Despite a recent resurgence of interest in pain mechanisms, research efforts have thus far failed to achieve a level of understanding that even begins to approach our knowledge in other sensory systems. Thus, efforts to devise new and effective treatments for pain have generally failed (p. 238).... The situation is perhaps even more complicated in animal subjects, since, in nonhuman subjects, it is not possible to obtain verbal subjective reports (p. 240).... The pain literature is filled with hundreds of different techniques ... for measuring responses to noxious stimulation in animal subjects (p. 250).... It is obvious that no method available is without serious limitations (p. 251).... One cannot with absolute certainty conclude that a stimulus is either painful or not painful on the basis of the probability of that stimulus eliciting an escape response (p. 273).... One cannot, therefore, with confidence describe reductions in response to noxious stimuli as analgesia.... This is an old problem in analgesic testing, with no evident solution given the experimental techniques available at the present time (p. 274).

The infliction of pain in laboratory animals will be discussed further in this paper. Suffice to say that two monumental practical problems exist for the animal researcher in this area: a) knowledge about pain in animals is very rudimentary and still basically inferential; and b) there are serious problems in cross-species extrapolation of the effects of anesthetics, analgesics, and tranquilizers.

Behaviorally Active Drugs

Levine, et. al. (1971) concluded, "During the brief history of treating psychiatric depressed patients with drugs, therapeutic efficacy has almost always been developed from clinical experience—usually by accident." Baldessarini (1975) noted:

> The behavioral effects of drugs in the experimental situation was often very different from the effects observed clinically. An outstanding example of this phenomenon is that large acute doses of most anti-depressants tend to produce sedation in normal laboratory animals, and it has been very difficult to devise reliable laboratory behavioral tests to screen potential new anti-depressant drugs. Another problem is that most of the so-called "animal models of affective (mental) illness" are more nearly models of sedation or stimulation, thus making it very tricky to make predictions about human clinical responses based on animal behavior (p. 74)

Shapiro (1982) observed that, "Most of the 'major tranquilizers' which control some psychotic disorganization were discovered in human contexts, either clinical and epidemiological studies or 'accidental' discovery—not in animal studies."

Chlorpromazine (Thorazine) is given special notice by Miller (1985) as one beneficial by-product of animal research in the treatment of schizophrenia. This is a debatable attribution in view of the record that the phenothiazine class of drugs (of which chlorpromazine is the best known example) was used originally at the turn of the century as antibiotics (Kuker-Reines 1982). Chlorpromazine itself was initially developed for use as a sedative. Its "anti-psychotic" properties were not discovered until the early 1950s, and then by the use of astute clinical observation, not by laboratory research, even though (as always) efficacy was tested on animals. While there is no doubt that the use of chlorpromazine (and other psychoactive drugs) has made a major contribution in the symptomatic treatment of serious psychological disturbances, one must remember that such substances are palliative not curative. Furthermore, while chlorpromazine is not associated with the development of tolerance, dependence or withdrawal, the drug comes with a host of unpredictable, serious, and sometimes irreversible side effects.

Effects on Early Experience

Miller (1985) cites the animal work of Wiesel and Hubel (1965) as, "showing that various forms of visual deprivation or conflict between images from the two eyes causes permanent deficits in visual connections in the brain. As a result of this work, pediatricians are paying far more attention to the very early detection and correction of visual defects in infants."

In response to such claims, Drewett and Kani (1981) commented:

> Such claims are now commonplace, yet it is difficult to see what new principle of clinical importance derives from these findings. The animal

> work originates with Wiesel and Hubel (1963) and Hubel and Wiesel (1965); but it was by then already well established in clinical practice that there was a critical period in the development of the human visual system.... Indeed, Wiesel and Hubel (1963) themselves point out that the difference between the effects of deprivation in kittens and adult cats is "a difference one might have expected from the profound visual defects observed after removal of congenital cataracts in man, as opposed to the absence of blindness on removal of cataracts acquired later in life;" and Hubel and Wiesel (1965) that, "it is recognized that squint in a child must be corrected in the first few years of life if capability of using both eyes in binocular vision is to be retained." So the fact that there is a critical period in the development of vision, and its clinical implication, that visual defects should be detected and corrected as early as possible, did not derive from this work on animals. It was already known (pp. 191-192).

A similar, and more disturbing, set of inflated claims is Miller's praise for the deprivation and social isolation research of Harlow, et al. (1965). Considered as a whole, it would be difficult to find a more traumatic series of experiments than those inflicted by Harlow and his associates at the University of Wisconsin primate laboratory. The "ingenious" (some would say diabolical) techniques Harlow used to produce extreme psychopathology are well known and need not be dwelled upon here. The best rebuttal to Miller's scenario that these researchers were humane individuals who advanced clinical understanding of child abuse is to let them speak for themselves. As Harlow once confessed in a moment of candor (*Pittsburgh Press Roto*, October 27, 1974), "The only thing I care about is whether the monkeys will turn out a property that I can publish. I don't have any love for them. Never have. I really don't like animals. I despise cats. I hate dogs. How can you like monkeys?" (Pratt 1976). Elsewhere, Harlow and Suomi (1977) addressed the question of the clinical relevance of this work:

> Some researchers have pointed out the similarity between elements of the isolate monkeys' behavior and specific behavior patterns exhibited by autistic human children. Anyone who has had the opportunity to observe both autistic children and isolate monkeys would feel compelled to consider them as examples of similar phenomena—particularly with respect to stereotypic rocking activities. Does this mean that, keeping in mind the basic behavioral differences between the species, the social isolation syndrome in monkeys serves as an effective model of childhood autism? We doubt it. It is our belief that the social isolation syndrome in monkeys can serve as an adequate model for only one human disorder—the human total isolation syndrome.... If one could systematically separate human infants from mothers at birth and maintain them for the first two to four years in physical and visual isolation from other humans, the infants would probably exhibit the same reactions as monkeys reared in isolation (p. 145).
>
> Of what use are the data obtained from depressed monkeys for clinicians currently working with depressed patients? We have a considerably

> more difficult time establishing a strong case [for such use] since so much monkey work to date has been based upon existing human data and theories (p. 173).

As with other behavioral research with animals, in my judgment, the Harlow experiments did not substantially advance clinical knowledge in the sense of providing new key concepts. Basically, they simply demonstrated that psychopathology in animals can be produced by the same factors already known or suspected of producing it in humans. At best, this type of research mimics and follows human research. At worst, as in this case, Harlow ironically reconfirmed the importance of love to personal health by utilizing gross abuse, demonstrating (some might say) a profoundly warped sense of what love is all about.

Deficits in Learning and Memory with Aging

Miller (1985) makes a case for using animals in work related to memory loss, as in Alzheimer's disease. The logic is curious in that animals are said to make good models of human aging because, "Many animals age much more rapidly than people—rats approximately thirty times as fast." Miller enthusiastically proclaimed, "These animal models of memory defects with aging are providing powerful means for analyzing experimentally some of the mechanisms... that play a role in the memory deficits."

As before, we would do well to broaden our search in the professional literature for a more sobering perspective on the utility of laboratory-based research in the field of memory. Tulving (1979) had this to say:

> After a hundred years of laboratory-based study of memory, we still do not seem to possess any concepts that the majority of workers would consider important or necessary. If one asked a dozen or so randomly selected, active memory researchers to compile a list of concepts without which they could not function, one would find little agreement among them, particularly if one excluded terms referring to experimental operations and data. Similarly, if one compares different textbooks of memory, one discovers that there is little overlap among their subject indexes. It seems that important concepts of one author can apparently be dispensed with by another (p. 27).

Loftus, et al. (1985) recently noted that Neisser (1982) came to a similar conclusion:

> Recently, Neisser (1982) registered his dissatisfaction with the orthodox psychology of cognition, and particularly with the study of memory. To him, the field has little to show for a hundred years of effort, perhaps because it always avoided interesting issues.... The time has come, Neisser believed, to investigate questions of interest in more naturalistic settings. To paraphrase him, just as the naturalistic study of animal behavior has proved to be more rewarding than traditional research on "learning," so a naturalistic study of cognition may be more productive than its laboratory counterpart (p. 179).

Prevention

Miller (1985) asserts that principles of learning (based on animal experiments, of course) have been "useful" and "helpful" in designing programs of primary prevention, specifically citing projects aimed at reducing the number of children who start smoking. To suggest that smoking is an area where animal research has led to "breakthroughs" in the clinical problem for people is more wishful thinking:

> In spite of the documented dangers of smoking, 54 million Americans smoke tobacco (HEW 1976) and smoking therefore remains the greatest public health hazard in the United States. Unfortunately, no treatment technique has consistently been shown effective for the treatment or prevention of smoking. In fact, it has been estimated that only about one-half of smokers who participate in smoking cessation programs are able to abstain by the end of the program and, of these, only one-third continue to abstain during the following year (Hunt and Bespalec 1974). Interestingly, it has been estimated that 95% of the 29 million individuals who have stopped smoking since 1964 have done so without professional help (National Cancer Institute 1977) (AATBS: *Abnormal Psychology* 1984, p. 32).

Sexual dysfunction

Although not specifically cited by Miller (1985), this is an important area for obvious reasons. Drewett and Kani (1981) expressed some themes which can be constructively applied in this area as well as the others just reviewed:

> What we think is remarkable here is the extent to which the very large body of behavioural work on animals has not had any major clinical pay-off in the treatment of human sexual problems. The research workers who have made major contributions here have been those pioneers who have worked directly on human sexual behaviour, particularly the zoologist, Kinsey (Kinsey et al. 1948, 1953) and the gynecologist and social psychologist Masters and Johnson (1966, 1970). It is certainly true that research on the sexual behaviour of mammals contributed to the early development of the field.... But we are inclined to think that psychologists and others who are now genuinely interested in advancing medical progress in this area ought to be working directly on the human case, and not on animals.... What has been lacking has simply been a sufficient investment of time and effort. To some extent this may have been a result of too great a concentration on work on animals (p. 183).

General Summation

The preceding section offers no pretense of an exhaustive review. Among the lessons it does provide, however, are the suggestions that, like any special interest group, the vivisection lobby in psychology is prone to hyperbole in overstating the case, exaggeration of the clinical application of this work, and selective restructuring of the history of psychology for purposes of elevating animal research to a level of practical utility it does not merit. This is by no means a new conclusion. Heim (1979), Ryder (1975), Dalen (1969) and others have arrived at similar positions. Echoing the appeal of Drewett and Kani (1981), I would contend, "It is these same facts that ought, we feel, to make psychologists more unwilling than they are to carry out experiments that cause suffering to their animal subjects; here, as so often elsewhere, the most creative response to criticism may be to listen to it."

The Psychology of Animal Psychologists

Ironically, I have often found myself defending animal researchers from brazen accusations of "sadism" and of inflicting "torture" upon animals. Such characterizations are overly sensationalized and, in my judgment, simply *wrong*. I have too much respect for most of my colleagues in psychology and too much appreciation for the complexities of this issue to arrive at such a banal diagnosis. There are, however, important psychological factors at work here which should be discussed because they shed light upon the experimenter him/herself and thereby upon the issue in dispute.

Psychologists are generally adept at devising clever techniques to test hypotheses with great precision. Unfortunately, our training generally does not leave us very skilled at generating important or interesting hypotheses to test. Unlike other areas of research, psychologists cannot afford the pretense of being objective, detached observers. This is because, unlike the situation in the physical sciences, psychologists cannot turn a blind eye to their own behavior during the research process without ignoring the most direct psychological data available. In trying to mimic the physical sciences, psychology has seized upon the use of so-called animal models because, among other things, it facilitates the fictional gap between the researcher and the object of his/her research.

Bannister (1981) discussed this issue in terms of "reflexivity," i.e., self-awareness of the researcher as something more than a "detached," "objective" collector of data:

> Animal psychology offers its practitioners a domain within which they can personally and publicly avoid the issue of reflexivity in all its forms. It has served as an undercover way of introducing and maintaining mechanical models in psychology because it is easy to be mechanistic about animals but more difficult to be mechanistic about one's fellow human beings. Not surprisingly, the current wave of humanistic psychology which insists that we see human... concerns, received much of its initial impetus from a rejection of "rat" psychology. Working within the socially remote world of animal experimentation has sheltered many psychologists from the kind of political questioning to which psychology is now rightly subject.... Part of the urge to evade the reflexivity issue stems from a desire to mimic, in a concretistic way, the natural sciences: to earn for ourselves the title of "scientist" and be rewarded with the

> prestige attached to that title. Thus psychologists have sought the kind of "precision" which they see as being the hallmark of science. We have sought the appearance of precision by hiding tenuous argument behind elaborate, statistical design (quoting figures, whose conceptual referents are doubtful, to the third decimal place) and by using impressive instrumentation. However, so long as our experiments involve people, our peers, with their capacity to outwit and seduce us and to see beyond the experiment, then our precision is often set at nought. If we use speechless animals—our infinitely manipulable *property*—then we can achieve a kind of spurious precision: we can be precise within the confines of our experiment even though the wider implications of the experiment are enormously imprecise (pp. 314-315).

As the so-called "talking animal," it is also hard to overestimate the importance which language has on this insidious conditioning process. Consider, for example, the word "animal." The word itself is frequently used in a derogatory sense, to mean sub-human, filthy, or debased. The term "beast" is even more explicit in this regard. There are many other common examples where animal names are used intentionally as insults, e.g., pig, swine, vermin, rat, weasel, skunk, jackal, jackass, chicken, turkey, goat, wolf, snake, lark, bird-brain, bitch, ass, etc. If one looks hard enough, one will find samples of animal phrases used in a complimentary way. For example, "wise as an owl," "brave as a lion," or "busy as a beaver." But for every such example, many more counter-examples which reflect the rule are to be found, e.g., "shouldn't happen to a dog," "go ape," "stubborn as a mule," "crocodile tears," "this place is a zoo," "crazy as a loon," "smells fishy," "dumb bunny," "bull-headed," etc.

As Bowd (1980) has written, the specialized vocabulary of experimental psychology is also an important factor in creating and maintaining attitudes toward laboratory animals. There is a certain hygienic illusion in using euphemisms like "organism" or "model" instead of dog, "aversive stimulus" instead of punishment, "deprivation" instead of starvation, "phonate" instead of scream, "agitate" instead of struggle, and "sacrifice" instead of kill. Ironically, it is generally considered unscientific and anthropomorphic to attribute emotional or intellectual states to laboratory animals, even though the very rationale of psychological research presumes that the causes of animal behavior are analogous to the causes of human behavior. Consequently, in the psychological literature, one often sees words like pain, fear, intelligence, insight, sadness, curiosity, etc., placed within inverted commas. This is supposed to signify that these words should not be taken literally, but rather are needed to avoid the inconvenience of trying to describe animal behavior without any reference to the animal's subjective experience. The net effect of the customary linguistic style in the scientific literature is to maintain a nonscientific distinction between human animals and nonhuman animals. Set in the context of prevailing philosophical assumptions about animals (to be discussed elsewhere), such linguistic detachment allows the otherwise sensitized researcher to dispassionately discuss traumatic manipulations that would be considered heinous if performed on a fellow human being.

As an academic discipline, animal researchers-in-training or in practice are subject to not so subtle pressures noted by Bowd (1980), as follows:

> In addition to language practices, psychology students are persuaded to accept prevailing attitudes toward animal research by a variety of social forces. Peer pressure and the attitudes of professors categorize squeamishness and sentimentality as unscientific, it being implied that such natural emotional reactions are irrational while the ability to suppress them is not. The graduate student who for ethical reasons may choose not to subject animals to painful experimental procedures may find fewer doctoral programs available. Finally, there are subtle prejudices within university psychology departments such that experimental animal research is frequently considered more basic and is invested with a prestige that is denied more applied study (p. 205).

Evasion of reflexivity, sanitized language, peer pressure and other factors often result in extraordinarily self-serving public posturing by the animal researcher. Even more important, the private self-image of such individuals is characteristically of similar quality. Lockwood (1984) made the following astute observations:

> One of the reasons why the animal welfare movement elicits such a visceral response from the opposition is that we are challenging the self-image of many researchers. They have convinced themselves that they are the intellectual light and salvation, and whatever suffering they might produce is for the greater good of mankind. Bernard Rollin has summarized their view as "Leave me alone, I love my dog and I'm curing cancer." Often they have labored hard and long to build a shell of insensitivity that makes their basic routine possible. Frequently, I believe, these defenses have been constructed at great personal and social cost and we cannot expect them to be shed easily (p. 10).

One of the important insights of social psychology is that physical abuse is more likely to occur when the victims are anonymous and physically separated from their oppressors. Uniform-looking laboratory animals which are then isolated from the investigators foster such a situation. Utilization of sophisticated laboratory equipment has a similar impact. The original questions which promoted a line of research can be overshadowed by the techniques and hardware available for studying them. Speaking from years of personal experience, Ulrich (1984, unpublished paper) observed that many behavioral researchers hardly ever see the animals themselves. Instead, they become preoccupied with the *data* produced by the animals via pressing levers, pecking keys, running mazes, etc. Investigators write about animals in journals and read about animals but hardly ever interact with them.

Many researchers are not so much interested in animals as with the computerized, sterilized equipment which brings in reports on the animal's behavior. Pratt (1980) forcefully makes the point, "What they seem to be interested in are the distortions, the pathology of behavior: either the fragments which remain after surgical or other mutilations have destroyed the marvelous wholeness of a functioning organism, or the reflex jerks teased out by any of the myriad of prods, punishments, or pleasures which the ingenuity of a researcher can devise."

Any analysis of the psychological motivations of animal researchers would be incomplete without reference to the pressure to publish. Peters and Ceci (1982) noted that the "publication count" can have important consequences for entire departments in terms of reputation, the quality of graduate students and faculty, and the awarding of competitive grants. In a excellent recent analysis of the general issue (not specifically addressed to the animal research controversy), Mahoney (1985) declared:

> Publication, for example, lies at the very heart of modern academic science—at levels ranging from the epistemic certification of scientific thought to the more personal labyrinths of job security, quality of life, and self-esteem.... Our academic science departments are active participants in the maintenance and inflation of "publish or perish" policies (cf. Conference Board of Associated Research Councils 1982). Teaching excellence, creative thinking, and all manner of other valuable attributes will do little to earn security in academic science if they are not accompanied by published payment to the piper of tenure (p. 30).... This observation highlights the important role played by publication in the recognition, selection, and nurturance of an idea or research theme. Those scientists who successfully publish their work are not only insuring the survival of their ideas, but they are also enhancing their own chances for obtaining employment, making vertical professional moves, and receiving grants, promotions, and tenure. They are, in other words, protecting and projecting their personal careers primarily through the vehicle of publication (p. 31).

Protecting and projecting their personal careers through publication of animal research can sometimes translate into a militant self-righteousness and resistance to dialogue, qualities at complete odds with the academic tradition of free inquiry and debate. One such personal experience occurred as a graduate student at the University of California, Los Angeles. In response to my call for an extended colloquium on animal research, one departmental researcher responded in the following fashion:

> Thank you, but I choose not to participate because I think the discussion would be a waste of time. You wish to abolish animal experimentation for personal motives, and for these very reasons, I wish to pursue animal research in the traditional scientific and medical model. The issue is polarized, the rhetoric is flatulent, and the debate would be self-serving and futile.

> Pain, injury, disease, privation and stress are imposed upon animals by pet owners, sportsmen, farmers, butchers, industrialists and developers, as well as animal researchers. Human population growth and hunger are destroying habitats and wiping out species after species. Abolition of experimentation upon laboratory animals would not reduce this carnage one whit.
>
> You may lament this biological view in all sincerity, but you and your pet cat sit atop the food chain and partake of its banquet directly and indirectly. The real trick is to find a place at the table, and not on it. But, please spare us the after-dinner speeches (J. Garcia, 1981, personal communication).

Although the proposed colloquium had clearance from both the colloquium committee chairman and the acting departmental chairman, the event never took place because the animal researchers in the department simply refused to participate. Contrary to their presumed expectations, the passage of time has (fortunately) not made "the problem" go away.

Broad and Wade (1982), in a well-documented book on fraud and deceit in the halls of science, made the following comment which provides an excellent characterization of scientists as persons:

> Scientists are not different from other people. In donning the white coat at the laboratory door, they do not step aside from the passions, ambitions, and failings that animate those in other walks of life. Modern science is a career. Its stepping-stones are published articles in the scientific literature. To be successful, a researcher must get as many articles published as possible, secure government grants, build up a laboratory and the resources to hire graduate students, increase the production of published papers, strive to be awarded a tenured post at a university, write articles that may come to the notice of committees that award scientific prizes, gain election to the National Academy of Sciences, and hope one day to win an invitation to Stockholm (p.19).

The APA: Principles and Practice

> Many safeguards operate to assure that laboratory animals receive humane and ethical treatment.... The American Psychological Association and other scientific professional associations have codes of ethics prescribing humane and ethical treatment of research animals, to which all members must conform. APA and other associations are currently strengthening and upgrading these requirements significantly and establishing more stringent standards of review by research committees.... The American Psychological Association has been committed to the welfare of animals and their humane use in research for more than 60 years.... APA's Committee on Animal Research and Experimentation (CARE) was established in 1925. It has continuously strengthened and upgraded APA's Ethical Code and standards for animal use and care.... All APA members engaging in animal research must ensure "appropriate consideration for the comfort, health and humane treatment" of laboratory animals (APA pamphlet 1984).

It must be noted that the APA Committee on Animal Research and Experimentation (CARE) notwithstanding, never once in APA's history has an APA member been sanctioned in any form for alleged unethical treatment of animals. Representatives of the 250 APA-member Psychologists for the Ethical Treatement of Animals (PsyETA) have noted that historically the CARE committee has been heavily invested in protecting the animal scientist rather than the animals.* CARE has actively been promoting the use of animals (e.g., via publication of "exemplars" of positive research). Complaints to CARE have been rare (due to the cumbersome and risky reporting process) and rarer still have they been actively investigated.

Since 1981, the APA Committee on Scientific and Professional Ethics and Conduct (CSPEC) has had the responsibility for inquiry into charges of animal abuse, although CSPEC has no specific expertise in this area. CSPEC's most significant action to date has been to absolve an APA member (Edward Taub) of ethical wrongdoing—in spite of the fact that the National Institutes of Health considered the Taub case serious enough to permanently revoke his grant based on substandard veterinary care provided to deafferented monkeys. Taub was initially convicted for cruelty to animals under Maryland State law (later overturned on a technicality, not on merit, by the Maryland Court of Appeals) and to date the APA has awarded Taub $16,000 for his legal expenses. No cases of "failure to ensure welfare of animal research subjects" have been investigated by CSPEC for 1983, 1984, or 1985 to date.

APA's current *Ethical Principles for the Care and Use of Animals* was adopted in 1979 and incorporated in 1981 into APA's *Ethical Principles for Psychologists* as Principle Ten. It reads in part, "The investigator ensures the welfare of animals and treats them humanely. Laws and regulations notwithstanding, the animals' immediate protection depends upon the scientist's own conscience." To sample the quality of both the APA's safeguards and the "conscience" of investigators, a complete survey was done of APA-published animal research for the first half of 1984 (complete results available from this author). This survey was deliberately limited to very recently published research since this presumably represents APA's current attitudes, policy and interpretation of "humane." Among the procedures to which animals were subjected were:

a) up to sixty seconds of inescapable shock (Minor and LaLordo 1984);

b) up to 360 shocks in 1.1. hour (Anisman et al. 1984);

c) up to 47.5 hours of of water deprivation (Poulos and Hinson 1984);

*Psychologists for the Ethical Treatment of Animals (PsyETA). Contact: Kenneth J. Shapiro, c/o Psychology Department, Bates College, Lewiston, Maine, USA 04240.

d) food deprivation producing 75 percent of normal body weight (Kaplan 1984a);

e) repeated contact with a 126 degree F hotplate (Ross and Randich 1984);

f) prolonged social isolation (Capitanio 1984);

g) elicited fighting between females in labor and males (Mayer and Rosenblatt 1984);

h) attacks upon pups resulting in death (Mayer and Rosenblatt 1984);

i) severe motion sickness (Ossenkopp and Tu 1984);

j) exposure to loud bursts of sound (Wu et al. 1984); and

k) induction of intense fear (Mineka et al. 1984).

For the uninitiated, even a cursory glance through the *Journal of Comparative Psychology* or the *Journal of Experimental Psychology: Animal Behavior Processes* (both APA journals) can be a disconcerting experience for anyone at least moderately sensitive to animals' suffering. In my view, the problem is not *individual* acts of cruelty but rather *institutionalized* cruelty of which APA is only a small part. The following excerpts, in the words of the researchers themselves, do not reveal the deliberations of "cruel" people, rather they reveal a remarkably desensitized, detached, and emotionally chilling attitude toward their animal "models." In this regard, animal researchers in psychology are far from unique.

Most published research contains multiple experiments in each journal article. For the sake of continuity, no attempt was made here to differentiate between each and every experiment within a given published report. The key consideration is that, as the APA proudly says, all research published in APA journals must also conform to the *Ethical Principles*:

> The approaching animal would trample on the prone partner, mouth its ears and toes, run its teeth along its partner's backbone, gnaw on its skull, thrust against its back or simply sit on it, which usually resulted in grimacing, screaming, and clasping on the recipient's part (Capitanio 1984 p. 41).

> "Priming" a female hamster by allowing it one biting attack on a smaller, drug-treated target hamster significantly decreased its latency to attack a subsequently presented probe target. Conversely, the latency of attacks on the probe was increased, and the number of attacks decreased, if the subject was first "satiated" by allowing it 1 hour of ad-lib access to a target followed by a series of briefer target presentations (p.66).... In the attack-satiation condition, an MT exposure target was left in the subject's home cage for 1 hour during which time the subject could attack ad lib (Potegal and tenBrink 1984 p. 68).

> Each test was begun by placing one pup in contact with the female's body.... When a female was found to have bitten or killed the first pup, one additional pup was introduced (p. 179).... A further effect of

previous maternal experience was evident in tendencies to bite or cannibalize pups.... Pup killing also appeared more often among pregnant females (p. 183).... Many or most of the females showing aggressive nest defense and immediate responsiveness to older pups may have been in labor (Mayer and Rosenblatt 1984, p. 187).

Experimental evidence for motion sickness in non-human primates... and cats and dogs... is well established when vomiting is used as the criterion response (Ossenkopp and Tu 1984, p. 189).

Animals in one of these groups were maintained on a 47.5 hr. water-deprivation regime (Saline/Deprived), but animals in the other group had free access to water in the colony room (Saline/Satiated). Four animals died during this phase (Poulos and Hinson 1984, p. 82)

Informal observations of the rats' behavior in the present experiments indicated that substantial freezing behavior was acquired following repeated exposure to shock. However, this freezing behavior was only manifested during the temporal interval immediately preceding shock presentation. Following shock presentation, there was a substantial increase in motor activity, primarily reflected by jumping and rearing responses.... On the other hand, it is still possible that shock-induced increases in arousal in some fashion reduce the rats' ability to effectively attend to the painful thermal stimuli (Ross and Randich 1984, p. 135).

Experience with an uncontrollable aversive event severely interferes with subsequent performance in several species.... For example, following exposure to unavoidable and inescapable electric shock, rats perform poorly in aversively... and appetitively motivated tasks... lose out in a food competition dominance tests... and show enhanced signs of stress, including weight loss and stomach ulcerations (p. 168).... Rats apparently exude a unique odor during experience with powerful stressors. Stressed and nonstressed rats can discriminate between the odor of stressed and nonstressed conspecifics [same species]. ... Further, rats given prior experience with shock later avoid a place in which a conspecific has been shocked (p. 169).... Reasoning that it might take greater stress to produce an interference effect in such animals, we increased the number of pretreatment shocks from 80 to 100, and increased the difficulty of the test task by making the rat run further into each compartment of the shuttlebox to terminate shock (Minor and LaLordo, 1984, p.175).

The US was a 50-ms, 3-mA, 50-Hz AC shock delivered via stainless Autoclip wound clips positioned 10 mm apart and 10-15 mm posterior to the dorsal canthus of the right eye.... Each rabbit's right external eyelids were held open by No. 3 tailor-hooks mounted on a Velcro strap which fitted about the head. A muzzle-like headset, fitted securely about the snout, supported a transducer for detecting movements of the nictitating membrane. A small hook was attached to a silk loop sutured in the nictitating membrane of the rabbit's right eye.... During the course of the experiment, one animal in Group S150 died, and its data were discarded from subsequent analyses (Kehoe and Morrow 1984, p. 207).

> Whereas not a single failure to attempt to escape was evident in nonshocked mice, 4 mice that had been exposed to inescapable shock exhibited failures to attempt an escape response on more than 60 percent of the trials on the last test day. That performance deterioriated over sessions among mice that received inescapable shock is not particularly surprising (p. 232).... On the third day, half the mice received 360 inescapable shocks of 2 s duration (p. 234).... The motoric demands on the animal were increased (given that animals were required to retrace incorrect responses), hence permitting expression of the disturbances engendered by inescapable shock (Anisman et al. 1984, p. 236).

> All programming of experimental events and observations was carried out in the darkened experimental room.... At the end of the 15 min. of ledge exposure the barriers were removed, and the movable wall was pushed forward so that the ledge was now only 2.5 cm deep (not enough for the subjects to rest on). This wall movement also served to push the subjects onto the grid floor. During the next 75 min. subjects were exposed to a series of fifty 0.7-mA shocks (p. 309).... Thus an additional set of measures of fear.... has been shown to reflect the phenomenon of "fear from a sense of helplessness"... fear of the entire situation (grid floor and surrounding area) was being assessed in the fear test (Mineka et al. 1984, p. 310).

> Animals in this condition spend a large amount of time facing away from the magazine wall, because animals exposed to primary frustration are known to actively engage in behavior to escape frustrating stimuli (Rosellini et al. 1984, p. 357).

In an effort to assimilate current information on psychological research (and improve its public image), last year the APA mailed an "Animal Research Survey" to several hundred graduate departments of psychology. One of the reported findings was that 252,000 animals were used in American university psychology laboratories in 1983 (APA *Backgrounder 2* 1984). To many familiar with the field, this total seemed surprisingly low. Upon closer examination, it became apparent that, by design or by oversight, the total was substantially underestimated for at least the following reasons: a) the survey was mailed to only 650 graduate departments whereas there are approximately 4,000 colleges and universities in the U.S.; b) the survey did not include animals used in behavioral research in other than academic settings; and c) the survey (question # 7) did not ask for yearly totals of animals but rather was worded in such a way as to elicit information on standing totals. When the results of the survey were discussed by CARE representatives at the APA convention last year, these points were raised but the CARE Committee had no explanation. Curiously, when I later requested a hard copy of the APA survey, the form I was sent had "(per year)" typed in at the end of question 7. The less than professional manner in which this project was handled may lead some to question the validity of the survey results and perhaps the motivations of the survey takers as well.

The March 1985 APA *Monitor* reported that, "In an unprecedented step made necessary by the current political climate, Council [of representatives] adopted interim ethical guidelines for behavioral researchers who use animals in their experiments." The article also noted that, "In last minute letters to Council members, Neal Miller of Rockefeller University and Ethel Tobach of the Museum of Natural History in New York warned that the guidelines could unduly restrict scientists and did not acknowledge the importance of such research." Reviewing the new *Guidelines* themselves, it is hard to see why anyone would be concerned about them "restricting" anyone from anything. The only experimental procedure specifically prohibited in the eight-page document is, "Utilization of muscle relaxants or paralytics alone during surgery or other invasive procedures, without general anesthesia, is unacceptable, and should not be used for surgical restraint," a practice already forbidden in item number 4 of the current *Guidelines* ("Surgical procedures shall be performed under appropriate anesthesia"). The rest of the document is replete with qualifiers and loopholes such as: "when feasible," "only with justification," "used only when less stressful procedures are inappropriate," "undertaken judiciously," "only when the training objectives cannot be achieved in any other way," "alternatives should be considered," etc. The original draft of the new *Guidelines* did contain one highly progressive and eminently reasonable new principle, to wit, "It is recognized that certain extreme procedures may be inherently objectionable on ethical grounds." To the great dismay of many, the APA Council of Representatives dropped this enlightened provision from the draft accepted on an interim basis (personal communication, Kenneth Shapiro, Co-Coordinator, PsyETA). The Council plans to take final action on the new *Guidelines* in August, 1985.

Ethical Considerations

Ethical defenses of psychological research with animals (e.g., Miller 1983, unpublished paper presented at the 1983 APA convention; Coile and Miller 1984; King 1984) have relied heavily upon "straw man" tactics; i.e., set up the most extremist or even nonespoused arguments from the opposition and then knock them down. For example, King (Letters to the Editor, APA *Monitor,* April 1984) asserted that the animal advocate position is that, "Animals' rights are synonymous with human rights [and] animals have rights equal to humans." Clearly, the operational factor here is not equal *treatment* but equal *consideration* of relevant needs, interests,and capacities. No one is arguing that nonhuman animals have a "right" to vote, to obtain parking spaces, or otherwise be entitled to "rights" which are obviously incongruent with their own nature. What realistically has been stressed is that *all* animals have inherent interests in staying alive, being free from pain, and fulfilling their own unique evolutionary potentials. To automatically denigrate and disregard the fundamental interests of all other species in the exclusive pursuit of perceived human priorities is the quintessential essence of arrogance and selfishness.

To advocate animal rights in no way implies *absolute* liberty for animals any more than advocating human rights implies absolute liberty for people. Sudak (Letters to the Editor, APA *Monitor,* April 1984) illogically argues that, to avoid ethical inconsistency, animal rightists must allow animals to roam and breed indiscriminately. Respecting the rights of animals does not mean the abdication of human power, it means the exercise of human power in the spirit of humane stewardship. Enforcing animal birth control is entirely consistent with this spirit, particularly in light of the tragic pet overpopulation problem—a tragedy created in the first place by irresponsible human stewardship.

In a similar vein, Miller's (1983) address to the APA asserted:

> One obvious implication is that we should not eat meat, eggs, or milk, wear leather shoes or furs, or sleep with down bags or pillows. Killing animals for such purposes obviously is exploitation. If animals have equal rights, we should not kill those who destroy our crops nor even fence in our fields to keep them out—changes that, if universally forced by legislation, could precipitate a major crisis of starvation in the world. We even should not starve or poison the rats that, if left to multiply freely, could cause outbreaks of typhus and bubonic plague. (p. 6).

The strategy is clear. Miller attempts to show that, carried to its "logical" extreme, respecting the rights of animals is impossible because to do so would mean giving up all means of human self-preservation and self-defense. This line of argument is obviously fallacious. For example, using it one could rule out all human research by showing that, carried to its "logical" extreme, scientific freedom would trample on the rights of the individual. No responsible animal rights advocate of which I am aware has argued that absolute respect for non-human life is mandatory, or even possible (how does one take a shower without killing millions of bacteria?). From an animal rights perspective, the issue is simply one of minimizing the level of violence and compulsive exploitation, or "getting off the backs of the animals" to the greatest extent possible.

Miller and his colleagues do make a key point, however, in noting out that an animal rights position does imply radical changes in the life-style of most individuals and of humanity as a whole, i.e., the exploitation of laboratory animals must be seen in a *cultural* context. Animals have been oppressed and abused in virtually all areas of human activity: for food, for furs, for "sport," for movies, etc., areas which cannot even make a pretense of "necessity." It is no coincidence that every vivisector I have met also eats animals.

Ironically, it seems to be widely accepted among animal researchers that keeping animals in captivity and eventually killing them are of no moral significance in themselves. Bannister (1981) has observed, "We can do things to them which we never consider ethical to do to people. Animal experimentation is lauded as a solution for ethical problems." This attitude is abundantly evident in Miller's (1985) article: "Other experiments on stress, which ethically can be carried out only on animals...;" "Other experiments on animals that would be extremely difficult, impossible or unethical to conduct on people...;" "...recent behavioral research, which ethically could be done only on animals...;" "...neuroanatomical, biochemical, hormonal, and drug studies can be carried out that, although not painful, would be unethical with people...."

Consequently, Miller (1985) is completely dispassionate and with clear conscience in referring to such traumatic procedures to animals as: "nausea-inducing agents...;" "...if animals were deprived of the sensations from a limb by cutting sensory nerves from it...;" "...used a mouse colony designed to produce stress by conflict among the mice for food, water, and space...;" ".... increases the susceptibility to experimentally induced infections, to experimentally implanted cancers...;" "...the after-effects of unpredictable, uncontrollable shocks...;" "...a promising model for at least one type of human depression...;" "...analyze in more detail the anatomical damage and the permanent hearing losses... produced by exposure to various durations and types of loud sounds...;" "...behavioral tests for the suppression of pain-elicited responses...;" "...test new drugs for addictive potential...;" "...conditioned withdrawal symptoms can be elicited...;" "...complete deprivation of visual stimulation for a critical period in the infant chimpanzee's life caused the adults to show severe visual defects...;" "...separation of infant monkeys from their mothers and playmates during an early critical period in their development could produce striking and apparently permanent deficits in their social behavior, as well as certain neurotic and psychotic symptoms...;" "...infant monkeys who have been deprived of adequate mothering grow up to become mothers who neglect and abuse their children...;" "...experiments on effects of giving alcohol and other drugs to pregnant animals...;" "...experiments on various animals on the change in sex behavior that appear at puberty as a result of prenatal exposure to sex hormones...", etc. Furthermore, Miller feels no need to justify animal suffering through a cost-benefit analysis and argues against, "the fallacy of requiring that any specific experiment that causes animals to suffer must be justified by a cost-benefit expectation of directly producing a sufficient reduction in human suffering." Apparently, all's fair in love, war, and vivisection.

In a sensitive article by Sarason (1984), the author observes:

> When we speak approvingly, respectfully, and with awe about the benefits of science and technology, should we not temper our enthusiasm by the fact that those benefits in part derive, however serendipituously, from a long history of catastrophe, carnage and misery? Has the price been too high? (p. 477)... The scientific-technological communities have been forced to recognize that no less important than what they study is how they utilize people and other animals as subjects. Initially, the response of these communities was quite negative. They viewed their critics as bleeding hearts who did not appreciate the gifts given them by science and technology or who did not understand the trade-off problem. The amount of good society derived from the customary conduct of inquiry far exceeded the harm inflicted on some people and animals. To tamper with untrammeled inquiry would be injurious to societal improvement. Today, a large part of these communities has come to see that they had been insensitive to the fact that in their roles as scientists and technologists they had to be governed by criteria deriving from society's view of what was good or bad for its citizens. In short, there were or should be restrictions on the freedom of the conduct of inquiry (p. 481).

Dumont (1976), in an article on behavioral research (not specifically focused on animal work), captured the essence of the researcher's mentality in noting that, "There is no malice in it. In fact, its most characteristic feature is the absence of ideology and moral judgment. It is a collection of perfectly decent professionals and administrators hustling their tenures... and being unconcerned with the consequences of their collective behavior."

The *Oxford English Dictionary* defines *humane* as "gentle or kind in demeanor or action; civil; courteous; friendly; obliging; marked by sympathy and with consideration for the needs and distresses of others; feeling or showing compassion or tenderness." This definition is consistent with the use of the word humane as it is generally applied to human subjects as well as with commonsense usage of the term. I believe that many types of animal research also merit the adjective humane, e.g., clinical studies, noninvasive lab work, and ethological or naturalistic observations. Vivisection, however, is another matter. In the laboratory environment, the theoretical definition of humane is to limit the suffering to the level required to complete the objectives of the research or testing. If the objectives are to induce heart disease, or to inflict cancer or diabetes, or to produce depression or even severe pain, this is still defined as "humane." I suggest to you that, at best, this constitutes a degraded and invalid use of the word "humane." At worst, it is hypocrisy and self-deception of the highest order. I also question the use of the word "humane" in view of the grossly minimal standards for animal care required by law, and the woefully inadequate enforcement of these laws (Giannelli 1985).

Animal research is also defended as being "necessary." I have noticed that "necessity" has a way of expanding to fill the volume supported by available funding. I think the word "necessary" is basically a cop-out and an ineffectual attempt to escape responsibility for our collective behavior. The use of animals in research is a long-standing social policy. One may support that policy or one may oppose it, but at least it should be honestly acknowledged that, to the extent we have become dependent on animals for research, we have made this choice with our eyes wide open. The word "necessary" is also inappropriate because it implies that we could not stop this practice even if we wanted to. Breathing is necessary. Sleeping is necessary. Eating and drinking are necessary. Vivisection is a *choice*, and to growing numbers of us, a most unfortunate and unjustifiable choice.

While ethical considerations apply across the spectrum of vivisection, the problem is particularly acute in behavioral work. Rowan (1984) asserted:

> The psychologist must confront ethical questions that stem from the *essential* elements of his or her research, unlike the biochemist or physiologist, who may be interested in muscle function.... We thus come to the psychologist's paradox. Since we should, if consistent, confer moral worth according to some property (or properties) of the organism's nervous system, then the more suitable the animal is as a model of the human psyche, the greater should be the attention to the ethical issues relating to the research. The paradox boils down to this—the better the animal is as a model of the human psyche, the more restricted its use should be (p. 139).

Drewett and Kani (1981) raised a similar point in arguing that, "It is also here, of course, that the central moral question raises itself most acutely; for the same evolutionary insights that lead us to believe that there can be no radical discontinuity in psychological functions ought also to make us wonder whether it is proper to continue to treat them as radically different in morals." Rollin (1985) observed that, "... in studying the effect of such phenomena as fear, pain, grief, the psychologist has precluded the possibility of providing pharmacological relief... because such drugs would mask the phenomenon being studied. These unpleasant experiences form the substance of such experiments, and are not simply the unfortunate by-products of research."

Bowd (1980) has been a leading advocate of ethical reform in this area. He identified two basic arguments offered by defenders of animal vivisection: a) "It is reasonable to sacrifice the interests of animals in order to satisfy the interests of human beings;" and, b) "Animal interests may be disregarded for the advancement of knowledge or in the interests of science." Rollin (1985) contends that, "... moral questions—even this one—... are not simply matters of taste and opinion. A person's ethical beliefs are subject to rational examination and may be found incoherent, inconsistent, self-contradictory, ambiguous and so on, in just the same way as any other beliefs. The chances are... these discrepancies are more likely to be found in moral beliefs than elsewhere." Rollin notes several of the differences frequently cited between humans and animals (e.g., we have "immortal souls," we are at the top of the "evolutionary ladder," we are more powerful, we are rational, we use language, etc.). He then makes the telling point, "But merely citing differences is not enough; the differences must also have *moral relevance*." Using the example of human rationality (ignoring for the moment the fact that humans can also behave in a highly irrational fashion), Rollin then observes:

> But what is the moral relevance of rationality? Doubtless one needs to be a rational being to be a moral agent or actor in order to be held morally responsible for what one does. But one surely does not need to be rational to be an object of moral attention and concern—consider children, infants, the insane, the senile, the comatose, the retarded, and so on. Furthermore, if rationality is the key feature in making something worthy of moral attention, why is so much of our moral concern devoted to aspects of human life have nothing to do with rationality (p. 923)?

Singer (1975) defined the word "speciesism" as, "A prejudice or attitude of bias toward the interests of members of one's own species and against those of members of other species." Historical analogies have been drawn between speciesism and other forms of arbitrary discrimination, such as racism and sexism. Psychologists at least acknowledge these other forms of prejudice because, in theory at least, they represent undesirable and deviant social attitudes. On the other hand, speciesism is as invisible to most of us as is water to a fish. We live in a sea of speciesism. It is the norm, the unchallenged standard which seemingly constitutes the natural order of things. To challenge this perspective, to doubt that "people *always* come first" is very unusual, although not actually abnormal in a clinical sense.

Psychology has often been accused, unfortunately but I think fairly, of fostering some of the most painful and misguided animal experiments. It is not that the scientists are necessarily sadistic, but rather that the present system results in great suffering. Scientists are usually not trained for or inclined to ethical thinking, and science itself (being neutral in such matters) cannot always be relied upon to supply reasonable ethical restraints on animal research. In my judgment, the inherent callousness of most current animal research has also had unfortunate psychological and intellectual consequences for people—for the researchers themselves, for generations of students encouraged to trade empathy for inquiry, and for humanity as a whole.

Segal (1982) issued a strong appeal for ethical retrospection in this area:

> Yet we seem never to question our treatment of laboratory animals and the brutalizing effect of some of our practices on ourselves and our students.... It is only a small step from ignoring the welfare of animals to ignoring the welfare of people.... If we do not model a strong

> moral sense of the sacredness of life, we can hardly expect better of our students.... Most animal welfare proponents *do* understand the value and the needs of science (indeed, many are scientists themselves, speaking from personal experience).... They ask for an end to wanton and unthinking cruelty.... Is *this* experiment necessary? Does it needlessly replicate earlier work? Could our students learn from a demonstration rather than a crudely-done experiment of their own? Could the experiment be done with an earlier-evolved species? fewer subjects? a lesser intensity of shock? with appetitive rather than aversive stimuli? with a lesser degree of starvation, social or sensory isolation, confinement, restraint, or mutilation? For how many days, weeks, months, or years should one animal be required to serve science with its pain or suffering?... Does expedience justify animal suffering? (p. 115)

Lockwood bemoaned the fact that the phrase, "ethical restraints on animal research," often leaves the uncomfortable implication that the main concern of reformers is telling people what they cannot do. Lockwood concluded, "But having an ethical point of view can open many doors, adding validity to studies of animal consciousness, cognition, intelligence, and the diversity of relationships that exist between human and animal. Having an ethical point of view restrains nothing that is truly in the spirit of sound and creative scientific inquiry."

Alternatives to the Status Quo

In recent years, a large number of articles have appeared which have both critiqued contemporary psychology's overreliance on laboratory-encapsulated research and offered suggestions for both more humane and more externally valid ways of doing things. In an article on the roles of naturalistic observation in comparative psychology, D.B. Miller (1977) took note of a problem that has gotten worse with time, "The literature is becoming increasingly inundated with examples of the importance of species variables in designing, conducting, and interpreting laboratory experiments.... Comparative psychology has a great deal to gain by orienting its research around the animal in its world." Tunnel (1977) discussed an expanded definition of field research:

> When the psychological researcher operationalizes the dependent measures, the treatment, and the background setting in real-world terms, his investigation may yield findings that might never have been obtained otherwise. The total effect of operationalizing all variables in real-world terms is greater than the effect of employing any of the three naturalistic dimensions singly. Not only are unexpected findings often obtained, but the findings are generally stronger, more convincing, and more highly valued by the research community. In short, the research is more meaningful.(p. 430).... Although the problem of external validity is not fully soluble, naturalistic studies do possess more potential for achieving greater generalizability than do laboratory studies, simply because the former are conducted in real-world contexts,

> to which all research ultimately seeks application (p. 434).... Learning to recognize naturalistic dimensions and learning to exploit them will require some reeducation among psychologists to the end that the response of entering the lab when one is stimulated by a research question becomes less automatic. The real world can become the primary laboratory, with recourse to experimental laboratories as the problem dictates. Ultimately, psychology seeks basic understanding of natural behaviors, natural treatments, and natural settings. They should be actively exploited in our research from the very beginning (p. 436).

In one of the most astute and compelling articles of its kind, Petrinovich (1979) discussed the concept of "probabilistic functionalism." Owing to its direct contribution to the issue at hand, the article is deserving of quotation at length:

> Our application of this [scientific] method has led us to overrely on the laboratory-encapsulated, simple linear process model that prevailed in the older physical sciences. The strict reliance on these procedures seems not to be expanding our range of understanding, and this has caused serious consternation among some who study those aspects of psychology that must, by definition concern themselves with behavior in a context.... This turn of events is even more distressing when one realizes that an adequate paradigm was developed by Darwin in 1859.... There has been concern expressed recently regarding the ability of the science of psychology to deal with significant behavioral issues at an adequate level of complexity. This concern has taken the form of questioning the adequacy of traditional experimental research procedures for yielding generalizations beyond the particular experimental paradigm.... I am convinced that the time has come for us not only to question the degree of reliance that has been placed on the systematic research paradigm but to call for its overthrow to the extent that anyone attempting to generalize to representative situations on the basis of data gathered within a systematic framework should be compelled to justify the generalization. In short, this is a call for a scientific revolution in the Kuhnian sense (Kuhn 1970). (p. 373).

> The point is that unless variables are represented proportionally to their frequency of occurrence in the situations to which we want to generalize, we cannot establish the probable importance of variables in controlling the behavior of organisms (p. 374-75).... The generality of psychological principles is diminished seriously by failing to sample situations. Because of this failure we have little information concerning the situational determinants of behavior and know little about the manner in which organisms use the resources of the situation to support behavior patterns (p. 376).... If we are to understand the behavior of organisms it will be necessary to extend the basic definition of psychology to read similarly to that suggested by Brunswik: *The science of organism—environment relationships* (p. 378).

> The narrow laboratory-derived "laws" of the learning theorists have been found to be inadequate to apply to the instances of broader situational generality.... The essential artificiality of the laboratory and the usual lack of any essential relationship of the laboratory setting to an organism's adaptive capacities do violence to the integrity

> of behavioral units. Since both the brain and behavior evolved as organized functional entities, we must understand the integrity of these entities before we can understand the mechanisms regulating them (p. 383).... If the situations are not representative, if our subjects are not representative, and if our behavioral samples are not representative, then no analytic method is of much value—no matter how sophisticated we might be in its use.... Theories of behavior must be developed within the context of the environment, since it is the environment that provides both the stimulus and the response supports for behavior. Only when the capacities of the organism are considered as a part of the ecological setting can behavioral laws of adequate generality be developed (p. 388).

Although I am opposed to the exploitation of animals in the name of science, it should be abundantly clear that we can learn a lot from animals (and should) without removing them from their natural environments or acting against their interests. There are situations, however, when ethological or field research is inadequate for the subject of inquiry and laboratory research may be in order. This is not, of course, to say that we are entitled to do something aversive to animals simply because there is no other way to get the information. One cannot justify pursuing an experience using the circular logic that, without pursuing the experience, one could not have it. Nor are good intentions enough. Noble intent ought to be considered necessary but not sufficient ground for pursuing any type of research—especially on subjects incapable of giving informed consent. At times this may be less than convenient or expedient, but its justification rests not with its convenience or expediencey, but rather by virtue of the unnecessary suffering it avoids.

Granted that there are justifiable laboratory procedures which: a) are noninvasive; and/or b) done for the *direct benefit* of the specific animals involved, what general recommendations might one offer to make the laboratory environment more humane as well as productive? Lockwood (1984) presented some excellent suggestions, here summarized:

1) Study the history and philosophy of the scientific method.

Good science begins with a good question, followed by keen observations; avoid becoming a "behavioral data collector" of inert and stagnating information simply because it can be readily analyzed and quantified.

2) Fit the technology to the question, not vice versa.

Don't allow the technology to dictate the methodology; profound questions may be explored in elegantly simple ways; consuming large amounts of electricity, paper and animals' lives is not very imaginative.

3) Get your hands dirty.

Study your animals up close and personal, not simply the data they generate; appreciate the difference between discovering behavior of interest vs. inducing behavioral oddities; focus on studies *with* animals rather than experiments *on* animals.

4) Don't be afraid of empathy and anthropomorphism as sources of hypotheses.

Simplistic or mechanistic interpretations are a long way from understanding; precise predictions of sterile behavior are irrelevant; empathy allows one to make more meaningful predictions which can be empirically tested.

5) Provide your subjects with suitable environments.

The animal facilities should be designed around the needs of the animals, not the convenience of the caretakers; enriched environments stimulate a wealth of diverse behavior you'd otherwise never discover.

6) Don't be afraid of anecdotes as a source of hypotheses.

Anecdotes tell us about the range of animal abilities and experiences.

7) Appreciate the individuality of animals.

Creative questions come from being alert to the subtleties of behavior; individuality is biological reality.

8) Examine your motives and self-image.

Stop playing the role of "noble scientist;" find the source of your defensiveness toward criticism.

9) Keep your sense of humor.

If you've lost touch with the inconsistencies and absurdities so common in the behavior of humans and other animals, you're missing a lot of fun as well as inventive observation.

10) Keep your sense of awe.

The greatest deterrent to creative thought is the belief that you know it all.

We have considered the alternative of studying animals in real world environments, touched on the ethical advantages of clinical research done to benefit the animals themselves, and reviewed suggestions for bringing creative kindness into the laboratory. All of this is good, but we must eventually face up to the fact that, to learn about the psychology of people, one needs to study people. This is surely no revelation. Even animal research advocates who defend the practice to the hilt concede that over ninety percent of current behavioral studies are based on people. (APA *Backgrounder 2.* 1984). It should come as no surprise to learn that, in general, the best alternative to the use of animals in psychological research is *ourselves*. This is fair and fitting given that we are supposed to be the beneficiaries of such research. By its very nature, such research is inclined to be both more relevant and more ethical. The proliferation of human subject protection committees and greater attention to issues of informed consent are exceedingly healthy developments. What is needed is an analogous (don't read "identical") set of ethical standards for animal research, not the current lip-service and paper shuffling that pose and posture as "*Ethical Guidelines*."

As psychologists, we must also be particularly concerned with psychological alternatives; recognition that vivisection is a choice, not an imperative; ceasing to regard animals as laboratory "tools" or simply means to self-serving human ends; rather, appreciating that animals are fellow sentient beings with interests and needs of their own which should be respected; and a genuine reexamination of our attitudes about ourselves, including the tough admission that historically *Homo sapiens* have always greatly overrated our sense of being "the chosen," a sort of species version of "manifest destiny."

In terms of improvements in human health, both medical and psychological, there is increasing recognition that primary prevention is our greatest alternative. Hamburg (1982; former president of the National Academy of Sciences' Institute for Medicine; in Cohen 1985) observed:

> We have missed valuable opportunities to reduce our burden of illness by underinvesting in programs for disease prevention and health promotion. Over the last decade, it has become increasingly clear that cardiovascular disease, cancer, stroke and accidents—which together account for nearly 75 percent of deaths annually—are intimately linked to a variety of health damaging behaviors ranging from smoking to drunk-driving to sendentary lifestyles. Yet policy has not matched understanding: while support for disease prevention is growing, it is miniscule compared with the support given to high technology care (p. 214).

In a very recent article for *American Psychologist*, Senator William S. Cohen stated, "Until now, only an insignificant fraction of our resources—less than 2 percent of the total amount spent for health care—has been devoted to keeping people well.... Many health care professionals are convinced that the next major breakthrough will come not from the research laboratory, but through changes in our individual lifestyles" (Cohen 1985).

Concluding Remarks

Psychology is an honorable profession, and the vast majority of my colleagues I believe to be honorable persons. The "sins" of the behavioral animal researcher are particularly disturbing to me, not because they are so different in quality from other types of animal abuse (they aren't), surely not because they constitute in quantity the greatest amount of cruelty (they are only a tiny part of the problem), but mainly because I am grieved to see my beloved profession glorify and engage in behavior so unbecoming of *civilized* humanity.

I believe the most valuable things we have learned through animal research are insights into the human mentality. These insights have arisen from direct analysis of researchers at work, not from tenuous extrapolations to ourselves based on animal behavior in highly artificial laboratory environments. We have learned that otherwise compassionate people can become remarkably desensitized and detached from the suffering they inflict upon animals. We have learned that highly intelligent people can be engaged in the most trivial or eccentric research yet convince themselves that their work is important. We have learned that, as a species, we can be remarkably uncivilized, aggressive and selfish.

If there is one key word which, for me, sums up human "speciesism," that word is *arrogance*. Our attitude and behavior toward other animals is rooted in unjustified human arrogance; that is, in unchallenged assumptions regarding human superiority, uniqueness, and self-importance. This rather sweeping hypothesis is supported by any honest backward glance at our historical self-portraits. The major scientific revolutions have progressively dethroned *Homo sapiens* from a fictional place of unique creation. The Copernican revolution showed us that we are not situated at the center of the universe. The Darwinian revolution showed us that we are biologically related to other earth animals. The Freudian revolution demonstrated that our behavior is powerfully influenced by unconscious and irrational aspects of the psyche; and the Einsteinian revolution even pulled out from under us our assumptions about absolute space and time. Despite the staggering importance of these scientific revolutions, for the most part, we still behave as if we were the "*Special Darlings*" of the universe, ecologically and ethically central to creation.

A major irony of speciesism is that all the available evidence to be found in the temple of science contradicts the "Special Darling" theory. The hardest of hard physical sciences, physics, teaches us that at the atomic and subatomic levels, the matter which constitutes the human body is made of the same basic particles and subject to the same primal forces, as are all other types of matter. On the cosmic scale, the evidence is even more impressive. We now realize that the earth itself occupies an inconspicuous position in the Milky Way galaxy which consists of over 100 billion stars. Our galaxy itself is only one of more than one billion observable galaxies. One of our "closest" neighbors is M 31, the Andromeda galaxy. M 31 is only 2.2 million light years away; that is, thirteen million trillion miles, or 13×10^{18} miles. Our Milky Way, M 31, and sixteen other galaxies are roughly clustered together in what is affectionately called "the local group." As its name implies, the "local group" is only one of the many clusters of galaxies,some estimated to be two to three billion light years away. The most distant energy sources yet discovered are quasars, estimated to be five to fifteen billion light years away. Obviously,these dimensions are completely unimaginable to our little minds. Perhaps that partly explains why the message of our triviality doesn't get absorbed, doesn't make the headlines. I am always impressed by those cosmological calendars we have all seen—where January 1st is scaled to represent the beginning of the known universe and December 31st represents today. On such a scale, the earth was born in September and humanity-come-lately came on the scene a few seconds before midnight on December 31st.

The point I am trying to capture is that if ignorance ever served to justify our arrogance, our speciesism, that excuse is no longer valid. The arrogance of vivisectors, to me, represents a particularly vile anachronism, a throwback to the days when we didn't know better. Having only lately clawed our way to the top of the food chain, humanity is still drunk with power. On earth, at least, we have become the unchallenged "*Planetary Bullies*."

I am constantly finding ironies in my analysis of speciesism. One of the most important is that we are not "pure" speciesists by any means. By that I simply mean that as a species, we are remarkably disunited and brutal toward each other. How can any species which has never known the absence of war, which allows tens of millions of its own kind to starve to death every year, how can such a species pretend to be "humane" and "civilized"? Scientific advancement, including medical and psychological technology, is, of course, a highly desirable objective. But all the animal research in the world won't save us from the number one threat to our health—*ourselves*. In my judgment, speciesism is a symptom of this underlying collective pathology, a pathology which is more serious now than ever before because of our lethal technological power for self-destruction. At one stage in human evolution, the full exercise of human power was essential to our continued survival. However, in the modern era of nuclear weapons and ecological erosion, the full exercise of human power is incompatible with our continued survival. The over-exercise of our strength has become manifestly self-defeating. We should, further, remember that the Darwinian "survival of the fittest" does not mean "survival of the strongest." Ultimately, those species most fit and therefore most likely to survive are those most in harmony with their environment.

In a recent and timely article on open scientific exchange and the growth of knowledge, Mahoney (1985) issued a poignant reminder to his colleagues which I wish to pass on to mine:

> Ours is a privileged profession, indeed, and that very privilege demands a corresponding sense of responsibility and commitment. As we come to more deeply appreciate that one of the cardinal features of science is its perennial openness—its freedom to grow—it is to be hoped we will examine the most salient constraints on that openness. Whatever paths and policies we pursue in our quest for knowledge, however, we can only hope to grow by remaining open to change, and that, in itself, is a most formidable challenge. (p. 37).

As uncomfortable or incomprehensible as it may at present be to some, the changes which I and others in the animal rights movement seek are profoundly *pro*-human. It is not a simplistic question of whose interests, humans vs. animals, should come first. All of life's interests must be considered together as the organic unity that it is. No one needs to prove their compassion for people by condoning cruelty to animals.

As the community mental health movement was spurred by desire to address and correct those social conditions which facilitate stress and psychopathology, as a clinician I feel a professional obligation to address and correct those cultural conditions which frustrate the enormous potential of our self-actualization as a species.

In my judgment, vivisection is a grave social evil because it fosters the worst in human nature; our arrogance, aggressiveness, selfishness, callousness, and our sense of alienation from the rest of nature. It is all the more problematic because it is promoted by the intellectual elite, professional scientists pursuing their craft for the presumed welfare of humanity, leaders who are in a position to shape the society of our children and the world of their children's children. Even if one does not accept this assessment, it is clear that the essence of ethical behavior is a system of self-restraints in the pursuit of one's perceived self-interests.

We must remind ourselves that *scientific* progress is not invariably *human* progress. The continued expansion of human knowledge at the cost of human character is a pathetic trade-off which, if continued, will eventually destroy the civilization we glorify. At present, there appears to be decreasing prospects that humanity will ever make peace with itself. Many say, this being the case, how can you expect humanity ever to make peace with the rest of the animal kingdom? There is hope for animal liberation because it also represents human liberation, freeing ourselves from the ages-old dependence on animal sacrifice. There is also hope for animal liberation because other animals do not represent the threat to us which we do to each other. As a species, with good reason, we distrust and fear each other far more than we distrust and fear other animals. The only animal which threatens to push us away from the dinner table is man himself. Perhaps, just perhaps, there is hope for facilitating the peace process by first deescalating our aggression against the other, less warlike, species which inhabit this fragile earth.

References

Ainsworth, M.D.S. 1969. Object relations, dependency and attachment: A theoretical review of the infant-mother relationship. *Child Dev.* 40:969-1025.

Anisman, H., Hamilton, M. and Zacharko, R.M. 1984. Cue and response-choice acquisition and reversal after exposure to uncontrollable shock: Induction of response severation. *J. Exper. Psych.: Animal Behav. Processes.* 10(2):229-43.

APA *Backgrounder.* Public Information Office. 1984. *The use of animals in psychological research.*

APA *Backgrounder 2.* Public Information Office. 1984. *The use of animals in psychological research.*

APA *Monitor.* March 1985. p. 14.

APA (pamphlet). 1984.*Behavioral research with animals.*

APA Summary Report for Journal Operations. 1983. *Amer. Psych.* 39(6):689.

Arzin, N.H. and Thienes, P.M. 1978. Rapid elimination of enuresis by intensive learning without a conditioning apparatus. *Behav. Therapy.* 9:342-54.

Association for Advanced Training in the Behavioral Sciences. AATBS Staff. 1984. *Abnormal psychology.* 3:1-87.

Bakan, D. 1972. Psychology can now kick the science habit. *Psych. Today.* March.

Baldessarini, R.J. 1975. Amine hypotheses in affective illness. In: Mandels, J. ed. *The Psychobiology of Depression.* New York: Spectrum Publishers.

Bannister, D. 1981. The fallacy of animal experimentation in psychology. In: Sperlinger, D. ed. *Animals in Research: New Perspectives in Animal Experimentation.* New York: John Wiley and Sons. pp. 307-17.

Baron, J. 1971. Is experimental psychology relevant? *Amer. Psych.* 26(8):713-6.

Basmajian, J.V. 1963. Control and training of individual motor units. *Science.* 141:440-1.

Beck, A.T. et al. 1979. *Cognitive Therapy of Depression.* New York: Guilford.

Becker, J. 1984. *Behavior modification.* In: 1985 review course for the national licensure in psychology by the Association for Advanced Training in the Behavioral Sciences (AATBS). 1:1-42.

Bevan, W. 1982. In: Sarason, S.B. 1984. If it can be studied or developed, should it be? *Amer. Psych.* 39(5):477-85.

Bowd, A. 1980. Ethical reservations about psychological research with animals. *Psych. Record.* 30:201-10.

Bowlby, J. 1969. *Attachment and loss.* Vol. 1: Attachment. New York: Basic Books.

Brewer, W.F. 1974. There is no convincing evidence for operant or classical conditioning in adult humans. In: Weimer, W.B. and Palermo, D.S. eds. *Cognition and the Symbolic Processes.* Hillsdale, New Jersey: Lawrence Erlbaum Assocs.

Broad, W. and Wade, N. 1982. *Betrayers of the Truth.* New York: Simon and Schuster.

Capitanio, J.P. 1984. Early experience and social processes in rhesus macaques *(Macaca mulatta)*: I. Dyadic social interaction. *J. Compar. Psych.* 98(1):35-44.

Chomsky, N. 1959. Review of *Verbal Behavior* by B.F. Skinner. *Language.* 35:26-58.

Chomsky, N. 1968. *Language and Mind.* New York: Harcourt, Brace and World.

Cohen, W.S. 1985. Health promotion in the work place: A prescription for good health. *Amer. Psych.* 40(2):213-6.

Coile, D.C. and Miller, N.E. 1974. Comment: How radical animal activists try to mislead humane people. *Amer. Psych.* 39(6):700-1.

Coleman, J.C. and Broen, W.E., Jr. 1972. *Abnormal Psychology and Modern Life.* 4th edition. Glenview, Illinois: Scott, Foresman and Co. pp. 149, 627.

Dalen, P. 1969. Casual explanations in psychiatry: A critique of some current concepts. *Brit. J. Psychia.* 115:129,132.

Demarest, J. 1983. The ideas of change, progress and continuity in the comparative psychology

of learning. In: Rajecki, D.W. ed. *Comparing Behavior: Studying Man Studying Animals.* Hillsdale, New Jersey: Lawrence Erlbaum Assocs. pp. 143-79.
Drewett, R. and Kani, W. 1981. Animal experimentation in the behavioral sciences. In: Sperlinger, D. ed. *Animals in Research: New Perspectives in Animal Experimentation.* New York: John Wiley and Sons. pp. 175-201.
Dumont, M. 1976. Social science vs. privacy. (letter). *J. Humanis. Psych.* 16(3):81. Summer.
Ellis, A. 1962. *Reason and Emotion in Psychotherapy.* New York: Lyle Stuart.
Endler. N. and Magnussen, D. 1976. Toward an interactionist psychology of personality. *Psych. Bulletin.* 83(5):968-9.
Fletcher, G.J. 1984. Psychology and common sense. *Amer. Psych.* 39(3):203-13.
Franks, C.M. 1969. *Behavior Therapy: Appraisal and Status.* New York: McGraw-Hill.
Gadlin, H. and Ingle, G. 1975. Through the one-way mirror: The limits of experimental self-reflection. *Amer. Psych.* 30(10):1003-9.
Gangsei, D. 1983. *Community psychology.* In: 1985 review course for the national licensure exam in psychology by the Association for Advanced Training in the Behavioral Sciences (AATBS). 4:1-35.
Giannelli, M.A. 1985. Sacrificing animals in experiments: Vivisection excesses in modern medicine. *Cogitations on Law and Govt.* 2(4):75-83.
Giorgi, A. 1970. *Psychology as a Human Science: A Phenomenologically Based Approach.* New York: Harper and Row.
Hamburg, D. 1982. In: Cohen, W.S. 1985. Health promotion in the workplace: A prescription for good health. *Amer. Psych.* 40(2):213-6.
Harlow, H.F. 1974. In: Pratt, D. 1976. *Painful Experiments on Animals.* New York: Argus Archives. p. 89.
Harlow, H.F., Dodsworth, R.O., and Harlow, M.K. 1965. Total social isolation in monkeys. *Proceed. Nat. Acad. Sci. USA.* 54:90-97.
Harlow, H.F. and Suomi, S.J. 1977. Primate models of depression. In: Seligman, M.P. and Maser, J.D. eds. *Psychopathology: Experimental Models.* San Francisco: W.H. Freeman Co.
Heffernan, J.A. and Albee, G.W. 1985. Prevention perspectives from Vermont to Washington. *Amer. Psych.* 40(2):202-4.
Heim, A. 1979. The use of animals in experimental psychology. Speech given to the International Association Against Painful Experiments on Animals, West Berlin.
Henry, J.P. and Stephen, P.M. 1979. An animal model of neuropsychological factors in hypertension. In: Yamori, Y., Lovenberg, W. and Freis, W. eds. *Prophylactic Approach to Hypertensive Diseases.* New York: Raven Press. pp. 229-307.
Hunt, H.F. 1964. Problems in the interpretation of experimental neurosis. *Psych. Reports.* 15:27-35.
James, W. 1890. *The Principles of Psychology.* New York: Henry Holt.
Kamiya, J. 1969. Operant control of the EEG alpha rhythm and some of its reported effects on consciousness. In: Tart, C. ed. *Altered States of Consciousness.* New York: John Wiley and Sons. pp. 489-501.
Kaplan, P.S. 1984a. Importance of relative temporal parameters in trace autoshaping: From excitation to inhibition. *J. Exper. Psych.: Animal Behav. Processes.* 10(2):113-26.
Kaplan, R.M. 1984b. The connection between clinical health promotion and health status: A critical overview. *Amer. Psych.* 39(7):755-65.
Kehoe, E.J. and Morrow, L.D. 1984. Temporal dynamics of the rabbit's nictitating membrane response in serial compound conditioned stimuli. *J. Exper. Psych.: Animal Behav. Processes.* 10(2):205-20.
Keller, F. and Schoenfeld, W. 1950. *Principles of Psychology.* New York: Appleton-Century Crofts. p. 399.
Kelly, J.A. 1985. Psychological research and the rights of animals: Disagreement with Miller. Comment submitted to *American Psychologist.*

Kimble, G.A. 1984. Psychology's two cultures. *Amer. Psych.* 39(8):833-9.
King, F.A. 1984. Animals in research: The case for experimentation. *Psych. Today.* Sept.: 56-58.
Koch, S. 1969. In: Gadlin, H. and Ingle, G. 1975. Through the one-way mirror: The limits of experimental self-reflection. *Amer. Psych.* 30(10):1003-9.
Kubie, L.S. 1939. The experimental induction of neurotic reactions in man. *Yale J. of Biology and Medicine.* 11:541-5.
Kuker-Reines, B. 1982. *Psychology Experiments on Animals: A Critique of Animal Models of Human Psychopathology.* Boston: NEAVS.
Kvale, S. 1973. The technological paradigm of psychological research. *J. Phenom. Psych.* 92:175-212.
Lazarus, A.A. 1971. *Behavior Therapy and Beyond.* New York: McGraw-Hill.
Levine, J., Schield, B. and Bouthilet, L. eds. 1971. *Establishing the Efficacy of Psychotropic Agents.* Public Health Service. Publication #2138. p. 101.
Lineberry, C.G. 1981. Laboratory animals in pain research. In: Gay, W.I. ed. *Methods of Animal Experimentation.* New York: Academic Press. 6:237-311.
Lipsey, M.W. 1974. Research and relevance: A survey of graduate students and faculty in psychology. *Amer. Psych.* 29:541-53.
Lockwood, R. 1984. Kindness is creative. Paper presented at APA meeting, Toronto 1984.
Loftus, E.F., Fienberg, S.E. and Tanur, J.M. 1985. Cognitive psychology meets the national survey. *Amer. Psych.* 40(2):175-80.
London, P. 1972. The end of ideology in behavior modification. *Amer. Psych.* 27(10):913-20.
Mahoney, M. 1977. On the continuing resistance to thoughtful therapy. *Behav. Ther.* 8:673-7.
Mahoney, M.J. 1985. Open exchange and epistemic progress. *Amer. Psych.* 40(1):29-39.
Mancucella, G. 1984. *Learning theory.* In: 1985 review course for the national licensure exam in psychology by the Association for Advanced Training in the Behavioral Sciences (AATBS). 1:1-28.
Marks, I. 1977. Phobias and obsessions. In: Seligman, M.P. and Maser, J.D. eds. *Psychopathology: Experimental Models.* San Francisco: W.H. Freeman Co.
Maslow, A.H. 1954. *Motivation and Personality.* New York: Harper.
Mayer, A.D. and Rosenblatt, J.S. 1984. Prepartum changes in maternal responsiveness and nest defense in *Rattus norvegicus. J. Comp. Psych.* 98(2):177-88.
Meichenbaum, D. 1973. Cognitive factors in behavior modification: Modifying what clients say to themselves. In: Franks, C. and Wilson, G.T., eds. *Annual Review of Behavior Therapy, Theory, and Practice.* New York: Brunner/Mazel.
Meichenbaum, D. and Cameron, R. 1973. Training schizophrenics to talk to themselves: A means of developing attentional cues. *Behav. Ther.* 4:515-34.
Mellgren, R.L., Misasi, L. and Brown, S.W. 1984. Optimal foraging theory: Prey density and travel requirements in *Rattus norvegicus. J. Comp. Psych.* 98(2):142-53.
Miller, D.B. 1977. Roles of naturalistic observation in comparative psychology. *Amer. Psych.* March:211-9.
Miller, N.E. 1978. Biofeedback and visceral learning. *Annual Rev. of Psych.* 29:373-404.
Miller, N.E. 1980. Applications of learning and biofeedback to psychiatry and medicine. In: Kaplan, H.I., Freedman, A.M. and Sadock, B.J. eds. *Comprehensive Textbook of Psychiatry 1/III.* Baltimore: Williams and Wilkens. pp. 468-84.
Miller, N.E. 1983. Value and ethics of research on animals. Unpublished paper presented to the APA convention in Anaheim, California, August, 1983.
Miller, N.E. 1985. The value of behavioral research on animals. *Amer. Psych.* 40(4):423-40.
Mineka, S., Cook, M. and Miller, S. 1984. Fear conditioned with escapable and inescapable shock: Effects of a feedback stimulus. *J. Exper. Psych.: Animal Behav. Processes.* 10(3):307-23.
Minor, T.R. and LaLordo, V.M. 1984. Escape deficits following inescapable shock: The role of contextual odor. *J. Exper. Psych.: Animal Behav. Processes.* 10(2):168-81.

Mowrer, O.H. and Mowrer, W.M. 1938. Enuresis: A method for its study and treatment. *Amer. J. Orthopsych.* 8:436-59.

Ossenkopp, K.-P. and Tu, G.S. 1984. Motion sickness in quail: Body-rotation-induced conditioned fluid aversion in *C. coturnix japonica*. *J. Comp. Psych.* 98(2):189-93.

Paul, S.M. 1977. Models of madness: Animal models of schizophrenia. In: Seligman, M.P. and Maser, J.D. eds. *Psychopathology: Experimental Models.* San Francisco: W.H. Freeman and Co.

Peters, D. and Ceci, S.J. 1982. Peer-review practices of psychological journals: The fate of published articles submitted again. *Behav. and Brain Sci.* 5:187-95.

Petrinovich, L. 1979. Probabilistic functionalism: A conception of research method. *Amer. Psych.* 34(5):373-90.

Pion, G.M. and Lipsey, M.W. 1984. Psychology and society: The challenge of change. *Amer. Psych.* 39(7):739-54.

Potegal, M. and tenBrink, L. 1984. Behavior of attack-primed and attack-satiated female golden hamsters (*Mesocricetus auratus*). *J. Compar. Psych.* 98(1):66-75.

Poulos, C.X. and Hinson, R.E. 1984. A homeostatic model of Pavlovian conditioning: Tolerance to scopolamine-induced adipsia. *J. Exper. Psych.: Animal Behav. Processes.* 10(1):75-89.

Pratt, D. 1976. *Painful Experiments on Animals.* New York: Argus Archives. p. 164.

Pratt, D. 1980. *Alternatives to Pain in Experiments on Animals.* New York: Argus Archives. p. 311.

Rajecki, D.W. 1983. Successful comparative psychology: Four case histories. In: Rajecki, D.W. ed. *Comparing Behavior: Studying Man Studying Animals.* Hillsdale, New Jersey: Lawrence Erlbaum Assocs. pp. 67-107.

Rollin, B.E. 1981. *Animal Rights and Human Morality.* New York: Prometheus Books. p. 126.

Rollin, B.E. 1985. The moral status of research animals in psychology. *Amer. Psychol.* 40(8):920-6.

Romanyshyn, R.D. 1971. Method and meaning in psychology. *J. Phenom. Psych.* 2:93-114.

Rosellini, R.A., De Cola, J.P., Plonsky, M., Warren, D.A. and Stilman, A.J. 1984. Uncontrollable shock proactively increases sensitivity to response-reinforcer independence in rats. *J. Exper. Psych.: Animal Behav. Processes.* 10(3):346-59.

Ross, R.T. and Randich, A. 1984. Unconditioned stress-induced analgesia following exposure to brief footshock. *J. Exper. Psych.: Animal Behav. Processes.* 10(2):127-37.

Rowan, A. 1984. *Of Mice, Models and Men.* Albany: State University of New York Press.

Ryder, R. 1975. *Victims of Science.* London: Davis-Poynter.

Sarason, S.B. 1984. If it can be studied or developed, should it be? *Amer. Psych.* 39(5):477-85.

Segal, E. 1982. Editorial. *J. Anal. of Behav.* 38(2):115.

Segal, E. and Lachman, R. 1972. Complex behavior or higher mental process: Is there a paradigm shift? *Amer. Psych.* 27(1):46-55.

Shapiro, K. 1982. A review of the NIMH grant application entitled: Production and alleviation of depression (Stephen Suomi, University of Wisconsin). In: Kuker-Reines, B. *Psychology Experiments on Animals: A Critique of Animal Models of Human Psychopathology.* Boston: NEAVS. pp. 5, 38.

Shotter, J. and Gauld, A. 1971. The defense of empirical psychology. *Amer. Psych.* 26(5):460-6.

Singer, P. 1975. *Animal Liberation.* New York: Avon Books. pp. 7, 47.

Skinner, B.F. 1975. The steep and thorny way to a science of behavior. *Amer. Psych.* 30(1):42-49.

Smith, M.B. 1973. Is psychology relevant to the new priorities? *Amer. Psych.* 28(6):463-71.

Smith, M.B. 1978. Humanism and behaviorism in psychology: Theory and practice. *J. Humanistic Psych.* 18(1):27-36.

Suinn, R. and Richardson, R. 1971. Anxiety management training: A non-specific behavior therapy program for anxiety control. *Beh. Ther.* 2(4):498-510.

Tulving, E. 1979. Memory research: What kind of progress?: In: Nilsson, L.G. ed. *Perspectives on Memory Research.* Hillsdale, New Jersey: Lawrence Erlbaum Assocs.

Tunnell, G.B. 1977. Three dimensions of naturalness: An expanded definition of field research. *Psych. Bulletin.* 84(3):426-37.

Wade, N. 1982. Smart Apes, or Dumb? *New York Times.* (essay). 30 April.

Weimer, W.B. and Palermo, D.S. eds. 1974. *Cognition and the Symbolic Processes.* Hillsdale, New Jersey: Erlbaum Assocs.

Wertheimer, M. 1972. *Fundamental Issues in Psychology.* New York: Holt, Rinehart, and Winston. p. 194.

Wolpe, J. 1976. How laboratory-derived principles of learning have conquered the neuroses. In: *Psychopathology of Human Adaptation.* New York: Plenum Press. pp. 291-306.

Wu, M.-F., Krueger, J., Ison, J.R. and Gerrard, R.L. 1984. Startle reflex inhibition in the rat: Its persistence after extended repetition of the inhibitory stimulus. *J. Exper. Psych.: Animal Behav. Processes.* 10(2):221-8.

ALTERNATIVES TO AVERSIVE PROCEDURES WITH ANIMALS IN THE PSYCHOLOGY TEACHING SETTING*

Jeffrey A. Kelly

Department of Psychiatry and Human Behavior
University of Mississippi Medical Center
2500 N. State Street
Jackson, MS 39216

Introduction

Every college undergraduate learns in his or her first introductory course that the aims of scientific psychology are understanding, explaining, and predicting behavior. How students are taught about behavior varies depending on the area of psychology involved. But within some major psychology subfields—behavior analysis, learning, experimental, and physiological psychology—teaching students about behavior often means instruction and observation in *animal* behavior. In some cases, students are asked to study the principles of animal behavior for their own sake. More commonly, however, animals are used in teaching or laboratory settings because they are assumed to be models which serve as approximations for analogous behavior in humans.

The treatment of research animals by behavioral scientists has received substantial and increasing scrutiny by both the public and professionals who are concerned about animal welfare. The principle focus for most of this attention has been the treatment of experimental animal subjects in biomedical or behavioral *research* studies and, to a lesser degree, those animals subjected to toxicity and consumer products testing. Much less attention has been directed to the welfare of animals used in *teaching* settings. It is unclear how many animals are used

Portions of this paper were presented to the Annual Meeting of the American Psychological Association, August, 1984 in Toronto.

each year in undergraduate and graduate psychology department teaching laboratories, but the number appears very substantial given that most colleges and universities have animal laboratories; most use animals extensively in such courses as learning, behavior analysis, and experimental and physiological psychology; and most encourage advanced students to conduct independent projects primarily for their educational value.

While concern for animal welfare in behavioral research, biomedical research, and toxicity testing certainly demands attention, reducing the pain and suffering of animals used in teaching may be more easily attained than accomplishing that same end in some other contexts. As we will see, this is because there are alternatives in instructional settings for reducing the number of experimental animals used, for reducing their suffering, and for replacing the use of animals in aversive demonstration without compromising educational objects (see Russell and Burch 1959). Further, because no new scientific knowledge is generally gained in teaching demonstrations, there is less justification for permitting pain and distress to animals. As a result, an aversive procedure defensible in a critical research study might well be improper to use in a teaching demonstration.

In this paper, we will consider the treatment of laboratory animals in psychology instruction and will focus on practical alternatives to traditional practices that cause pain and distress to animals. While the discussion will draw on psychology for examples, many of the issues apply equally to the instruction of students in other courses of study, including medicine, veterinary medicine, biology, and physiology.

Animals, Ethics, and Psychology Teaching

Some psychological experiments employing animals pose few ethical concerns because the studies do not involve aversive conditions. Behavioral observation studies, naturalistic observations that do not interfere with animals' normal behavior, and conditioning studies that do not entail aversive procedures or the induction of severe deprivation states (e.g.,water, food, social, or sensory deprivation) are relatively free of ethical concerns, subject to certain qualifications. The qualifications chiefly concern whether the animals are housed and maintained with adequate consideration of their physical, social, and emotional needs, and whether induced deprivation states are sufficiently mild so as to allow students to study motivation without creating distress to the animal. Although these qualifications sound straightforward, in fact they involve rather complex issues. For example, a teaching demonstration of positive reinforcement—i.e., showing students that a rat will learn to bar press for food on some schedule—is not an ethically problematic procedure on the surface. However, how *long* that rat is food-deprived before the demonstration begins can determine whether the teaching demonstration is actually humane. While investigators are recognizing that the severity of food, water, or other need deprivation is an ethical issue (Segal 1982) and, by inference, that past demonstrations have often used overly harsh deprivation levels, we know little about the point at which deprivation becomes inhumane and unnecessarily severe.

In similar fashion, there is a growing recognition that the conditions under which animals are maintained involve issues which extend well beyond feeding and watering the animal, and keeping its cage clean (Lockwood 1984). Animals have broader social and emotional needs that must also be taken into account in their housing. While an instructional procedure may involve no aversive conditions at all, if the animal is housed in a way that neglects its needs for environmental stimulation, the project is ethically troublesome. While there is a considerable literature documenting the social/emotional needs of various higher animals, it is rare for animal housing facilities to take these needs into account.

Ethical issues become even more pronounced when students are asked to perform procedures that clearly cause pain to animals. The kinds of aversive procedures to which animals are subjected in psychology teaching laboratories are, unfortunately, wide and varied. Classical conditioning with aversive stimuli; employing learned helplessness analogue paradigms; administering drugs; surgically ablating or lesioning; inserting and implanting invasive measurement instruments; and invasively altering sensory capabilities are aversive procedures that students commonly observe or perform on living animals.

Proponents of allowing (or requiring) students to learn about behavior by conducting such aversive exercises defend the practice on several grounds. Their arguments fall into several categories and include: (1) the conduct of animal studies, including those which cause pain, is necessary to train scientists; (2) there is no acceptable alternative to "hands-on" experimentation; (3) aversive procedures with animals represent one of the few ways to demonstrate the effects of certain behavioral phenomena; and (4) teaching demonstrations with animals already have sufficient controls to ensure the welfare of animal subjects. Let us consider these arguments and existing alternatives to them.

Animal Welfare and Student Welfare

The usual first focus of our ethical attention when animals are subjected to aversive procedures is on the welfare of the animal. That is, of course, an appropriate focus when animals are shocked, ablated, lesioned, operated upon, or otherwise caused pain. But it is also appropriate to inquire into the potentially negative effects to students who are asked to watch or perform such procedures.

A substantial body of research demonstrates that exposure to violence or other aversive experience gradually leads to densensitization, numbing, and an emotional acceptance of that experience. For example, persons shown films of violence or bloody human battle exhibit fairly rapid attitudinal shifts towards acceptance and toleration of violence (Thomas et al. 1977). There is no reason to think that psychologists or psychology students do not experience the same attitudinal shifts in our laboratories and classrooms. By exposing students to animal pain, or by accustoming students to *causing* pain to animals, we may be desensitizing them to the fact that they are hurting living beings and we may inadvertently be promoting students' tolerance or acceptance of inhumaneness. Rollin (1981), for example, describes an incident in which a student asked what should be done with some rats at the end of a teaching experiment. The student's professor had the young man watch as the professor held the rat and rapped its head against the side of a table, breaking the animal's neck. The student was taken aback by the sight and said so. The professor, according to Rollin, responded by coldly suggesting that the young man "might not be cut out to be a psychologist" if he were going to be so sensitive.

In this incident, we can identify several desensitizing factors at work. First, as the student continues his lab work, he will become emotionally desensitized to events that he formerly found troublesome. As students become used, not just to killing animals in a violent way, but also shocking, invading, operating on or otherwise maiming them, the emotional impact of doing so is gradually lessened until those actions become commonplace and emotionally unarousing.

Moreover, the social influence of a professor legitimizing, modeling, and instructing a student to perform aversive procedures is also powerful and likely to produce student compliance. Quite a number of years ago, Milgram (1963) demonstrated that professorial influence and authorization were sufficient to cause students to personally administer what they thought were extremely painful electric shocks to another person. When a student is trying to be "scientific," hoping to please a professor, and when the recipient of pain-infliction is an animal rather than the perceived human in Milgram's study, shifts towards inhumaneness in student attitudes, values, and ethical sensitivities are even more likely.

We often become professionally indignant when the media publishes photographs of research animals immobilized, implanted, maimed, and in pain. The public is startled, shocked, and often upset when they see such photographs. As psychologists, our response is often to dismiss public reaction by saying something like, "They really don't understand what we are doing," or "They haven't been exposed to the methods and benefits of this research." However, what we may really be witnessing is a discrepancy between professionals who have desensitized themselves to an animal's pain and a public which is appropriately sensitive to animal distress.

In our role as educators, should we try to desensitize students to pain? Should we be reassuring students in our undergraduate and graduate labs that it is perfectly acceptable for them to shock or experimentally operate on animals just so they can see some known behavioral phenomenon firsthand? That is often what we do, and often we do it without much thought at all. The implicit messages that we may inadvertently be teaching students are that "Cruelty in the name of science is okay,"* "It's only a rat and it will be dead next week anyway," or, even worse, "The end justifies the means."

Thus, the issue of animal welfare in the teaching setting also raises the issue of student welfare. If teaching practices do reduce humane sensitivity, we may also be at risk for producing students who have become dulled not only to pain, but to empathy and observational acuity as well. Within the medical profession, observers have pointed out that all too many physicians have outstanding technical skills but appear desensitized to, and emotionally distanced from, their patients (Maddison 1978). They suggest that medical training directly fosters this problem by promoting the view that living beings are objects to be mechanistically studied, observed, or treated with as little emotional involvement as possible.

In psychology, we must be especially concerned about teaching practices that may hinder a student's capacity to develop characteristics such as accurate empathy, sensitivity, and humaneness, since these characteristics appear to be necessary to effective clinical practice (Truax et al. 1966). Because many students in undergraduate and graduate psychology labs will one day work with people, we should be working to increase sensitivity and humaneness, rather than destroying these characteristics.

Even within the animal laboratory setting, aversive procedures with animals may blunt students' observational and cognitive skills. High emotional arousal—anxiety—disrupts fine-grained observational acuity, cognitive performance, problem-solving, and recall (Janis and Mann 1977). If a student is upset by an aversive teaching exercise, that student's ability to learn from the demonstration is also lessened. On the other hand, if a student is desensitized to, and unaffected by, an

---

*The message that cruelty in the name of science is somehow different than cruelty to animals on a city street has been conveyed not only to students but also, evidently, to legislators. Many ordinances specifically exempt certain activities in universities and research facilities from prosecution under local anti-cruelty statutes.

animal's pain, that student may actually become a less skilled observer of behavior. Reese (1984) has pointed out that by allowing students to somehow "pretend" that animals are inanimate or insensitive objects—a precursor, it would seem, to intentionally hurting them—we encourage students to misperceive and distort other aspects of what they observe. In doing so, the objectivity on which good science relies is undermined.

Finally, in a broader view, we live in a world that seems too often characterized by insensitivity, inhumanity, and a lack of concern and empathy for other beings. The extent to which sensitivity to animal welfare facilitates sensitivity to human welfare is not yet well-established, but such a linkage is both plausible and probable. From this broader perspective, behavioral scientists *especially* should be addressing ways to increase students' humane sensitivity and should never try to extinguish it.

Alternatives to Aversive Demonstrations

If we accept as desirable the goal of reducing the number of animals subjected to pain in order to educate students, both for the animals' sake and the students' sake, the next task becomes one of developing instructional alternatives. To see how alternatives can be developed, let us first consider what we try to accomplish when teaching psychology, including experimentally-oriented classes.

In most psychology course work, we want students to gain knowledge, information, and the ability to form hypotheses, rather than personal skill or expertise in using a technique. For example, we want students to understand the key *principles* of conditioning and learning, not to learn how to operate a conditioning chamber or to shock rats. We want students to understand and appreciate *principles* of neurological functioning and the physiological bases for behavior, not to master the skill of operating on an animal.

Is it really necessary for students to shock animals in order to learn the fundamentals of avoidance conditioning or classical conditioning? Must students implant electrodes or ablate and lesion animals to learn principles of physiological psychology? Almost certainly not, especially if they are undergraduate or graduate students who are not preparing for careers in physiological research. Students studying psychology need to understand and appreciate the *principles* of behavior; the vast majority will never need to master specific techniques that cause pain to animals. In most teaching demonstrations and student practice with animals, the use of the animal is but a means to an end—knowledge—and there may be better and certainly more humane ways to reach that end.

What are some methods for teaching students behavioral principles that do not entail aversive procedures with animals? Since there is already an enormous data base on most behavioral phenomena, asking students to read, listen, and think critically about behavioral principles is still a viable way to teach. Students can study and discuss phenomena like aversive classical conditioning, sensation/perception processes, and neurological functioning comprehensively, accurately, and at a higher conceptual level than they could while performing isolated laboratory experiments with animals in these areas. Computers can be used to present graphic, lively, visual portrayals to illustrate physiological/neurological processes more clearly than experiments using living animals without sacrificing interest value. There are also known laboratory alternatives to some aversive procedures. For example, students can conduct classical conditioning studies with paradigms using unconditioned positive rather than aversive stimuli, a fact psychologists sometimes forget. Even within the operant literature, students can choose among many different methods to reduce behavior which do not involve punishment or aversive stimuli (see Reese 1984).

On those rare occasions when a pain-causing phenomenon must really be seen to be understood, a teacher can videotape the procedure once with a single animal and show the tape on all subsequent occasions rather than demonstrate the phenomenon "live" or ask students to perform it on many animals again and again, semester after semester. Observation of a videotape, in lieu of actual practice of an aversive technique, may carry a number of teaching advantages. Tapes can focus on a specific feature of interest, tapes can be replayed by the student and re-observed,and a skillfully-made videotape may prove educationally superior to clumsy, hands-on practice with a living animal. Branch and his colleagues (Branch et al. 1984) have successfully used interactive videotapes to replace certain live animal demonstrations in veterinary education; similar applications can be made in areas such as psychology, medical education, and physiology.

Those who defend the status quo of allowing students to conduct aversive procedures with animals typically cite several justifications for the practice. These justifications involve the long tradition of student experimentation with animals, a belief that students cannot otherwise acquire observational/experimental skills, and the view that students must personally conduct aversive experiments in order to fully understand the phenomenon they are studying.

With respect to the tradition argument, it requires only cursory reflection to see that many widely-accepted traditions from the past today seem crude, archaic, and curious. It used to be accepted tradition to sacrifice animals and humans to the gods, to burn "witches" at the stake, and to drain suspect humors from the bodies of emotionally-disturbed persons. Gradually, people realized that these traditions were unnecessary, invalid or inhumane, and they were abandoned. In an era of enlightened attitudes towards animal welfare, the practice of allowing students to hurt animals in order to see some phenomenon that is already perfectly well-known seems equally anachronistic. The practices that guided student training in the past are not necessarily those that need to be followed in the present, especially if we take seriously our professed professional commitment to improving animal welfare.

With respect to the argument that students cannot acquire observational and hypothesis-forming skills without conducting animal experiments, two points can be raised. First, it is possible for students to conduct many animal behavior projects in a humane, ethical manner; it is projects which cause pain to animals or which fail to genuinely respect their physical, social, and emotional needs that are of concern. A whole array of nonaversive, noninvasive experimental observational procedures are available to teach students about animal behavior and help them appreciate, rather than exploit, animals (Riss and Goodall 1977; Lockwood 1984). Second, to suggest that students cannot learn to think and hypothesize about a phenomenon without conducting a laboratory investigation may reflect inadequacies in the way we teach students to reason. A student who understands state-of-the-science findings about nervous system functions should not need to personally lesion rats or cats in order to generate predictions about the effects of CNS injuries on behavior.

This, in turn, leads to the final contention of many animal research "traditionalists," that students somehow learn "better" with hands-on experience. If our aim as teachers is to teach well, and if we also seek to better respect animal welfare, there is a pressing need to develop, empirically test, and publish the results of teaching procedures that do not involve pain to animals or that require fewer animals than traditional approaches. For example, students could be taught about aversive classical conditioning by (1) shocking rats and observing conditioning effects, (2) watching a videotape of the same procedure, or (3) reading about, listening to classroom discussions about, and responding to programmed instruction questions about conditioning principles. These three instructional strategies range from being highly aversive to animals, to involving no pain to animal subjects. The dependent measures in a teaching method study of this kind could include an assessment of knowledge and understanding of the key principles one wants students to grasp, as well as the duration of instructional effects and the impact on students' ability to generalize their knowledge to human phenomena.

If students learn as well or better under a teaching alternative that does not cause pain to animals, practical and empirically-based strategies for more humane teaching can be developed. Even if students are found to learn somewhat better under the lab study, it remains the burden of psychology teachers as a professional group to demonstrate that those learning benefits clearly outweigh the costs, in pain, endured by the animal. Given the degree of public interest in animal welfare, and given the negative attention behavioral and biomedical investigators receive on this matter, solid research producing alternatives to aversive teaching procedures should prove fundable, publishable, and of wide interest to educators in psychology, medicine, veterinary medicine, biology, physiology, and other areas.

The Utility of Animals as Human Analogues in Teaching Demonstrations

Virtually all introductory psychology texts tell their readers that animals are used as subjects in studies involving procedures that cannot be ethically or easily conducted using human subjects. Shapiro (1983) has pointed out that those same textbooks rarely deal with the ethical questions that arise when animals are used. By omission, they implicitly seem to convey to students early on that "anything goes" ethically so long as a project's subjects are not human. Even beyond the matter of ethics, however, is the issue of whether teaching demonstrations with animals that are intended to approximate some human phenomenon really do justice to the phenomena we want our students to understand.

The extent to which psychologists are willing to generalize findings from animal behavior studies to human behavior (and thereby assume the validity of animal behavior analogues) depends considerably on the theoretical orientation of the psychologist. Within certain schools—behavior analysis, behavior therapy, and approaches stressing the biological bases of behavior, for example—the generality of behavioral principles across species is rather widely accepted. In contrast, theories which stress cognitive, dynamic, phenomenological, or humanistic variables are less likely to accept the premise that animals serve as reasonable analogues for important areas of human behavior.

A discussion of the validity of generalizing animal research findings to analogous human phenomena is beyond the scope of this chapter. The issue of generalizability depends greatly on the specific behavior in question, the history and individual makeup of the animal used in a study, artificial or unnatural constraints placed on the animal's behavior, the degree to which species-specific influences are present, the extent to which a class of behavior is mediated by cognitive or verbal factors that operate only or primarily in humans, and so on. However, with respect to demonstrations of the kind usually conducted in a psychology teaching laboratory, (1) phenomena which students observe using an aversive procedure with an animal are often easily understood without the demonstration; and (2) complex human phenomena can often be more directly studied by having students conduct projects with humans. Let us consider, especially, this second point.

An area of research that has been popular over the past decade concerns "learned helplessness" (Seligman 1978). This research, which evolved in the laboratory, entails highly aversive procedures such as extensive shock history to induce helplessness in experimental animals. There have now been many hundreds of animal analogue studies, student demonstrations, undergraduate honors projects, theses, and dissertations on learned helplessness, all of them intentionally creating pain and chronic, unalleviated distress for the experimental animals under study.

Interest in learned helplessness is understandable, in part because this phenomenon does appear salient for conceptualizing certain depressive disorders in humans. However, the persistence of animal studies and student laboratory teaching demonstrations of learned helplessness illustrates that an animal analogue can become extended far beyond the human construct it is intended to approximate: while there is consistency of findings among *animal* studies of learned helplessness, even proponents of this line of research concede that generalizing those animal findings to *humans* has proven difficult and inconclusive (Seligman 1978). One obvious reason for this problem is that animals represent a poor analogue for the helplessness phenomena because depression undoubtedly includes cognitive labeling processes, anticipations, cognitive expectancies, and complex affective variables that operate in humans but probably not in most other animals.

Rather than teaching students about learned helplessness by having them shock animals to induce helplessness and then observe the animals' behavior in some task that may be inhumane and further distressing (e.g., determining how long it takes a "helpless" rat to give up swimming and drown), we must develop more inventive, realistic, and valid demonstrations. There are many examples in the research literature of human paradigms to study behavioral phenomena for which we historically relied on aversive demonstrations with animals. For example, learned helplessness can be studied, not with animals, but by using task failure or frustration paradigms with human subjects; response suppression can be studied by having students develop behavioral self-management contingencies to modify their own bad habits; conditioning projects can, with inventiveness, allow students to use themselves as subjects. By utilizing such experimental human paradigms, it is possible to reduce unnecessary pain to animals, produce higher quality teaching demonstrations, and allow students to better see and appreciate key behavioral/motivational principles as they occur in people. Such human paradigms can teach many of the same observational, experimental, and conceptual skills as the aversive animal studies they could replace.

There is little to be gained, and much to be lost, by encouraging, assigning, or even permitting students to conduct aversive procedures with animals. The vast majority of psychology students—certainly all undergraduates and virtually all graduate-level students—can be taught behavioral and experimental procedures, can be exposed to the kinds of knowledge we expect them to learn, and can hone their observational skills without ever hurting an animal, depriving an animal of its needs, or behaving inhumanely. While promoting animal welfare and student welfare in these ways will require the adoption of alternative methods of instruction at both introductory and advanced levels and will require the bucking of some traditions, it can be done. The end result will not compromise educational objectives but can produce a more sensitive and ethical professional for the future.

There is, however, a small group of advanced students who will be preparing for professional careers that specifically involve animal research. These might include graduate students in physiological psychology, animal experimental psychology, and similar areas. While graduate students in these areas represent a very small and apparently declining percentage of the total number of advanced psychology students in our universities (American Psychological Association 1985), they are an important group. By enhancing the sensitivities towards animal welfare among those students who will be the laboratory teachers and animal researchers of tomorrow, many of the insensitive or inhumane practices which exist today can be eliminated. How can we promote better sensitivity for graduate students in these specialized areas?

Shaping Humaneness Among Graduate Students in Animal Experimental Psychology

Not long ago, I conducted a small, nonrandom survey of some advanced graduate students who had done supervised laboratory work with animals, chiefly aversive conditioning and neurosurgical experiments. I asked each student if he or she had seen the APA Ethical Standards for the treatment of laboratory animals posted in the lab (American Psychological Association 1981). All had. I then asked whether these standards were ever discussed with them, or whether the students had personal discussions with their faculty supervisor concerning ethical and humane issues in dealing with animals. Other than hearing advice to "keep the cages clean, and keep the animals fed and watered," none of the students recalled any discussion about humane issues. Not *one* of the students reported exposure to any structured teaching on ways to minimize pain or distress in animals, and none had been taught the desirability of using minimal levels of shock or deprivation, methods of reducing the number of animals used in experiments, or about analgesics and their effects. Not a single student I surveyed said that she or he had any awareness of how to house animals in such a way as to meet their social, stimulation, or psychological-emotional needs.

It was evident that these students had remarkably little exposure to ethical and humane issues even though each was engaged in projects that caused pain to laboratory animals. While the students were acquiring technical laboratory skills, there appeared to be no transmission of humane values or expertise from faculty to students. Under such circumstances, it would be indeed surprising if these students did not develop the same ethical "blind-spots" as their mentors. A national survey of ethics teaching in psychology conducted by Trautt, Reed, and Scheider (1983) suggests the students I had talked with were not unusual. Trautt et al. (1983) found that 72 percent of graduate programs in experimental psychology did *not* routinely train students in professional ethics, and that 83 percent had no formal procedure for students to demonstrate knowledge of ethics.

As one starts to label an advanced student as a researcher or a research assistant, as graduate students in animal behavior conduct their supervised research or theses or dissertations, the same ethical and humane responsibilities that affect a faculty member come to bear on his or her student. Unfortunately, while psychology has been quite strong in teaching students technical skills for working with animals, it has been very weak in teaching the ethical issues which arise in that research.

In a humane academic world, a faculty member would be keenly cognizant of animal welfare issues and would model, teach, and shape the same sensitivities in his or her students. Not only would humane sensitivity be encouraged, but a student would be expected to exhibit the specific skills, competencies, and knowledge necessary for treating research animals in an ethically responsible manner. Unfortunately, a number of factors operate to hinder this ideal scenario. Many experimental faculty researchers are themselves unaware of key issues in animal welfare and of new alternatives to the traditional research methods that *they* themselves were first taught. Some researchers react defensively to any suggestion that animals have been treated inhumanely in the past and deserve better treatment in the future. And, the same emotional desensitization and cognitive rationalization to animal pain discussed earlier in relation to students most certainly affects many faculty researchers to an even greater degree. Faculty, like most people who are invested in their work, tend to perceive (and perhaps to inflate) the potential benefits of their projects, and may unintentionally minimize or misperceive a project's limitations or even its inherent inhumaneness. The contention that researchers can, and often do, overestimate the importance and underestimate the limitations of their work is certainly not restricted to researchers in animal behavior. Most journals, publishers, conferences, and funding agencies in all scientific areas rely on expert reviewers to impartially evaluate manuscripts or proposals, and rejection rates of 80 to 90 percent are common among major scientific journals. If a journal rejects 90 percent of all manuscripts, one could argue that 90 percent of the time, external judges evaluate a study's limitations to be more serious than does the study's author. If we acknowledge these factors as possibilities, the need to ensure better ethical/humane education for advanced students in animal behavior is also evident.

There are many potential vehicles for enhancing humane values and skills in graduate students who plan career work with animals. A psychology department could develop a course in animal research ethics and require the course as a prerequisite to any laboratory activities. Such a course might address not only standard animal care, but also include broader discussion of ethical issues, consideration of alternative research strategies to those which cause pain to animals, presentation of methods for meeting the social-emotional-psychological needs of various animal species, discussion not only of the benefits of a research project but also the costs in pain that might be endured by animal subjects, and related topics. For a course of this kind to be viable, it would require evenhanded input from concerned animal laboratory researchers, ethicists, scientists with a background in animal welfare and animal rights, humane advocates, ethologists, veterinarians, and others. For the course to be successful, it should provide a vehicle not just for discussion and information transmission, but should also produce change in the way animals are viewed and treated, and in the way research is conducted.

A second vehicle for decreasing animal maltreatment is an effective institutional animal care review committee. While many psychology departments and research institutions have such committees, their role and safeguarding function varies widely. Too often, animal care committees are composed of animal researchers or faculty with a vested interest in the type of projects being evaluated, rather than persons who might knowledgably and impartially evaluate proposals with an eye to safeguarding the welfare of animals. Further, while review committees ordinarily consider whether a project adheres to existing but limited statutes concerning housing, feeding, and animal procurement, committees rarely deal with other substantive ethical and humane issues. These issues include evaluating whether a project will primarily replicate previous work, result in relatively unimportant findings, utilize more animals than necessary or use a procedure that could be replaced with a less invasive one, subject animals to distress with little potential scientific benefit, adequately address the social-emotional well-being of the animals, or utilize a large sample statistical design that could be replaced by a sophisticated "small n" design. Committees may avoid these important issues because they require making judgments and may result in dissension. However, the very purpose of a review committee *is* to critically review, judge, and evaluate; to the extent that a committee fails to deal with key humane issues and primarily "rubber-stamps" protocols, it also fails to perform a legitimate and necessary function.

Animal use committees should influence not only faculty researchers, but also graduate students in animal behavior. Training ethical researchers requires that students learn to anticipate and address humane issues while a study proposal is being developed. A properly-constituted, stringent, questioning review committee can help to establish contingencies that will shape more ethical and humane treatment of animals in teaching settings.

Finally, individual faculty must broaden their teaching functions to explicitly instruct students in humane issues. The role of a professional mentor is an important one for influencing the values, practices, and sensitivities of students, especially at a doctoral training level. To the extent that faculty researchers are themselves sensitized to animal welfare issues, they will be better able to transmit those sensitivities to their students. Reese (1984), for example, has developed a detailed questionnaire that must be completed by students before they can initiate any project using animals. The questionnaire requires the student to state how animal care needs, broadly defined, will be met; whether animals will suffer any distress; what will be done to prevent or eliminate that distress; how the number of animals to be studied can be reduced; and which alternative, noninvasive methodologies can be employed. Discussion of these issues by a student and a faculty member will not automatically ensure that animal welfare needs will be met unless there is also a strong commitment to improving humane treatment of animals and a willingness to alter research paradigms to promote it. On the other hand, it is very unlikely students can be ethically sensitized without discussion and guidance of the kind advocated by Reese (1984).

Teaching Students in Psychology: A Curriculum Sensitive to Animal Welfare

Let us summarize and review how a psychology teaching program that is humane towards animals might look and how instructional change can be accomplished. The first step in bringing about animal welfare reform is for a department to critically assess the number and kinds of animals employed in teaching and instructional/student research projects; the courses or projects in which animals are used; the reasons animals are used in those courses and projects (e.g., to have students learn behavioral principles by conditioning rats); and the invasiveness or severity of procedures to which animals are subjected. With respect to this latter issue, Shapiro (1984) has pointed out the need to develop a reasonable, workable system for estimating the pain level or aversiveness to animals of various laboratory procedures. At present, there is no widely-used invasiveness rating scale, although one has been described (see Ross 1981) and is being used in Australia. By estimating empirically levels of invasiveness or pain, it will be possible to estimate the relative distress caused by different procedures. For example,an observational study of animals in a naturalistic environment suitable for that species would likely be considered noninvasive or, say, a "1" on a 10-point severity scale. Projects that entail the use of aversive stimuli, severe deprivation, surgery, drugs, and other invasive procedures would be rated higher on the severity scale. By classifying procedures in this way, it will be possible to direct attention on developing alternatives to those procedures, altering procedures to reduce their invasiveness, or requiring stronger justification for their use.

A second step towards developing a more humane curriculum is establishing strictures on various practices and, concomitantly, developing instructional alternatives to replace unacceptable procedures. For example, a department might establish a policy that students will not conduct projects, and faculty will not perform demonstrations, that entail shock, surgery, or severe deprivation to animals in undergraduate courses or in most graduate courses. (As noted earlier, there is a need for better objective guidelines concerning both the invasiveness of laboratory procedures and the point at which deprivation of food, water, sleep, or stimulation needs becomes inhumane.) It would rest with the individual or collective faculty to develop alternative methods to teach students the principles about which they would have learned from the demonstration. Here, reading or classroom discussions; the use of computer-assisted or audio-visual materials; a demonstration not creating distress for animals; or some other human experiential project could be used as instructional alternatives.

Third, explicit policies and more effective safeguarding mechanisms can be developed to address those relatively specific occasions when aversive procedures with animals are justified. Such occasions might be theses or dissertations by students specializing in areas of psychology such as animal learning and physiological psychology, or student assistance on a faculty member's research. Several safeguarding mechanisms (including a course in animal welfare and research ethics, review committee scrutiny, and justification/invasiveness reduction planning) have already been discussed. Others, including ongoing review committee monitoring of faculty research, can promote more humane treatment of animals by both faculty members and students. Departments that take seriously the mandate for improved animal welfare could establish contingencies and provide academic recognition for faculty and students who develop and implement research and teaching alternatives that reduce the number of animals used, reduce the aversiveness of laboratory procedures, or replace the use of living animals altogether in various studies.

Finally, the conditions under which animals are maintained merit attention in the humanely-sensitized psychology department. Faculty and students who work with animals have an obligation to become familiar with their preferences for social contact with other animals, the environmental stimulation, and the habitat conditions needed—or enjoyed—by any animals maintained in a laboratory vivarium. The practice of housing animals in a manner that is convenient and inexpensive for humans, but distressingly barren for the animals, is ethically unacceptable to psychologists concerned with animal welfare. Several researchers have described the creation of naturalistic, environmentally-enriched housing settings for laboratory animals (Reese 1984; Segal 1983), and there are ample sources of information concerning animals' habitat preferences both in the ethology literature and through consultation with national humane organizations.

The focus of this paper has been the teaching of students in psychology. However, similar problems for animal welfare exist in the way we have traditionally taught medical students, veterinary students, and students in other behavioral/biological sciences. In each of these areas, animals often endure painful, invasive procedures solely for the purpose of showing students some already well-known phenomenon.

The alternatives we have discussed throughout the paper apply not only to teaching psychology students, but to teaching students in these other areas as well. For example, many traditional instructional practices using animals in medical education—having students observe physiological effects, observe toxicity effects, and "practice" surgery on animals—could be replaced by alternative teaching methods that would eliminate the use of living animals in some cases or greatly reduce the number of animals subjected to unnecessary pain in other cases (Branch et al. 1984). The benefits of exploring and implementing teaching alternatives in medical, veterinary, and biological science education are the same as those discussed earlier; animal welfare would be improved and student ethical/humane sensitivities would remain intact rather than be deadened. In addition, the more practical issues of cost and public image are increasingly salient. As communities and states enact legislation reducing the availability of cheap pound-seized animals, and as the public becomes aware of unnecessary, inhumane use of animals, there is a further impetus to develop new ways of teaching. While some would argue that living animals must be subjected to distress in order to train physicians, veterinarians, and others, this contention is questionable and probably reflects American tradition rather than educational necessity. In Great Britain,for example, nontherapeutic procedures are rarely performed on living animals during the training of veterinary students (Rollin 1981).

Summary and Conclusions

The treatment of animals within educational, research, and training institutions has received growing scrutiny both by the public and by scientists concerned with animal welfare. As in many "movements," we have seen to date a strong tendency to polarize issues involving animal welfare into extreme positions. Some animal rights proponents argue against the use of animals for any scientific purpose; scientists, on the other hand, often defend the status quo of animal experimentation and deny the existence of fundamental ethical issues arising from it. Yet, from these polarized viewpoints can come the potential for dialogue that will result in both better science and the more humane treatment of animals. Recent symposia on animal welfare at major scientific meetings are a sign, tentative but promising, that the treatment of laboratory and research animals is beginning to change.

Change is possible quite quickly in the way animals have been used as "teaching tools" for students in psychology and in other academic areas. Technologies and educational alternatives already exist which, if used creatively, can eliminate the tradition of hurting, distressing, and maiming animals for the purpose of showing students behavioral phenomena. In those few instances when advanced students in a specialty area must use invasive procedures—and these instances should be rare—we can have available safeguards to better ensure animal welfare, to decrease the level of aversive procedures that are employed, and to greatly reduce the number of animals subjected to distress. Throughout this paper, such alternatives and protective mechanisms have been discussed.

The mandate to improve animal welfare in the teaching setting will require changing practices that have become traditional and longstanding. Retrospective justifications ("We have always done this with animals and it has led to great advances..."), as Shapiro (1984) has pointed out, do not tell us that a particular practice was the only one available, that it was the best practice, or that it should be continued in the future. Rather than defending the historical status quo, behavioral scientists and educators should take the lead in developing and evaluating new humane teaching and animal protective alternatives.

If successful, alternatives like those discussed here should produce clear, measurable effects. In a humanely-sensitized educational program, the frequency of procedures that could be considered aversive will be substantially reduced in all courses and independent study projects. As teaching alternatives replace many "live animal" demonstrations, the number of animals being secured will decrease. Course requirements in animal welfare and animal research ethics will appear in departmental course listings. Animal care committees, rather than approving proposals almost carte blanche and evaluating them based on the usual narrow criteria of cage space and food, will be broad-based in composition and will assume an active animal welfare advocacy role. Committees will require study modifications and statistical changes to reduce the number of animals used; will decrease the use of aversive procedures; and will reject proposals lacking sufficient merit, creating excessive distress for animals, or using procedures that are inherently objectionable. In a humanely sensitized department, animal housing facilities will look different. If fewer animals are being used, fewer will need to be housed; those that are housed will live under carefully-created conditions that very much resemble the animals' preferred habitats and meet their social-emotional, as well as physical, needs. The point here is that improvement in the treatment of animals in teaching settings will ultimately be reflected not just in talk about animal welfare, but by actual, visible, measurable change along dimensions such as these.

To a large extent, initial pressures for reform in the way that animals are treated in behavioral and biomedical areas have come from humane, animal welfare, and animal rights groups outside the scientific community.* However, for change of the kind discussed here to take place, it will be necessary for those of us in the academic community to explicitly recognize an obligation not only to teach and conduct research, but also to create conditions that ensure better animal welfare than is the case presently. By developing, examining, and implementing new teaching approaches that do not cause pain for animals, we will be in a position to teach students just as scientifically as always, but more humanely as well.

While most pressure for humane reform has arisen outside the scientific community, animal welfare groups within various professions also exist and have advocated reform. These groups include Psychologists for the Ethical Treatment of Animals (PsyETA), the Scientists Center for Animal Welfare (SCAW), the Animal Legal Defense Fund and others.

Acknowledgments

The author extends appreciation to Felicia Ford for her research assistance, and to Jane Peters, Janet S. St. Lawrence, Evelyn Segal, and Kenneth Shapiro for their comments concerning an early draft of this paper.

References

American Psychological Association. 1981. Ethical principles of psychologists. *American Psychologist.* 36:633-8.

American Psychological Association. 1985. Unpublished data reporting on the results survey of admissions to experimental psychology doctoral programs in the United States.

Branch, C.E., Robertson, B.T., Smith, E.P. and Vaughan, J.T. May, 1984. Interactive video in veterinary medical education: An alternative to live animal experimentation. In: *Proceedings,* American Veterinary Computer Society, College of Veterinary Medicine, Mississippi State University, Second Symposium on Computer Application. pp. 219-22.

Janis, I.L. and Mann, L. 1977. *Decision-making: A Psychological Analysis of Conflict, Choice, and Commitment.* New York: Free Press.

Lockwood, R. August, 1984. Kindness is creative. Presentation to Psychologists for the Ethical Treatment of Animals. American Psychological Association Annual Meeting. Toronto.

Maddison, D.C. 1978. What's wrong with medical education? *Journal of Medical Education.* 12:97-102.

Milgram, S. 1963. Behavioral study of obedience. *Journal of Abnormal Social Psychology.* 67:371-8.

Reese, E.P. August, 1984. Teaching sensitivity to animal welfare will make students better scientists. In: Bernstein, E. (Chair). Ways to minimize pain and suffering for laboratory animals. Symposium at American Psychological Association Annual Meeting. Toronto.

Riss, D. and Goodall, J. 1977. The recent rise to the alpha rank in a population of free-living chimpanzees. *Folio Primatol.* (Basel), 27:134-51.

Rollin, B.E. 1981. *Animal Rights and Human Morality.* Buffalo, NY: Prometheus Books.

Ross, M. 1981. The ethics of experiments on higher animals. *Social Science in Medicine.* 13(F):51-60.

Russell, W.M.S. and Burch, R.L. 1959. *The Principles of Humane Experimental Technique.* London: Methuen.

Segal, E. 1982. Editorial. *Journal of Experimental Analysis of Behavior.* 38:115.

Segal, E. August, 1983. Discussant comments. In: King, F.A. (Chair). Use of primates in behavioral and biomedical research. Symposium presented to the American Psychological Association. Anaheim, CA.

Seligman, M.E. 1978. Learned helplessness as a model of depression: Comment and integration. *Journal of Abnormal Psychology.* 87:165-79.

Shapiro, K. 1983. Personal communication reporting on an informal survey of 25 introductory psychology textbooks.

Shapiro, K. May, 1984. Cost-benefit analysis: Critique and complements. Paper presented to the Association for Behavior Analysis Annual Meeting. Nashville.

Thomas, M.H., Horton, R.W., Lippincott, E.L., and Drabman, R.S. 1977. Desensitization to real-life aggression as a function of exposure to television violence. *Journal of Personality and Social Psychology.* 35:450.

Trautt, G.M., Reed, J.G. and Schneider, J.A. 1983. Teaching of ethics in psychology: Results of a national survey. Paper presented to the Eastern Psychological Association Annual Meeting.

Truax, C.B., Wargo, D.G., Frank, J.D., Imber, S.D., Battle, C.C., Hoehn-Saric, R., Nash, E.H., and Stone, A.R. 1966. Therapist empathy, genuineness, and warmth and patient therapeutic outcome. *Journal of Consulting Psychology.* 22:331-4.

ANTHROPOMORPHISM IS NOT A FOUR-LETTER WORD*

Randall Lockwood

The Humane Society of the United States
2100 L Street, NW
Washington, D.C. 20037

In recent years animal experimentation in American psychology has been subjected to harsh criticism from inside and outside the discipline (Bannister 1981; Giannelli, this volume; Griffin 1976, 1984; MacDonald and Dawkins 1981; Rollin 1981). The critics have warned of a loss of both an ethical framework and a creative spark in contemporary psychology. It is no secret that much of what passes for good science in psychology is trivial, boring, repetitive, and inhumane. I think that many of the factors that stifle creativity in this field are the same ones that lead researchers to conduct studies that are ethically impoverished. Conversely, I believe that an empathic and humane viewpoint often encourages scientists to ask valid scientific questions that are fresh, challenging, and beneficial to human and non-human animals alike.

How did psychology, particularly American comparative psychology, get into this sterile and often cruel rut? I would like to examine that question by briefly reviewing the history of the field and my own experiences as a student in this area.

When I first entered the world of the scientific study of animal behavior almost twenty years ago, I was given the distinct impression that it was time to put away my teddy bears and memories of Disney films and acquire the cold, hard, "objective" eye of the scientist. My textbooks were quite clear about the dangers of viewing animals in any other way:

---

*This paper is based on invited presentations at the Conference on the Perception of Animals in American Culture, National Zoological Park, Washington, D.C., November 1983 and the American Psychological Association, Toronto, Canada, August 1984.

> We cannot see into the animal's mind any more than we can see into that of any of our fellow humans, but that doesn't prevent us in both cases from thinking that we can. The animal may seem sad or happy, but we cannot infer that this is the case from the way that we ourselves might feel in the same situation. To do so is to indulge in anthropomorphism—seeing man's shape in all things—and this is the *cardinal crime* (emphasis mine) for the animal observer (Broadhurst 1964, p. 12).

Another text from this same period warns:

> Sometimes we fall into the *dangerous pit of anthropomorphism* (emphasis mine) (which literally means "formed like a man") or the tendency to think of animals as if they were human (Breland and Breland 1966, p. 3).

Most animal scientists are directly or indirectly instructed to avoid any hint of anthropomorphism, yet it is an approach that is invariably applied by scientists and lay people alike. Science may have gained some objectivity in discarding this common view of animals, but it has gone overboard in its rejection of the concept of the continuity of human and animal experiences. I hope to outline how an anthropomorphic perspective can be applied in ways that are a service to science and the animals themselves.

Early accounts of animal behavior were both anthropomorphic and anthropocentric. Animals were seen as existing only for man's benefit, or to provide him with some moral lessons about the power and potential wrath of God or gods. Prior to the nineteenth century most natural histories were anecdotal and largely erroneous. The deficiencies made it difficult to equate the study of animal behavior to the quantitative sciences such as physics, chemistry, and astronomy, which were experiencing dramatic growth and vigor during this period.

Charles Darwin made extensive but careful use of anecdotal reports in many of his greatest works. His descriptions of behavior were also highly anthropomorphic. He wrote, for example:

> Dogs exhibit their affection by desiring to rub against their masters... I have also seen dogs licking cats with whom they were friends. This habit probably originated in the females' carefully licking their puppies —the dearest object of their love—for the sake of cleansing them (Darwin 1872, p. 118).

Darwin's anthropomorphism is partly based on literary style. We must remember that he was a best-selling author, with the first edition of *Origin of Species* selling out in a single afternoon. But Darwin's language also reflected his firm belief in the continuity of life, including a continuity of mental experiences.

A major concern during the 1870s and 1880s was the evolution of the human mind. Thus there was a comparable interest in the mental abilities of animals. Scientific journals of the era were flooded with letters reporting striking observations on the mental abilities of animals (Boakes 1984).

Many of Darwin's later contemporaries were eager to join the ranks of the "legitimate" physical scientists and were critical of the anthropomorphic approach. Darwin's initial entry into respectable scientific circles had been based primarily on his rather dry geological writings. His most anthropomorphic book, *Expression of the Emotions in Man and Animals* (1872), was largely ignored by the scientific community for many years.

Prior to his death in 1882, Darwin chose George Romanes as his intellectual successor and entrusted to him the task of compiling his vast correspondence relating to the mental abilities of animals. Sensing the swing to the methods of the physical sciences, Romanes expressed fears that his book on this topic, *Animal Intelligence* (1882), would be considered small improvement on the works of the "anecdote mongers." His predictions proved correct. His work has been unjustifiably ignored including his insightful notion of "ejection," the idea that we can infer the mental state of animals having some similarities to ourselves by reflecting on our own mental states under similar conditions.

In 1894, one of Romanes' students, C. Lloyd Morgan, released his *Introduction to Comparative Psychology.* The book echoed many of Romanes' ideas and stressed the importance of *both* subjective and objective approaches to understanding the mentality of animals. However, Morgan's book is most remembered for a simple statement on method which, taken out of context, became the guiding light for American biologists and psychologists. This idea, now immortalized as "Morgan's Canon," was brief and deceptively simple. He wrote:

> In no case may we interpret an action as the outcome of the exercise of higher psychical faculty if it can be interpreted as the outcome of the exercise of one that stands lower in the psychological scale.

Over the years this has generally been interpreted to mean that one should not refer to "intelligence," when the concept of "instinct" will suffice and that one should examine clearly identifiable reflexes and simple behaviors, rather than search for an understanding of animal or human "mind."

Like many statements in science that have achieved the status of dogma, Morgan's Canon had the effect of both freeing psychology from some of its pseudoscientific trappings while, at the same time, slamming the door on some of the most interesting questions possible.

Most of the major figures in the study of animal behavior from 1890 to the 1950s embraced Morgan's idea. Pavlov (1927) wrote that animals should be studied as "physiological facts, without any need to resort to fantastic speculations as to the existence of any possible subjective states... which may be conjectured as an analogy with ourselves."

In America, John B. Watson set the tone for animal research for the next forty years when he proclaimed the official position of Behaviorism. He wrote that "'States of Consciousness', like the so-called phenomena of spiritualism, are not objectively verifiable and for that reason can *never* become data for science" (Watson 1924).

As some have described it, this is the point where psychology, having already lost its *soul,* proceeded to lose its *mind.* Given the choice between accepting the possibility of mind and emotion in animals and man, and trying to build a theoretical framework around that, or denying the importance of subjective experiences, most psychologists chose the latter. A direct outgrowth of this approach was the proliferation of mechanical models of animal and human behavior that have been demeaning to both (Bannister 1984).

It is unclear exactly what we are being protected from by avoiding anthropomorphism. For the last 100 years the implication has always been that anthropomorphism is bad science, but what does that mean? A primary purpose of scientific method is to enable us to make valid predictions about the world. The better our science, the better the forecasts we are able to make. Physics, astronomy, and chemistry have been revered for their ability to make nearly infallible predictions. Biology has lacked this level of precision, but is still strongly predictive. Psychology has generally failed this test quite badly except for predictions made under conditions where the behavioral options are severely limited. It is for this reason that it is often not even considered a "science," even in its position within academic hierarchies.

If anthropomophism generates bad science, or science that is worse than that offered by alternative behavioristic approaches, then that should mean that the hypotheses we generate based on assuming things like animal emotion, intelligence, feeling, intention and so on, will be very inaccurate. But modern interpretations of Morgan's Canon, Pavlov's pronouncements and the position of Behaviorism tell us not to even bother asking the questions! To many animal scientists, the study of animal consciousness, animal emotion, or animal suffering is a contradiction in terms, like a scientific study of the soul. I find it hard to accept as "scientific" any philosophy that automatically excludes entire areas of inquiry.

In an attempt to avoid any taint of anthropomorphism, the research of Pavlov, Loeb, Watson, Skinner, and their contemporary ideological descendants often takes the form of precisely measured studies of trivial events. There has been, and continues to be, a fascination with studying areas of animal behavior that lend themselves to precise, objective, and often remote measurement. This is not so much because these events are intrinsically interesting or even theoretically important, but often simply because their measurement is *possible!* The result has been a body of "research" that represents the expensive measurement of the irrelevant and the painful elaboration of the obvious.

In the 1940s and 1950s, while American psychologists followed a largely Behaviorist tradition, ethologists in Europe were rediscovering many of the Darwinian traditions. Tinbergen's methods were the result of a desire to understand the entire pattern of an animal's adaptations to its natural environment, as well as the desire to study mechanisms of behavior without damaging the animal in any way. He described his procedures as "physiology without breaking the skin" (Tinbergen 1958). Lorenz, Tinbergen, von Frisch, and others performed naturalistic observations and natural experiments, all in accordance with accepted scientific method. However, they felt free to discuss their results, as Darwin had, with reference to animal minds, intentions, and feelings.

As with Darwin, part of this was for literary effect. Like Darwin's *Origin of Species,* Lorenz's books *King Solomon's Ring* and *On Aggression* became best-sellers. But the anthropomorphic tone of these books reflected a very different philosophical viewpoint from that found in the writings of most American comparative psychologists. It was one that had been neglected for some time in this country. Lorenz made it clear that his anthropomorphism was not to be confused with soft-headed sentimentality:

> Believe me, I am not mistakenly assigning human properties to animals; on the contrary, I am showing you what an enormous inheritance remains in man to this day (1952 p. 152).

Ironically, one outgrowth of ethology's popularity in the 1960s and 1970s was the proliferation of "zoomorphism," the widespread application of concepts of animal behavior to human motivation and behavior. While the intellectual stock of this approach has declined dramatically, it has been followed by the more systematic application of principles of inclusive fitness to human and nonhuman behavior by contemporary sociobiologists who are often comfortable with freely interchanging terms drawn from studies of both human and animal behavior. Despite this renewed interest in the continuity of human and nonhuman experiences, the fear of anthropomorphic interpretation has still kept the study of the mental and emotional experiences in animals outside the reach of most mainstream psychologists and biologists.

The continuing aversion to anthropomorphism is partly due to confusion about the actual meaning of the term. Few students of behavior take the time to consider what it is they are supposed to be avoiding. Thus they tend to avoid any thinking or writing that seems to touch on parallels between animal and human mental events. At this point it is important to clarify some of the different meanings that the term "anthropomorphism" can have. In this way we might understand the almost irrational ends to which scientists have gone to avoid it.

I find it useful to distinguish between several different kinds of anthropomorphism. The first I call *allegorical anthropomorphism*. This would apply to descriptions of animal behavior that are not intended to be taken as biological fact. These descriptions use animals to make some point more appealing, or to conceal identities. This would be the form of anthropomorphism we see in most fables and literary or political allegories such as *Alice in Wonderland* and *Animal Farm*. This form is entertaining and, since it does not presume to portray biological reality, it is essentially harmless. The dangers lie in extending the allegory to the forms of anthropomorphism below.

A second form comes closest to what we commonly think of as anthropomorphism. This would encompass instances of people who dress their pets in human clothes, feed them human treats, or in other ways, superimpose their own desires on the animal's requirements. I prefer to call this *personification* since the animal is treated as a person with needs identical to those of the humans with whom it interacts. As above, there is no appreciation of the biological needs or adaptations of the animal. The animals are being used to portray some personal, perhaps symbolic, message.

A third form, which I call *superficial anthropomorphism*, characterizes much of the pre-Darwinian natural history writings. In this case the animal's behavior or temperament is interpreted on the basis of superficial qualities that are unrelated to those that are actually involved. For example, we might interpret the "kissing" behavior of gourami fish to indicate affection since it bears a superficial resemblance to the human pattern. Similarly we might interpret the retracted lips of a chimpanzee's fear grimace or submissive grin to be an indication of pleasure. Such anthropomorphism is bad science since it leads us to make inaccurate predictions.

A fourth variety can be termed *explanatory anthropomorphism*. This approach offers circular definition of behavior using terms drawn from human motivation. The fallacy here is in thinking that we have explained an event by giving it a name. Take the example of a dog owner who leaves one dog alone at home while taking another for a walk. He returns to find garbage strewn around the living room and attributes this behavior to "spite" or "revenge" on the part of the dog that was left behind. How do we know that the behavior was spite?... because the behavior was spiteful! Unfortunately, it is not only non-scientists that employ such logical circularity in assuming that behavioral phenomena are explained because they are named. Psychiatry and the study of human intelligence have had a long history of such nominal fallacies.

All of the above approaches have serious shortcomings as tools for science. They either make no attempt to understand the animal in its own world, or they overlook the need to verify the accuracy of the explanation in a systematic way. The title of this article suggests that I consider some anthropomorphism to be of potential benefit to science and the animals that it studies. This brings us to the form of anthropomorphism I hinted at in describing the work of Darwin, Romanes, modern ethologists, and some other contemporary scientists. I refer to this as *projective anthropomorphism;* the use of our personal perspective on what it is like to be a living being to suggest hypotheses about what it is like to be another living being of our own or some other species.

This process is a form of projection, the mental activity that makes our life as social beings possible. Our most basic problem in dealing with other organisms is that we can never fully experience the world as it is perceived by another. I have no immediate way of knowing what it is like to be one of my students, my wife, Ronald Reagan, my cat, a wolf, a whale, or a fly on the wall. But the essence of consciousness is using self-knowledge to try to predict and interpret the behavior of others. Normal human beings must constantly generate hypotheses about what it might be like to be someone else in order to regulate their social interactions. Many of us also frequently attempt to understand what it would be like to be some*thing* else. If we are successful in empathizing with others and projecting our own feelings onto the situations faced by others, then our predictions will be accurate. If the predictions fail, our hypotheses must be reevaluated.

Ethologists have long recognized the concept of "Umwelt," the unique perceptual world of each species and individual, and have considered the understanding of a creature's Umwelt to be a central goal of scientific inquiry (Uexkull 1957). This kind of empathic introspection was implied in the writings of Darwin and Romanes and is elegantly summed up in an early text on animal behavior by Margaret Floy Washburn (1917, p. 24):

> When a being whose structure resembles ours receives the same stimulus that affects us and moves in the same way as a result, he has an inner experience which resembles our own... we may extend this inference to the lower animals, with proper safeguards, just as far as they present resemblances in structure or behavior to ourselves.

We have to keep two things in mind when applying this idea. First, our projection of mental events must be considered to be hypothetical. To be a sound scientific hypothesis it must be falsifiable. There must be some objective data that could be collected that would confirm or deny the accuracy of our interpretation. Such an experiment might be quite complex, or it might be as simple as allowing an animal a choice between two different situations. Second, we must keep in mind the "proper safeguards" alluded to by Washburn.

Let's examine these safeguards in detail. For the entire process of projective anthropomorphism to be of scientific value, there must be some analog of the experience of others in our own repertoire. If I enjoy a particular book about natural history then I can predict with some certainty that a friend who has exhibited a parallel interest will also appreciate the book. However, it would probably be erroneous for me as a nonparent to approach a mother who has just buried a child and say "I know how you must feel." I have known grief, but I doubt that my experiences have given me a pattern of responses and emotions that are fully analogous to what the parent is experiencing. Thus I cannot really predict how she wil respond to being left alone, comforted, etc. A similar problem arises when trying to fit our behavioral framework on the experiences of animals. Niko Tinbergen recognized his inability to relate to the experience of incubation on the part of a herring gull. He described the event as:

> ... monotonous, at least for the observer who, missing any incubation instinct in himself, has some difficulty in understanding the satisfaction which a bird presumably feels when just sitting on eggs (Tinbergen 1953, p. 134).

How are we to judge when there is the potential for some analogy between our own mental experiences and those of another species? One potential source of support for such parallels is the study of the physiological substrates of these experiences. As we gain an increasing understanding of the anatomical, physiological, and pharmacological events that underlie the experience of emotional states in animals and man, we are constantly forced to realize the extent of close parallels in a wide variety of animals. The neurotransmitters and other biological elements implicated in such human experiences as pain, depression, stress, and anxiety are remarkably widespread throughout the animal kingdom. Indeed many critics of contemporary animal psychology (e.g., Giannelli,this volume; Singer 1975) have alluded to the central ethical fallacy of much of this research. Simply stated: if animals used to model the human experience of pain, fear, depression, anxiety, helplessness, and other maladaptive states do not experience these conditions themselves, then their use as models is scientifically unjustifiable. If they do experience such states, their use is morally and ethically unjustifiable.

A second methodological safeguard we can use in applying an anthropomorphic perspective is to pay attention to the context in which a behavior occurs. When dealing with other people we find that our predictions tend to fail when we do not know the events that preceded the behavior that we are trying to understand. Such errors are most likely to occur in dealing with people from different cultural backgrounds. Similarly, anthropomorphism fails when we are insensitive to the biology, ecology, and evolutionary history of the animal, as well as its individual life history (concerns that are usually of no interest to the majority of American psychologists).

When my colleagues and I released a pack of captive-raised wolves into the Alaska wilderness, many people suggested that the animals would immediately vanish, based on their own predicted response to release from confinement. In fact, the wolves returned each night for nearly a week to sleep in the temporary cage in which they had been allowed to recover from their journey. Similarly, nearly all of the Arctic foxes released from a fur farm by protesters returned to their small cages within a few days (MacDonald and Dawkins 1981). Neither of these events is surprising when one considers the life history of the animals and the fact that confinement, for these animals, had a life-long association with food and safety. Obviously neither event should be construed as evidence that captivity is not stressful for either wolves or foxes, only that the initial release from captivity is more stressful than captivity itself for those animals that have never experienced anything else. Dawkins (1980) specifically notes the need to take an animal's past environmental history into consideration when interpreting the results of experiments that involve allowing chickens to select to live in standard battery cages or larger quarters.

To summarize, anthropomorphism must be applied with certain restraint. We must have reason to believe that there is potential for analogous experiences and we must have a good understanding of the animal's ecological, evolutionary, and individual history. Then we are free to use our empathy to make a prediction, which we must then evaluate. If the prediction holds up, I feel that this constitutes scientific evidence for the validity of the initial anthropomorphic assumption. We are then in a position to make increasingly more refined predictions, and from this construct a clearer understanding of what it is like to be some other human or nonhuman animal. This is essentially the process we use on a daily basis in building our friendships and other social relationships. It is a process that is almost universally employed but largely unconsciousness to us. It is precisely these properties that have made such an approach unattractive to most American psychologists. That view seems to be changing.

Recently many of the concepts that entranced Darwin and others of his era, such as animal intelligence and emotion, have returned to scientific prominence (see below). This has been brought about by a number of factors. First, ethology's rapid rise in popularity in the 1960s and 1970s resulted in a considerable infusion of fresh ideas into many American studies in animal behavior. Textbooks no longer speak of the contrast between European ethology and American comparative and physiological psychology, but instead point out the productive exchange of ideas. This has resulted in greater emphasis on studies that make reference to the adaptive value of behaviors witnessed in the laboratory and has made possible the serious investigation of the mental capacities of animals.

Secondly, the growth in power and sophistication of both the environmental and humane movements during this same period has produced scientists and non-scientists who are increasingly sensitive to both the biological relevance and the ethical basis of research. This change has not always been a rapid one, since charges of sentimentality and anthropomorphic thinking have frequently been leveled at the more compassionate members of the scientific community. Our society finally seems to be learning that one *can* separate methodology and ideology. An empathetic scientist, having selected a question he or she finds interesting, can gather data in accordance with the strictest tenets of scientific method.

A third factor has been the growing dissatisfaction with the predictive powers of hard-core Behaviorism in dealing with both higher human functions, such as problem solving, and naturally occuring animal behavior. Despite the claims of practitioners of this form of science, its applications to real-world issues have proven to be very limited.

We have not simply come full circle back to 1872. Today's scientists do not discuss anger, jealousy, nobility, and joy in all manner of insects, birds, and mammals in the same uncritical fashion as those of the nineteenth century. As Marian Dawkins (1980, p. 1) points out:

> Present day studies on the mental experiences of animals are far more rigorous and experimental than they were in the nineteenth century. The lessons of Behaviourism have not been lost. Perhaps the study of mental events in animals has advanced precisely because it had to stand up to the Behaviourists and justify itself in the face of their criticisms.

The late C.W. Hume, founder of the Universities Federation for Animal Welfare, commented that no students of behavior would know what to look for if they did not, consciously or unconsciously, use subjective clues (Hume 1962).Let me briefly review a few of the areas of scientific inquiry that have been helped by an anthropomorphic perspective and a sensitivity to these subjective clues.

Animal Learning

The study of animal learning has been dramatically enriched by breaking out of the intellectual and ethical impoverishment of standard Behavioristic paradigms. Fresh approaches have been produced by returning to the realization that much of animal behavior is done *on purpose* and that animals are not only "aware" of the consequences of their actions, but often have expectations of what these consequences might be. As Griffin (1984) notes, "if consciousness is an illusion . . . it is a remarkably useful one." This view is still a minority opinion. "Methodological behaviorism" (Staddon 1983) remains the standard approach for American psychologists. To the question "are there really such things as beliefs and desires and so on?," this approach answers "Maybe... but who cares?"

Even among learning theorists antagonistic to the concept of animal rights there is recognition of the merits of anthropomorphism as a tool for understanding animal behavior. For example, John Garcia's significant contributions in the study of taste aversion learning in rats seem to have come, at least in part, from a willingness to try to understand the world as viewed by a scavenger that eats garbage and cannot vomit. He notes (Garcia 1981, p. 151):

> I always use anthropomorphism and teleology to predict animal behavior because this works better than most learning theories. I could rationalize this heresy by pointing to our common neurosensory systems or to convergent evolutionary forces. But, in truth, I merely put myself in the animal's place. I cannot think in the cryptic jargon of learning theory.

Animal Communication

As with animal learning, most studies of animal communication that were done just a few years ago focused on the objective and often tedious description of animal sounds and postures and their context. These signals were viewed as behaviors that were motivated by some basic biological need and responded to in some reflexive way. Recently there has been considerable interest in analyzing animal communication from the standpoint of the message that the animal *intends* to send, and the behavior that it *intends* (or perhaps "hopes") to elicit in the recipient. There has also been renewed interest in the extensive parallels across species in certain common signals that are conveyed in common ways. These objective studies have strongly vindicated many of Darwin's writings on animal expression, and have raised questions about even more complex cognitive abilities.

Comparative Psychopathology

The idea of using animals to model human psychiatric disorders was challenged for years because of the assumption that mental suffering required a "mind," and thus could not be considered to exist in "mindless" animals. It is this resistance to the concept of mental disorders in animals that, I think, forced Harlow and his associates to go to drastic extremes to produce animals that were very clearly abnormal.

Today, there is continued use of animal models, with greater emphasis on the alleviation of disorders rather than the induction of abnormal states. Still, further intellectual growth of this field has been hampered by the preponderance of researchers who use animal models but who remain unwilling to acknowledge that the mental experiences of their animal subjects parallels the discomfort and distress experienced by the humans that they allegedly mimic. There have been many rat and monkey models of depression, yet most researchers would consider it unnecessarily anthropomorphic to hypothesize that their subjects "feel depressed." Such a consideration could generate many fresh hypotheses about the nature of illness and the ways in which it can be alleviated. Even Harlow eventually recognized that a problem with comparative psychopathology was not its reliance on the concept of animal mind, but on the extent to which the animals could suffer as much as people. In reviewing his life's work he said (Harlow and Mears 1979, p. 218):

> Perhaps our greatest, most significant discovery is that human behavior generalizes to monkeys, whether or not monkey behavior generalizes to humans.

The Human/Companion Animal Bond

We are obviously most likely to be anthropomorphic about the animals that we deal with on a daily basis. It is partly for this reason that the study of the behavior of domestic animals became scientifically acceptable only in the last few decades. The formal scientific study of dogs and cats, our closest companions, has only become fashionable in the last few years (Katcher and Beck 1983).

For years, scientists have rejected farmers, livestock handlers, and pet-owners as a source of valid ethological questions, and have shunned observations of domestic animals in favor of expensive and time-consuming studies of exotic animals whose Umwelts are largely unknown. Once again Darwin was a noteworthy exception. He made extensive observations of his own pets and relied heavily on the reports of livestock breeders and handlers in developing many of his ideas about domestication.

Douglas Spalding, a contemporary of Darwin who later influenced Lorenz and the European ethologists, also lamented the lack of interest in domestic animals shown by animal behaviorists of his era. He noted that "the many extraordinary and exceptional feats of dogs and other animals seem to be constantly falling under the observation of everybody except the few that are interested in these matters" (quoted in Boakes 1984).

The growing appreciation of the mental abilities of domestic animals, and the nature of their emotional bonds to humans and each other has made possible the rich and vital field of the study of the human/companion animal bond. Still, far more money is being spent on studying the communicative behavior of exotic species than that of the dog, an animal that has shared our social world for over 12,000 years. I look forward to the time, not far off, when we can recruit pet owners into the ranks of objective observers of animal behavior and tap an enormous resource for understanding the interdependence of animals and man.

Applied Ethology

Another discipline that has benefitted from the scientific application of anthropomorphic ideas is applied animal behavior. This field seeks to use principles of ethology and comparative psychology to modify animal behavior or adjust environments to produce desirable behaviors. A few years ago the notion that animals in captivity or confinement might suffer from boredom, stress, loneliness, or similar conditions would have been considered sentimental anthropomorphism by veterinarians and "hard" scientists. However, a growing number of investigators find such concepts useful in generating hypotheses about how to improve captive environments.

As an example of this change of approach, consider recent trends in housing for the great apes. Chimps and gorillas in captivity often appear to be sad, bored, and lonely to both lay people and trained animal scientists alike. In the past this view could easily be dismissed as sentimentally anthropomorphic. But it can also be used as a working hypothesis without being hampered by the fact that we cannot directly "know" the animal's mental state. If we hypothesize that the animal is bored, and that this boredom is responsible for the various behavioral abnormalities we see such as listlessness, masturbation, regurgitation and refeeding, then we can also hypothesize that relief of boredom should relieve the symptoms. To evaluate the hypothesis we need only assess the results of enriching the animals' environment with toys, social companions, and other sources of stimulation. Such changes almost invariably result in the same kinds of improvements in animal behavior that we would predict on the basis of introspection into our own responses to captivity (Markowitz 1982).

A similar empathic approach has helped the study of misbehavior in companion animals. Borchelt (1983) has found it useful to regard many of the destructive behaviors shown by dogs to be the consequence of "separation anxiety." By attending to the cues that would exaggerate or reduce this hypothetical state, he has been able to design effective treatment programs.

Animal Welfare

It would have been unthinkable not so long ago to propose to conduct scientific studies of animal suffering. Today there is great concern about assessing animals' experiences of pain, and the response of animals to different conditions of care. This change has not simply been the result of increased sensitivity to the lobbying efforts of the humane movement. It is a true reflection of many scientists' realization that these questions, rooted in anthropomorphic projections, are timely, interesting, biologically valid, and morally significant.

In summary, I hope that I have clarified the difference between various forms of anthropomorphism and have illustrated its slowly growing respectability as a scientific tool. There will always be barriers to understanding other beings. It is a disservice to ourselves and to our fellow human and nonhuman creatures to regard any attempt at reaching out as being merely irrational or sentimental. If we make use of an *ideology* based on empathy and a *methodology* based on science, we cannot go far wrong. Hume (1962) outlines the costs and benefits quite clearly:

> If I assume that animals have subjective feelings of pain, fear, hunger and the like, and if I am mistaken in doing so, no harm will have been done; but if I assume the contrary, when in fact animals do have such feelings, then I open the way to unlimited cruelties... Animals must have the benefit of the doubt, if indeed there be any doubt.

References

Bannister, D. 1981. The fallacy of animal experimentation in psychology. In: Sperlinger, D. ed. *Animals in Research*. New York: John Wiley and Sons.

Borchelt, P. 1983. Separation-elicited behavior problems in dogs. In: Katcher, A.H. and Beck, A.M. eds. *New Perspectives on Our Lives with Companion Animals*. Philadelphia: University of Pennsylvania Press.

Boakes, R. 1984. *From Darwin to Behaviourism*. London: Cambridge University Press.

Breland, K. and Breland, M. 1966. *Animal Behavior*. Toronto: MacMillan.

Broadhurst, P.L. 1963. *The Science of Animal Behaviour*. Baltimore: Penguin Books.

Dawkins, M.S. 1980. *Animal Suffering: The Science of Animal Welfare*. New York: Chapman and Hall.

Darwin, C. 1872. *The Expression of the Emotions in Man and Animals*. (1963 reprint). Chicago: University of Chicago Press.

Garcia, J. 1981. Tilting at the paper mills of academe. *American Psychologist*. 36(2):149-58.

Griffin, D.R. 1976. *The Question of Animal Awareness*. New York: The Rockefeller University Press.

Griffin, D.R. 1984. *Animal Thinking*. Cambridge, MA: Harvard University Press.

Harlow, H.F. and Mears, C. 1979. *The Human Model: Primate Perspectives*. New York: John Wiley and Sons.

Hume, C.W. 1962. *Man and Beast*. Herts, U.K; The Universities Federation for Animal Welfare.

Katcher, A.H. and Beck, A.M. eds. 1983. *New Perspectives on Our Lives with Companion Animals*. Philadelphia: University of Pennsylvania Press.

Lorenz, K.Z. 1952. *King Solomon's Ring*. London: Methuen.

MacDonald, D. and Dawkins, M. 1981. Ethology—the science and the tool. In: Sperlinger, D. ed. *Animals in Research*. New York: John Wiley and Sons.

Markowitz, H. 1982. *Behavioral Enrichment in the Zoo*. New York: van Nostrand Reinhold.

Morgan, C.L. 1894. *An Introduction to Comparative Psychology*. London: Scott.

Pavlov, I.P. 1927. *Conditioned Reflexes*. (1960 reprint). New York: Dover Books.

Rollin, B.E. 1981. *Animal Rights and Human Morality*. Buffalo, NY: Prometheus Books.

Singer, P. 1975. *Animal Liberation*. New York: Avon Books.

Staddon, J.E.R. 1983. *Adaptive Behavior and Learning*. Cambridge, U.K.: Cambridge University Press.

Tinbergen, N. 1953. *The Herring Gull's World*. London: Collins.

Tinbergen, N. 1958. *Curious Naturalists*. London: Country Life.

Uexkull, J. von. 1957. A stroll through the world of animals and men. In: Schiller, C.S. ed. *Instinctive Behavior*. New York: International Universities Press.

Washburn, M.F. 1917. *The Animal Mind*. New York: MacMillan.

Watson, J.B. 1924. *Psychology from the Standpoint of a Behaviorist*. Philadelphia: Lippincott.

Alternatives

THE IMBALANCE BETWEEN EXPERIMENT AND THEORY IN BIOLOGY: THE NEED FOR THEORY-DIRECTED MODELING

M.L. Fidelman
D.C. Mikulecky

Department of Physiology and Biophysics
Medical College of Virginia
Virginia Commonwealth University
Richmond, VA 23298

Introduction

In biological and biomedical research, the vast majority of resources are focused on conducting experiments. Most of these experiments utilize animals. Only a tiny amount of resources is spent on theory and modeling. It is our contention and the basic theme of this paper that the imbalance between theory and experiment in biology produces very poor science. The implications of which are that many of the experiments conducted have little real scientific meaning or value and, therefore, go hand-in-hand with unnecessary animal use and suffering. Given the finite resources available for research, the redirection of significant resources from an almost entirely experimental approach into one with an emphasis on more theoretical and modeling activity will achieve a much better scientific result while considerably reducing the number of animals used in biological research.

Although the arguments developed here have a bearing on other issues as well, such as the optimum use of resources, future directions in the training of research biologists, etc., they have a very direct bearing on the rising awareness that the indiscriminant use of animals for any purely human purpose needs to be carefully reexamined. Without getting into the moral questions of whether animal research is justifiable (see Singer 1985), we will attempt, in this paper, to analyze the current philosophical structure of a field which consumes animals at a high rate.

For these reasons, it is important for everyone to have some understanding of the philosophical underpinnings of modern biological research—its history, its present, and its future. This paper focuses on the relationship between experiment and theory in biology and the role that modeling plays in the quality and strength of this interaction. It concludes with a discussion of a relatively recent development, Network Thermodynamics. We believe that Network Thermodynamic modeling and computer simulation is the next step in providing a comprehensive theoretical framework for describing complex, hierarchical biological systems and will have a profound impact on the future of biology.

The Scientific Method: Theory and Empiricism

Empiricism is distinct from other epistemologies (theories of knowledge) in its almost total reliance on sense experience as the ultimate source of knowledge. As an approach to science, it represents the search for knowledge based solely on experiment and observation. Much attention is therefore focused on methods for collecting and processing data with the inherent belief that this collecting activity will lead to recognition of patterns and relationships between observed events and ultimately to our understanding of the laws of nature (Mahoney 1976). In contrast to this completely experimental approach, there is what we will call "theoretical deduction" which is based upon the ability of the human mind to deduce relationships between abstract, often seemingly unreal or imaginary entities, usually represented by mathematics. This is the completely theoretical approach and as a scientific methodology seeks to gain knowledge by reasoning from known principles to an unknown or by seeking a set of general principles which can then be applied to explain the specific. Its language is mathematics.

The strength of empiricism lies in its concrete attachment to the physical reality of the system being studied. Its weaknesses become more apparent and severe as the complexity of the system increases. In biological systems, for instance, where we often face multiple interactive, dynamic, nonlinear processes embedded within complex structures, it becomes virtually impossible to intuit the basic principles and theoretical framework by which the system operates from just "looking at the relationships" in the data. In fact, without a theoretical framework to start from, it is highly unlikely that the "critical" experiments necessary to eventually achieve understanding will even be performed. On the opposite side, theoretical deduction can provide the rigorous mathematical framework for the development of basic principles leading to understanding. The weakness of disembodied theorizing, however, is the risk of total irrelevance, i.e., the mathematical formalism of the theory has little or nothing to do with the actual structures and processes in the system.

Given the match of the strengths and weaknesses of these two approaches, it should not be too surprising that the scientific method frequently offered as the best and most productive comes from the strong interaction of theory with experiment (Platt 1964; Murphy 1982). This brings us to the concept of a model. Jaynes (1976) tells us that the concepts of science are all concrete metaphors which serve to generate abstract concepts. He distinguishes between a theory and a model by pointing to the theory as a relationship of the model to the things a model is supposed to represent. For example, Bohr modeled the atom to resemble a miniature solar system. The theory would state *all* atoms are represented by this model. This may seem a subtle distinction and is certainly a subjective one, but nevertheless a useful one. Thus modeling may be thought of as the vehicle for the interaction between theory and experiment.

Classification of Models

It is important to realize that all biologists use models in formulating and interpreting experiments, whether or not they are consciously aware of it. Many models never become formulated beyond the state of pictures, diagrams or even merely being verbalized. Such inherently intuitive and nonanalytical descriptions we will simply call qualitative models. Models which involve specific mathematical descriptions will be divided into two main categories: empirical models and theory-directed models. By empirical, we mean a mathematical description of the input-output characteristics of a system that is *not* based on or derived from the actual structures and/or specific processes of that system. Empirical models are basically models of data and may be thought of as essentially either "black box" approaches or curve-fitting. Theory-directed models, on the other hand, are an attempt to mathematically describe the physical reality of a biological system at a sufficient level of complexity necessary to explain system behavior. While theory-directed models may have some empirical elements within them, they are ultimately directed towards developing a comprehensive theoretical framework for understanding *both* the holistic behavior of the system and the specific behavior and contribution of each of the component parts of the system. As opposed to models of data, theory-directed models are more models of systems and are sometimes capable of telling us something very important about reality without any specific experimental data. This is, obviously, the point of departure from pure empiricism.

Criteria for Judging Models

If models are the vehicle for the interaction between theory and experiment, then the "quality" of the model becomes critical to the quality of the science produced. It becomes very important, therefore, to understand in a general sense the strengths and weaknesses of these three categories of models.

A model should be communicable since science is a community activity. Qualitative models, particularly the diagrammatic and pictorial ones, certainly have this quality. They are also simple to formulate and use and easy to alter. These qualities may have something to do with their being the most common type of model used in biological research. As the systems they describe become more complex, serious problems arise with their specificity, clarity, and rigor. At times, we are asked to help an experimentalist develop a theory-directed type of model to replace the qualitative model that they have been using. We typically find that the processes and mechanisms alluded to in their qualitative model do not have clear and specific descriptions. Quite often we also find that necessary intermediate steps have been completely left out or essentially ignored, although these steps may play an important role in regulating the overall system behavior. The biggest weakness with qualitative models is that they are untested (except perhaps in the mind of their developer). In other words, it is never demonstrated that a particular model can actually produce the type of behavior that it is supposed to explain, let alone make accurate predictions about the system's behavior under new conditions. An excellent example of this problem was shown by Eisenfeld and DeLisi (1984). They examined, on the basis of qualitative stability and instability, a number of qualitative models in the literature which described immune response regulation. Not too surprisingly, they found that a number of apparently plausible models were unstable and therefore were not viable models for the observed behavior. Thus qualitative models tend to produce a weak or nonexistent interaction between theory and experiment.

Empirical models are for the most part readily communicable and not too difficult to use or modify, although they are less so than qualitative models. Unlike qualitative models, they possess at least mathematical rigor in their definitions and descriptions and they are testable. They are good at codifying and organizing in a rigorous way the data sets for a particular system. For example, measurements are made under a given set of conditions and the data is used to calculate a number of parameters in the model. The experimental conditions are changed, new measurements are made, and again the particular parameters are calculated. How these parameters change under different conditions establishes a uniform way of discussing and analyzing the data between different labs investigating the same system. There are a number of weaknesses with this type of model. The first is that these parameters do not relate to the specific physical reality of the system. Some of the mathematical techniques used in this type of model (for example, compartmental analysis and equivalent circuit analysis) have a real physical interpretation in some very simple systems. In more complex systems, however, they no longer correlate with real physical parameters. Unfortunately, there is still the tendency to blur or ignore the original assumptions and incorrectly give these parameters a literal physical meaning. Second, since the parameters do not map one for one with the real system, there is usually a great deal of hidden information (the real variables of the system) buried in these parameters. This is why these models cannot be used to accurately predict system performance under new conditions but only to codify data between known conditions. Last, but not least, is the general inability of empirical models to provide fundamental insights into the behavior of complicated systems or to provide a fundamental theoretical framework because they do not correlate with the specific physical realities of the system and generally rely on "equations of convenience" which have little or no real scientific basis. The use of such equations may, in fact, make the model susceptible to violating basic scientific principles, such as conservation laws or the second law of thermodynamics. So we conclude that empirical models, while having some advantages over qualitative models, are also inadequate for producing the necessary interaction between theory and experiment.

Theory-directed models, like empirical models, also have the mathematical rigor for specificity and clarity in defining hypotheses and are also analytically testable as to their behavior. Because they are an attempt to model the physical reality of the system, they are not as "data dependent" as empirical models. They can, therefore, predict system behavior under new conditions as well as predict values of experimentally inaccessible variables or parameters. They are capable of exposing the contradictions in hypotheses as well as the contradictions and/or incompleteness of data sets. Insomuch as they utilize mathematical descriptions based on or derived from basic scientific principles, they can provide the fundamental theoretical structure for identifying the "essentials" of the system and provide general insights and knowledge into the functioning of the system. Their biggest weaknesses have been with their communicability, their difficulty of use, and their inadaptability. These are not so much inherent problems with theory-directed models as they are with the specific mathematical and analytical techniques that have been available to develop them. The most common approach has been using differential equations and solving them. As the models become more complex, this becomes a formidable task; solutions, if they can be obtained at all, become less and less transparent and often must be analyzed by computer. Finally, if closed-form solutions are not available, the problem is usually subjected to some numerical analysis technique. Such models tend to be difficult to eliminate even if they are shown to be incompatible with data, due to the labor involved in their creation, and they also can be difficult to modify for the same reason. Such techniques also require much time and effort to learn and are difficult to master. What is needed is a new technique or approach that can overcome these problems. Along with Chua (1969), we believe it must be a compromise between simplicity and reality. Along with Thom (1975), we will often ask it to be qualitatively faithful before it is made to be quantitatively so. His point, which needs to be taken seriously, is that often the shape of a predicted curve has more significance toward acceptance or rejection of a model than whether or not the model's prediction goes through one or more actual data points. Also, if possible, it must be testable by the most stringent tests available. We will have more to say about model verification later. Pictorial representations have always had value. If we can have a pictorial representation which also provides a paradigm for the analysis of holistic behavior while relating the holistic behavior to the various functional parts, we will have succeeded. We submit that the method we call Network Thermodynamics can provide a common language to bridge the gap between experimental and theoretical biology (Mikulecky 1983). We will present later some of the reasons why we believe this to be true. In the next sections we will discuss the current attitudes and practices found in biological research and their historical perspective.

Current Attitudes and Practices

Researchers in physics and chemistry, for example, are compelled to become familiar with both theoretical and experimental approaches. In a physics department at any major university, one finds a reasonable mix of theoreticians and experimentalists. The experimentalists have the quantitative background necessary to understand the theories and are expected to use them in designing and interpreting experiments. Unfortunately, in the life sciences, empiricism is the most widely accepted epistemology with only a very small subset of practicing biologists adopting the theoretical approach to some extent. This imbalance between empiricism and theory in biology has produced a number of serious and interrelated consequences.

Foremost, perhaps, is the growth of a literature full of data with weak interpretation, if any at all. Yates (1979), a former editor of the *American Journal of Physiology*, refers to it as, "...the routine, data-loaded papers without strong scientific context that constitute the bulk of those published in any biological field." Another discouraging result of this imbalance in biology is a communication gap of immense proportions between experimentalists and theoreticians characterized in part by a sense of isolation, frustration, and even distrust. The manifestations of this are many, but there is one type in particular which illustrates the closed-mindedness which has become almost fashionable as well as the misunderstanding of the issues involved. Often, good-intentioned meeting organizers bring together theoreticians and experimentalists at a meeting in the hope of breaking down the communication barriers and establishing some sort of common ground. An event which is all too common at such meetings is that after hearing some theoretical presentation, an experimentalist will introduce the talk he or she is about to present with sincere reassurances to their counterparts in the audience that the presentation is *totally free of models and theory*! The speaker then proceeds to describe a model which is both weakly defined and untestable, believing that the trap was really successfully escaped. This is a cheap shot in a way, because the type of model the experimentalist was avoiding was special,and the one inadvertently presented was so poorly formulated that it hardly qualified. We must at least grant that the distinction being made was valid.

It is important to realize that these attitudes are prevalent among those who define modern biology by deciding where the funding will go and by deciding who will be hired, promoted, and tenured as well as what will eventually become part of the literature and what else will go unpublished. That certain ideas, approaches, etc., are excluded is a natural and obvious consequence of this imbalance. This leads to the tendency for those who seek to pursue theoretical biology to be forced to obtain funds and justification for their existence by modeling the data produced by the "true" investigators—a more or less subservient service role. They are not asked to create theory, merely to model data and to help get it published by giving it some appearance of having been done for theoretical reasons. There is the suspicion that often biology is chosen as a field of study precisely because it is lacking the mathematical and theoretical rigor that seems so difficult to master in the other sciences. Murphy (1982), in a presentation at a conference on the Genetic Basis of the Epilepsies, comments on "... the deplorable divorce, between science and mathematics, that took place within the century or so since scholars were first allowed to believe that it is possible to be a serious scientist with an unsullied ignorance of mathematics. This I hold to be a capital mistake, partly because ignorance of mathematics narrows perspective, but mainly because it betrays what is the great strength of science, the mutually correcting influences of coherence and rigor on the one hand and empirical fact on the other."

A more subtle result of this imbalance, but possibly equally as serious, is the creation of a kind of "work ethic" which places a high value on activity relating to data collection but little value on time spent "thinking" or developing theory. Many biological researchers are quite ready to learn some very difficult physical, chemical, engineering, and mathematical concepts in order to apply them to the design, testing, calibration, and use of instruments, but will think nothing of failing to do even the most rudimentary modeling of their hypotheses and collected data. This problem was stated very clearly by Rene Thom (1979) when he commented on the possibility of experimentalists in biology testing predictions from Catastrophe Theory models: "... I feel that we should not hurry for any 'experimental confirmation'; I think that a lot of theoretical thinking, of speculative modeling, has to be done before one might really *start* (our emphasis) to experiment to make a choice between models. Even so, it is doubtful that these experiments would interest very much present-day biologists, as they would be unable to understand their motivation. Quite likely, there is very little which can be done about the present situation: I agree with P. Antonelli (Transplanting a pure mathematician into theoretical biology, *Proc. Conf. on Math., Stat., and the Environment*. Ottawa 1974), when he states that theoretical biology should be done in Mathematical Departments; we have to let biologists busy themselves with their very concrete—but almost meaningless—experiments; in developmental biology, how could they hope to solve a problem they cannot even formulate?"

This work ethic is tightly coupled to the most crippling omission from the life of modern biologists, which is some guideline for judging quality. In the more "exact" sciences, mathematical theories provide a path from general truths to specific lines of investigation which are often absent or which are at best applied in the above-mentioned limited way in biology. The argument that it is justifiable to use animals in research because the research ultimately eliminates human (and sometimes animal) suffering depends very much on the *quality* of that research. There is certainly a legitimate case that can be made that the almost completely empiricist approach prevalent in modern biology cannot justify on the basis of quality the amount of money, resources, and animals that it consumes. The ethical aspects of using animals has been treated very adequately by others (Singer 1985).

A Brief Historical Perspective

The situation described to this point exists and it is the dominant means of doing biological and, especially, biomedical research today. How is it justified? How can it have happened? Gaylord Simpson once said that biology is the queen of all the sciences because it studies levels of complexity beyond those studied by physics and chemistry. It is the complexity of the living system that has been the reason so many biologists do not believe that the development of theory which was so integral in the practice of physics and chemistry could play the same role in biology. Theories for dealing with most systems simply failed to work in these complex systems. Both classical and nonequilibrium thermodynamics were chained to the "black box" approach to highly organized systems. It can be argued most strongly that for the understanding of most biological systems these approaches are both inadequate and inaccurate since they arose out of the conceptual framework of the analysis of so called "simple" systems: those which were homogeneous and relatively unstructured in their basic nature. To properly apply either classical or nonequilibrium thermodynamic reasoning to organized systems, it is necessary to apply them at the level of such homogeneous substructures and then use the proper method for combining the substructures into a functional whole. Often, what was to be called "theoretical biology" suffered from the problem of "throwing out the baby with the bath water." In order to get solutions, the mathematical and theoretical descriptions of biological systems were oversimplified to the point of no longer being a meaningful description of the real biological systems.

The old question of whether or not life can be described in terms of the principles of physics and chemistry has never been adequately answered. The illusion is that physics and chemistry are complete and all that biologists need to do is use their principles. Unfortunately, this is not the case. There is one strong philosophical idea underlying all of this: *reductionism*, the idea that by continuously subdividing a system to subsystems and then studying the subsystems in detail, the properties of the whole can be learned. Due to the dominant role of reductionism, there is a wealth of particle physics done at the expense of a macroscopic physics of highly organized systems. Chemistry through chemical physics and physical chemistry follows suit. Thus modern biology (as well as its predecessors) has one of two choices. Either we believe that reducing living systems to parts totally describable by physics and chemistry can explain everything or we resurrect vitalism. As in all paradoxes, there is a truth hidden. In fact, vitalism and the missing areas of modern physics and chemistry may be different ways of stating the same idea: living systems, among other, highly organized hierarchical systems, need a holistic approach based on a more holistic science, specifically one designed to deal with highly organized systems. The development of this science will be a breakthrough in physics and chemistry as well as biology. Meanwhile, theory and quantitative ideas are accepted as useful only insomuch as they help the reductionist drive to look at smaller and smaller pieces of the organism in the hope of understanding the whole more completely.

This process of reduction, so central to modern biology's mode of operation, is often attributed to Descartes and it is often called "Cartesian Reductionism." It is possible that if Descartes were alive today he would take strong issue with this identification. As well as being a philosopher, Descartes was also a biologist and mathematician. In his *Rules for the Direction of the Mind*, he exhorted that we need not investigate "what others have thought nor what we ourselves conjecture, but what we can *intuit* (our emphasis) clearly and evidently or deduce with certainty, for there is no other way to acquire knowledge." This, upon first examination seems to be a clear exhortation toward the empiricists' approach. However, the fact that he put so much stock in intuition must also be seen in the context of his ability to reason mathematically. Given this ability, he could easily see the need for the examination of the natural objects he sought to understand. But, where would he have been without the mathematical background? Later in the same work, he said, "Intuition is the undoubting conception of a pure and attentative mind, which arises from the light of reason alone, and which is more certain than deduction" (Kline 1980).

The so-called neo-romanticists, often identified with Theodore Roszak (Marx 1978), go far beyond this call for the use of intuition. Roszak (1979) speaks in terms of a holistic epistemology based on the use of human emotion as well as human reason to arrive at truth. While these views are generally vigorously rejected within the scientific community, we bring it up here because Roszak's holism is a reaction to the blind reductionism seen among so much of modern science and technology and as such makes a point which may be germane to the issue of animal rights. Roszak (1979) states, "... it became permissible for the scientist to admire the mechanical intricacy of nature, but not to love it as a living presence endowed with a soul and reflecting a higher order of reality. A machine can be studied zealously, but it cannot be loved." The suggestion is that the reductionist view allows its advocates to avoid facing the ethical questions by its mechanization and depersonalization of the objects of scientific investigation, especially those which are alive.

An Example

Before moving on to Network Thermodynamics, we would like to present an example to illustrate and summarize the various approaches that we have already presented. Suppose we present a television to a number of investigators (who have no previous knowledge of electronics) and ask them to explain how the TV works. The totally empiricist investigator would remove the back of the TV set and begin making measurements of currents, voltages, resistances, etc., ad infinitum. Given the complexity of a TV set (which is still far less than most biological systems), it seems extremely unlikely, if not impossible, that just collecting data will lead to an intuitive development of the network theory needed to understand the holistic behavior of the many subcircuits working together or the physics of the individual solid state components. The totally reductionist investigator might start by smashing the set with a sledge hammer and sorting out the pieces according to size, color, shape, where they end up after density gradient centrifugation, etc. They might then look at the carbon, silicon, and germanium crystals in an x-ray diffraction machine. However, a TV set, like many biological systems, is hierarchical in its organization. It can also be broken down along more functional lines, i.e., supplying power, amplifying signals, etc. The molecular or "cellular" detail may only be incidental to understanding its function from this perspective. While something of value may be learned about the components, it again seems virtually impossible to understand how the TV works by ignoring the "circuit schematic diagram." Finally, the investigator who totally uses theoretical deduction might watch the TV for a while and then go off and devise a very complicated, formal mathematical theory to explain how the TV works. While there may well be some very interesting general knowledge that can be gained from the theory, the chances that the theory will correlate well with what is actually going on inside the TV is again extremely remote.

We would hope that by this time it is apparent that the best approach is one which stresses the strong interaction of both theory and experiment. With this example we have the hindsight of knowing how the TV and its components work. We understand that network theory, electromagnetic theory, and solid-state physics are all equally necessary to fully comprehend how a modern TV works and perhaps we also have a sense of the experimental input that went into the development of these theories. The application of these theories to the design of new and very complicated devices is now done in the electronics industry with computers using circuit simulation programs. New ideas are first modeled this way *before* any bench work is done. When the model works, then the device is built and tested and it is only when *both* the model and the experimental device agree that the understanding is complete and it goes into production. With this process in mind, we proceed to Network Thermodynamics.

Network Thermodynamics Modeling and Computer Simulation

About a decade ago, two independent proposals were made (Peusner 1983; Oster et al. 1971) to utilize the techniques of network theory as a tool to study complex interacting physicochemical systems such as those encountered in the description of biophysical processes. The innovative step was the realization that the formal structure of network theory was a good representation for other physical theories—thermodynamics in particular. In Network Thermodynamics, the topology of interactive systems, such as those in biology, is represented by means of interconnected network elements which dissipate, store, supply, or convert energy. In its "purest" sense it is an expansion of thermodynamic reasoning which uses concepts of topology, mainly graph theory, to include the structure or morphology of a system in its thermodynamic properties. In simple language, it allows us to "put together" into a functioning whole a lot of pieces we may have observed as parts of a complicated, organized system. This model of the functioning whole allows us to investigate the relationships between the whole and its parts. In a time when reductionist thinking is so prevalent, this is a significant conceptual step.

Network Thermodynamics is the product of the combination of thermodynamics with topological methods. It is important to realize that Network Thermodynamics is therefore completely independent from electronics and electrical network theory. In fact, electrical networks, which provide an excellent example of how the marriage of topology with the properties of single elements can be so very productive, can be considered as a special case of Network Thermodynamics in its broadest definition. Given the influence of reductionism in the basic sciences, it is perhaps not too surprising that the development of macroscopic approaches to highly organized, hierarchical systems became the domain of the engineering disciplines and was developed there first. In fact, it should be reassuring that this new approach readily and naturally incorporates what has been done in the past. It is not necessary to unlearn what we already know to utilize the added power of the network approach to organization. It is simply a matter of putting our existing thermodynamic notions into a broader framework which liberates us from most of the old constraints. Once we recognize, for example, that transport systems in membranes are capable of being phenomenologically described by Fick's law or a few, more complicated, relations such as the Michaelis-Menten scheme, we have a class of objects which are capable of being seen as "wired together" in a particular way in each distinct living system. A pattern develops and a network theory of life processes quickly emerges in the same way that electronic network theory evolved.

In biology, we seek to identify and characterize functional units that are typically more elusive than those in a TV and often must rely more strongly on the obvious morphological or biochemical units as a starting point in our analysis. The same reasoning leads to the recognition of an alternative generalization of the closure and conservation properties we usually call Kirchhoff's laws when applied to electrical networks. By examining the way the flows traverse a compartmentalized tissue, a network of flows can be described which obeys a Kirchhoff flow law, and by similarly noticing that the driving forces for biological processes follow a closure property around closed loops in any system, a Kirchhoff's force law arises.

If we notice that the transporter in a biological membrane, the chemical reaction, and the electrical resistance are all alike in that they are governed by some flow-force relation and are responsible for dissipation in the system, we can begin to talk about a class of biological network elements which we might call "dissipators." When inertial effects are present, such as in the pulsatile movement of blood or its change of direction in a curved blood vessel, an inductive form of energy storage is present. In Network Thermodynamics, the point is that these objects divide a system into *thermodynamic* elements since they each handle energy in distinctly different ways and furthermore, there is a small set of categories of objects which exhaust the ways in which energy can be handled. Together with the topology, which includes the conservation and closure properties we can now call Kirchhoff's flow and force laws, the system is completely defined. What emerges is a clear, simple, rigorous way to analyze any system with complex structure, especially living systems. Thus, a living system can be visualized in terms of a schematic which consists of dissipators (resistors), storage elements (capacitors), and so on.

So far, the emphasis has been implicitly focused on the *formulation* of a description and analysis of the living system using Network Thermodynamics. This would only be a hope for the future if it were not for the progress already made, mainly in circuit theory, in providing for the analysis of such systems. For this purpose, a number of powerful computer simulation programs have been created and provide a means for such analysis. We currently use the circuit simulation program, SPICE2, to solve our biological networks. Eventually new programs will be created for biological simulation which will not require the translation of the system's "schematic diagram" into a pseudo-electrical language before they can be simulated. The use of these circuit simulation programs may lead to the notion that Network Thermodynamics is "merely analog computing." Analog models, according to Jaynes (1976), are not really scientific models in the sense that they do not necessarily act as a hypothesis for explaining or understanding the object of study. "Instead, the analog is at every point generated by the thing it is an analog of." If we accept this definition, it will be clear that the type of models we are discussing resemble analogs very closely, but indeed are mainly used to test hypotheses and do indeed aim at understanding or explaining the object of study. The scope and depth of Network Thermodynamics far exceeds analog computing.

Network Thermodynamic modeling techniques offer many unique advantages over other approaches currently in use. Network Thermodynamic simulation is easy enough to do to allow models to actually be investigated by their originators and discarded or modified with little loss in time or effort. Unlike techniques using only higher mathematics, the fact that Network Thermodynamics rests on schematic depictions of a system rather than an explicit formulation in terms of equations makes it far more accessible to the non-theoretician, while still retaining its complete mathematical rigor. It is intuitively easier to visualize physical processes using the drawings of network theory than the formalism of topology. The topology of networks adds a systematic method for specifying connections to the mathematics of physics and chemistry, which are basically poor in these relations. And most importantly, network theory provides algorithms for interconnecting and representing functional systems, whether linear or nonlinear, reciprocal or not, and allows an infinite number of possibilities to represent these systems on an organized basis. As such, networks serve to represent differential equations by discrete, computable algorithms. The availability of powerful (and cheap) circuit simulation computer programs, which can represent thousands of interconnected points, puts the power of network theory at the fingertips of practically anybody with an imaginative application. Specifically, some of the fields in which Network Thermodynamic modeling has begun to be used are the cellular pharmacokinetics of an anticancer drug, methotrexate (White 1979; White and Mikulecky 1982), filtration in the glomerulus of the kidney (Oken et al. 1981), whole body pharmacokinetics (Thakker et al. 1982), the effects of insulin on glucose transport and metabolism in adipocytes (May and Mikulecky 1982,1983), calcium uptake by the sarcoplasmic reticulum (Feher and Briggs 1982), volume and salt flow in the rat ileum (Fidelman and Mikulecky 1982) and kidney proximal tubule (Thomas and Mikulecky 1978), and hormone regulation of ion transport in cultured kidney epithelia (Fidelman and Mikulecky 1985).

Model Verification

One of the most brilliant scientists of our time was Aharon Katchalsky. He was one of the prime movers in the quest for a method for modeling the complex organization found in living systems. The quest for him as well as the quest for us ended with the discovery of Network Thermodynamics. Katchalsky was also a careful enough scientist to worry about the ability to create useless, unverifiable models. One of his fondest quotations was: "With four unknown parameters you can draw an elephant. With a fifth, you can also wag his tail."

This concern is, in part, a valid one. Fortunately, a large amount of work has now been done on the verification of models (Walter 1982: Carson et al. 1983; Mikulecky 1981, 1983). By model verification, we mean the evaluation of a model with respect to the uniqueness of its representation of the real system and to the one-to-one correlation of model parameters with the real system parameters at all the hierarchical levels in the model. So far, although this has already become a field in its own right, the scope of the results obtained is very limited. The kinds of models which are best evaluated by this body of work are linear compartmental models of small size. In some of our latest work, we try to show how Network Thermodynamics can bring in additional mathematical constraints on models to help characterize them more completely. Also, in those cases where more rigorous analytical methods fail, parameter estimation is possible by trial and error methods using simulation. Thus we can expect that Network Thermodynamics will continue to serve to help evaluate models both by analytical methods as well as simulation.

Concluding Remarks

In our discussion of Network Thermodynamics, we have focused more on the conceptual framework of this approach than on a practical "how to" guide. We refer the reader to Thakker et al. (1982), White (1979), White and Mikulecky (1982), May and Mikulecky (1982), and May and Mikulecky (1983) for some specific, and not too difficult examples of the application of these techniques. We would also welcome direct contact with anyone interested in learning more about using Network Thermodynamics. As a general rule, it is not our intent to become "expert modelers" for others, but to teach and assist those who wish to learn for themselves how to do theory-directed modeling using the Network Thermodynamic approach.

The predominance of empiricism and reductionism in modern biological and biomedical research has led to a situation where the finite resources available are mainly used to generate an overabundance of data with little, or no, real scientific meaning. This lack of a basic theoretical foundation in biology also produces little real scientific criteria for judging quality of research. In our opinion, the diversion of significant resources from experimental work into the development of theory and theory-directed modeling will achieve a much better scientific result from a considerably reduced number of experiments. It is our belief that in Network Thermodynamics we have the necessary framework to begin bridging the gap between theory and experiment in biology.

Acknowledgements

We extend our thanks and gratitude to Betty Lou LaJoy for her energy in being the catalyst behind the writing of this paper and for her insights into the importance of Network Thermodynamics in moving biological research in a new direction that will begin to be more compatible with animal rights. We would also like to thank Dr. Sheella Mierson for her asistance in reviewing this manuscript.

M.L. Fidelman is the recipient of a grant from the Whitaker Foundation.

References

Carson, E.R., Cobelli, C. and Finkelstein, L. 1983. *The Mathematical Modeling of Metabolic and Endocrine Systems: Model Formulation, Identification, and Validation.* New York: Wiley.

Chua, L.O. 1969. *Introduction to Non-linear Network Theory.* New York: McGraw Hill.

Eisenfeld, J. and DeLisi, C. 1984. On conditions for qualitative instability of regulatory circuits with application to immunological control loops. *Symposium on Mathematics and Computers in Biomedical Applications.* NIH Publication No. 84-2705, p. 13.

Feher, J.J. and Briggs, F.N. 1982. The effect of calcium load on the calcium permeability of sarcoplasmic reticulum. *J. Biol. Chem.* 257:10191-9.

Fidelman, M.L. and Mikulecky, D.C. 1982. Network thermodynamic modeling of isotonic coupled flows in the rat ileum. *Physiologist* 25(4):334.

Fidelman, M.L. and Mikulecky, D.C. 1985. Network thermodynamic modeling of insulin and aldosterone stimulation of Na^+ transport in cultured renal epithelia. *Biophys. J.* 47:445a.

Jaynes, J. 1976. *The Origin of Consciousness in the Breakdown of the Bicameral Mind.* Boston: Houghton Mifflin.

Kline, M. 1980. *Mathematics: The Loss of Certainty.* New York: Oxford.

Mahoney, M.J. 1976. *Scientist as Subject: The Psychological Imperative.* Cambridge: Ballinger.

Marx, L. 1978. Reflections on the Neo-Romantic critique of science. *Proc. Am. Acad. Arts and Sci.* 107(2):61-74.

May, J. and Mikulecky, D.C. 1982. The simple model of adipocyte hexose transport: Kinetic features, effect of insulin, and network thermodynamic computer simulation. *J. Biol. Chem.* 257:11601-8.

May, J. and Mikulecky, D.C. 1983. Glucose utilization in rat adipocytes: The interaction of transport and metabolism as affected by insulin. *J. Biol. Chem.* 258:4771-7.

Mikulecky, D.C. 1981. Further uses of network simulation. In: Kuczera, J. Grygorczyk, C. and Przestalski, S. eds. *Biophysics of Membrane Transport IV.* Wroclaw, Poland: Agricultural Acad. Part II. p. 209-35.

Mikulecky, D.C. 1983. Network Thermodynamics: A candidate for a common language for theoretical and experimental biology. *Am. J. Physiol.* 245:R1-9.

Mikulecky, D.C. 1984. Network Thermodynamics: A simulation and modeling method based on the extension of thermodynamic thinking into the realm of highly organized systems. *Math. Biosciences.* 72:157-79.

Murphy, E.A. 1982. Muddling, meddling, and modeling. In: Anderson, V.E., Hauser, W.A., Penry, J.K., and Sing, C.F. eds. *Genetic Basis of the Epilepsies.* New York: Raven Press. p. 333-48.

Oken, D.E., Thomas, S.R. and Mikulecky, D.C. 1981. A network thermodynamic model of glomerular dynamics: Application in the rat. *Kidney Int.* 19:359-73.

Oster, G.F., Perelson, A. and Katchalsky, A. 1971. Network Thermodynamics. *Nature.* 234:393-9.

Peusner, L. 1983. The principles of network thermodynamic theory and biophysical application. Lincoln, MA: Entropy. (Reprint of Ph.D. Thesis, Harvard Univ., 1970.)

Platt, J.R. 1964. Strong inference. *Sci.* 146:347-53.

Roszak, T. 1979. Science, knowledge, and gnosis. *Proc. Am. Acad. Arts and Sci.* 103(3):17-32.

Singer, P. 1985. Ten years of animal liberation. *N.Y. Rev. Books.* Jan. 17:46-57.

Thakker, K.M., Wood, J.H. and Mikulecky, D.C. 1982. Dynamic simulation of pharmacokinetic systems using the electrical circuit analysis program SPICE2. *Comp. Prog. Biomed.* 15:61-72.

Thomas, S.R. and Mikulecky, D.C. 1978. A network thermodynamic model of salt and water flow across the kidney proximal tubule. *Am. J. Physiol.* 235:F638-48.

Thom, R. 1975. *Structural Stability and Morphogenesis*. Reading: Benjamin.

Thom, R. 1979. "Answer to Cristopher Zeeman's Reply." In: *Dynamic Systems – Warwick, 1979*. New York: Springer-Verlag. Lecture Notes in Mathematics #468, p. 384-5.

Walter, E. 1982. *Identifiability of State Space Models*. New York: Springer-Verlag.

White, J.C. 1979. Reversal of methotrexate binding to dihydrofolate reductase by dihydrofolate: Studies with pure enzyme and computer modeling using network thermodynamics. *J. Biol. Chem.* 254:10889-95.

White, J.C. and Mikulecky, D.C. 1982. Application of network thermodynamics to the computer modeling of the pharmacology of anticancer agents: A network model for methotrexate action as a comprehensive example. *Pharmacol. Ther.* 15:251-91.

Yates, F.E. 1978. Good manners in good modeling: Mathematical models and computer simulation of physiological systems. *Am. J. Physiol.* 234:R159-60.

Yates, F.E. 1979. Comparative physiology: Compared to what? *Am. J. Physiol.* 237:R1-2.

APPLICATIONS OF LABORATORY TECHNOLOGY IN THE EVALUATION OF THE RISK OF RABIES TRANSMISSIONS BY BITING DOGS AND CATS

Donald C. Blenden
Manuel J. Torres-Anjel
and F.T. Satalowich

Epidemiology and Public Health
College of Veterinary Medicine
University of Missouri
Columbia, Missouri 65211

Introduction

While rabies is not a common disease in domestic animal species of the United States, potential exposures to rabies in the form of bites are very common and increasing. A nationwide study conducted among general hospitals shows that 1 percent of emergency room visits are for animal bites, of which 80-90 percent are inflicted by the dog (Callaham 1980). This figure is conservative, as the study did not include pediatric hospitals, the bite of victims that progress only to a physician's office, or those that receive no medical care at all. In Missouri alone, this study would infer about 1500 dog bites per year reaching only the general hospital. The number of dog and other animal bites across the country is unknown but may safely be assumed to be staggering in magnitude.

The risk of acquiring rabies from an animal bite is one of the important considerations in medical treatment. While a significant number of the many bites are inflicted by the dog, the Center for Disease Control (CDC) reports an approximate figure of only 153 confirmed cases of rabies in the dog for 1982 across the United States. This figure is down from a high of about 250 in 1980 (U.S. Department of Health and Human Services 1983). This means that there is an inordinant difference between the number of bites and the number of cases of dog rabies; but, who at the time of a bite incident, can determine which biting animal is the one carrying rabies? The bite victim *is* one of a staggering yearly number; the biting animal is *probably* one of the large number which bites, but does not carry rabies. But, which is which? At the time of the bite incident, decisions must be faced concerning whether or not to treat the bitten person against rabies, and although all necessary information is often not available, the decisions must be made and cannot wait. The same principle of assessment applies to an animal which is bitten by a potentially rabid dog or cat, although the end consequences differ somewhat.

A scientifically accurate method of determining the rabies risk presented by the bite of an animal is to examine its brain tissue by immunofluorescence microscopy, sometimes supplemented by the inoculation of brain tissue into white mice. Properly treated and examined, the tissue containing rabies virus will fluoresce when examined under an ultraviolet microscope and brain tissue not containing rabies virus will not fluoresce; mice inoculated with tissue containing rabies virus will develop rabies, and those inoculated with virus-free tissue will not develop rabies. Brain examination has been a time-honored way of determining whether an animal that bites is infected with rabies in order to determine the risk of the bite to the person or animal bitten. The accuracy of brain examination via immunofluorescence microscopy approaches 100 percent both in sensitivity and specificity.*

An alternative to this drastic procedure is to confine the biting dog or cat for ten days and immediately obtain a reliable diagnosis of any illness present at the time of the bite, or any which develops within the period of confinement. This procedure is based on experimental observations conducted in the early 1960's. These observations ascertained that the dog or cat that is incubating rabies may have virus in its saliva for a maximum of three to four days prior to the development of the first symptoms of the disease (Vaughn et al. 1963, 1965). Thus, the healthy-appearing dog or cat that produces a rabies-dangerous bite and is confined will almost certainly be sick with rabies within the ten-day period. If it does not develop illness during the period, it can be assumed that the bite was not a rabies exposure. While a few exceptions to this rule have subsequently been described (lowering slightly the sensivitity), they are regarded as rarities and changes in bite management for these rarities is not warranted. It should be stressed that a confinement procedure is acceptable only for management of bites inflicted by the dog and cat; our knowledge of rabies in other species is inadequate to allow us to expand this procedure to include them. Indeed, there is

*A detailed discussion of sensitivity and specificity of tests follows.

considerable reason to believe that other species (especially wild animal species) present an entirely different and increased risk. Thus, the confinement procedure for the dog and cat is another testing procedure approaching 100 percent in sensitivity and specificity.

A last alternative in the management of animal bites is to do nothing with respect to the potential of rabies exposure. While this is often the desire of the person responsible for the actions of the offending dog or cat, it can well be seen that the person or animal bitten is thereby placed into a category of much higher risk of contracting rabies from the bite. When bites are particularly serious and the risk of rabies is high, the bitten person is often started on antirabies treatment pending results of the confinement period. When the confined animal reaches the ten-day period in perfect health (with respect to rabies) it then becomes obvious that the initiation of treatment was unnecessary and can be stopped; but the risk in waiting to start is too high.

Today's alternatives in the handling of bites by the dog and cat are thus limited to those which either kill the animal, confine the animal (producing expense and a waiting period) or do nothing, the latter placing the person bitten at greater risk. All alternatives are characterized by great anxiety and emotional stress on the part of all parties involved. It is natural and necessary that serious bites are associated with increased pressures to conduct brain examination rather than confine the animal for ten days.

Until about twenty-five years ago, the dog was a principle reservoir of rabies in the United States, and the risk of dog bites transmitting rabies was consequently very high; indeed, the dog is still a principle reservoir worldwide. The main reservoir of rabies in the United States today has become the wildlife species, specifically the skunk, racoon, and several species of bat. The cat remains important as a biting species, and although these animals were not historically considered a significant reservoir of rabies, this situation is changing. The CDC reports that in 1981, the number of confirmed cases of rabies in cats (275) surpassed those in dogs (225) for the first time since 1975. Although the confirmed cases of rabies in both species have fallen in the ensuing years, the cat still leads the dog.

One attempt to improve the handling of bite cases has been accomplished in this twenty-five year period. That is the concept of "rabies-free areas," in which cases of rabies have not occurred in carnivores for a long period of time, and therefore the bites of carnivores carry greatly reduced risk of transmitting rabies (Marr and Beck 1976). Here, the difference between "very low" risk and "no" risk becomes important. Seldom can it be said that the rabies risk of a bite is absolutely zero; but it can be said that the risk of the bite transmitting rabies might be comparable to or lower than the risk of taking antirabies treatment, which, after all, is also very low, but not zero.

Improvements in the medical management of animal bites to prevent rabies have occured because of the improvement of vaccines used for humans, not in the prevention of the need for the vaccine. While the vaccines are infinitely improved, they are still expensive, not totally risk-free, and tend to escalate the anxiety of a bite situation rather than producing a pallative effect as they are a defensive tool.

Concurrent with the decrease of rabies in the dog, the importance of the dog as a biting species has increased greatly. As a result, today we have the situation wherein the dog is much more likely to inflict bites, and is less likely to transmit rabies, but the technology of evaluation of the risk of rabies from bites has remained essentially the same. We still decapitate, however humanely, large numbers of dogs and cats in order to examine their brain tissue. Again, this is scientifically adequate or even ideal *technology*, but seems to be a grossly exaggerated and insensitive *response*, when it is clear that the rabies risk has greatly diminished. It is easily determined after the fact which death was necessary and which was not, but there are large numbers of dogs and cats sacrificed annually in order to find the relative few that present the risk of rabies. It seems logical that the application of modern technology can markedly lessen the need for brain examination; such technology is now available.

Following the idea that the treatment response often seems to be exaggerated in regards to animal bites of humans, we have conducted research with an overriding goal to lessen the need for the killing (and perhaps even some confinement) of animals for bite evaluation. Towards this goal, we hope to develop or apply existing technology in order to lessen the need for this killing and to contribute to the alleviation of the tremendous emotional distress produced in persons with real or imagined exposure to rabies or those who suffer the loss of a valued animal in order to conduct an examination. Making widely available the new and existing technology so it can be employed in the routine assessment of animal bites can lend supplemental, objectively obtained evidence to the body of information used to develop judgements regarding the relative risk of dog and cat bites. While the application of laboratory methods can improve evaluations, it is no panacea. The methodology will not answer all questions, and will not save much money, but it should allow more accurate assessments to be made and eliminate the killing of many animals. It will also reduce the number of antirabies treatments considered to be necessary, and grossly decrease the anxiety levels which so often commonly accompany bites. The employment of these new methods which depart from traditions and the confidence which is conferred by upon them by time and usage, requires that one differentiate between, and act on, the basis of degrees of risk. It is also essential that the desirability of preserving, rather than destroying, animal lives when appropriate be adopted as a goal.

Today, the philosophy of brain examination most frequently is to justify why it should not occur. By adopting a positive attitude and employing laboratory methods to substantiate the opinions involved, the question then can become how brain examination is justified in each instance. To be perfectly clear, this discussion centers upon dog and cat bites only and applies to no other species. Indeed, realistically, brain examinations will not be eliminated entirely in the foreseeable future for any species, but the recent advances in technological knowledge should, in the long term, benefit both society and dogs and cats.

In addition to overcoming tradition, new technologies may encounter legal or regulatory obstacles. For example, many communities have ordinances requiring confinement and observation of biting dogs and cats for a period of ten days. Other ordinances require annual immunization of dogs and cats, but do not allow for the utilization of improved vaccines that produce two or three years duration of immunity. Such ordinances are slowly being replaced with those recognizing appropriate technological advancement. As our knowledge about rabies in wild animals indicates that the disease behaves differently in these cases, it is the sad reality that these bite incidences must still be handled in the traditional way. Considerable research must be done to determine the feasibility of new diagnostic technology when applied to wildlife, since laboratory assessment of the living wild animal may not answer the necessary questions, thereby endangering human life.

How Are Bites Handled Today?

Situation A: A dog* bites a person and promptly escapes, never to be seen again. What should be done?

The dog is gone, so no testing on it is possible. Unless the dog was accurately identified and its history known, the animal is a "stray." The only way to evaluate the probability of an exposure to rabies is for an experienced advisor to reconstruct the circumstances of the bite as accurately as possible. Any and all characteristics of the animal such as its species, its behavior or signs of illness at the time of the bite, evidence of provocation, any suggestion that the animal was known in the neighborhood to be a chronic "biter," knowledge of its vaccination status, the level of rabies infection in the community or many other factors which may help to assess the situation must be evaluated. Some situations can then be logically decided to be *low* in risk, others may be decided to be *high* risk ("low" risk can only rarely be interpreted to mean "no" risk). Most persons can decide for themselves on the level of risk they

*While the dog is used as an example, the discussion also applies to the cat.

wish to undertake *if* they are presented with factual and objective understanding of the situation. The decision to treat or not treat with antirabies globulin and vaccine then becomes a bit more automatic.

Unfortunately, expert advisory services on animal disease and behavior are not always easily available or even less commonly consulted. These services should be made more widely available (many state health departments do not employ a veterinarian) and used to avoid unnecessary treatments, risk, and expense. The expert advisor should be a physician and/or veterinarian who is experienced and knowledgeable of the subtleties of rabies. Many persons are treated unnecessarily (Schnurrenberger et al. 1969) because physicians do not have access to the needed advice concerning the animal, and the risk of *not* treating is perceived as too great.

Situation B: A dog bites a person, is clearly sick or acting abnormally, and is confined and available for examination.

The illness of the animal should be evaluated by a veterinarian as soon as possible. If the animal has a diagnoseable illness other than rabies, the chance of a concurrent infection with rabies is remote. If the animal was hit by a car or some such incident, one must question: why was it hit? It could have been hit because of inability to react properly due to illness, perhaps rabies. Unless the illness is diagnosed with great certainty, it must be assumed to be rabies until proven otherwise; undiagnosed paralytic or neurologic disease carries high risk. This means either confinement to see how the illness progresses (rabies will usually progress and worsen within two or three days) or immediate laboratory examination, or both. "Laboratory examination" today means an examination of the brain for evidence of rabies virus. If a veterinarian is not available to examine the animal, the risk of erroneous diagnosis increases.

Situation C: A healthy-appearing dog bites a person, is captured, and is known to be a friendly type of dog.

The aggressive behavior of the animal must be interpreted as *normal* (if the animal is mistreated, injured, otherwise stressed or threatened) or *abnormal* (abnormal behavior is an early sign of rabies). The interpretation of the behavior must be done by an experienced person and the "provoked" or "unprovoked" bite must be viewed as through the eyes of the dog or cat, not the person evaluating. As an example, an animal will bite because of invasion of what it regards as its territory, which will have nothing at all to do with its owner's property line. So, the unprovoked bite (abnormal behavior) must be regarded as caused by rabies until proven otherwise. The bite because of provocation can be considered normal behavior, and so the risk is considerably lower. However, animals can carry rabies virus in the saliva before they begin to show symptoms (three to four days in the dog and cat). Therefore, the provoked bite of the healthy animal can transmit rabies, although the relative risk of this is much lower. The animal delivering a provoked bite, while presenting less risk of transmitting rabies virus, should be confined for ten days. At the first sign of illness during that period, immediate diagnosis and (often) brain examination is needed.

The unprovoked bite is considered a rabies risk until proven otherwise, as the bite is then regarded to be a symptom of illness, and immediate brain examination is needed. In a mild bite situation, confinement and observation is sometimes appropriate but in a serious bite situation, the risk increases and decisive action is essential.

Situation D: A healthy-appearing dog bites a person, is captured, and is known to be an aggressive dog or habitual biter.

The aggressive behavior can be regarded as normal, and that behavior can be expected to be magnified if the animal is provoked. The risk of rabies transmission from a normally aggressive animal is perhaps less to the person bitten than a bite by a normally placid dog. By the same token, the aggressive dog is more likely to inflict more serious bites, which increases the risk of rabies infection if the virus should happen to be present. Even though the bite likely reflects normal behavior, there is still the risk of the animal carrying rabies virus the few days before it shows symptoms. This dog or cat should be confined for ten days and/or brain examined immediately. If confinement is elected, an immediate diagnosis and perhaps brain examination is mandatory if illness develops.

It is the bites of these two latter categories of healthy-appearing dogs that encompasses the majority of bites (excluding those where the animal escapes), and also have lower risk of rabies transmission than the bites of sick animals. From these groups there are tremendous numbers of animals that are (necessarily) confined and/or brain-examined. There is much room for subjective interpretations of these situations: what is abnormal versus normal, provoked versus unprovoked, healthy versus unhealthy, mild exposure risk (to the person bitten) versus serious exposure to rabies, and so on? We desperately need a better way to supplement and make objective determinations to reduce needless confinements and killings, while not sacrificing the safety of the persons bitten and exposed.

Consider also the following. The circumstances considered in determining whether or not a bite was provoked are almost always viewed by only a few persons, and those persons are often subject to tremendous influence of observer bias; e.g., the child who is unable or unwilling to accurately recount the event, or the defensive and devoted owner whose dog "can inflict no wrong." In either case, or the myriad of variations on the same theme, the description of the event is relayed less than objectively. This information is then recounted to another party, often a medical person, always with the best of intentions but often with high levels of anxiety. Thus, it is up to the medical professional to assure that adequate information is elicited, and to proceed with appropriate decisions with the best information that is available. Although only 2-30 percent of dog bites in urban areas are attributed to ownerless animals (Beck 1981), perhaps as high as 50 percent of bites in rural areas are from animals that cannot be identified or captured for observation. These animals present a dangerous situation, as they have a greater likelihood of having been exposed to wildlife vectors of rabies virus. Therefore, the history of the animal is often the only resource available in these cases upon which to base treatment decisions. The obviously sick animal presents a well appreciated and easily interpreted risk. The real problem situations commonly boil down to questions of relative risk of the healthy biting dog or cat being *subclinically* infected with rabies but fully capable of transmitting the disease.

Consider also the relative risk of the *provoked* bite of an *apparently healthy* dog in the following geographical areas:

a. New York City
b. rural Colorado (all rabies is rare in Colorado)
c. rural Missouri (canine rabies occurs sporadically)
d. a tropical foreign country (canine rabies is common)

It can be seen that the relative risk of the bites varies greatly (the basis for "rabies-free areas"); the bite of a dog in rural Missouri or in a foreign country must be considered a significant risk until proven otherwise. (It is clear that the geographical area in which the bite occurs must also be considered; this discussion focuses primarily on the United States.) Is the rabies risk of a given bite zero, 1:1,000,000, 1:1,000 or higher? The answer is seldom either zero or absolute. However, most anxiety stricken parents of even a severely bitten child can deal with the situation and decide upon the level of risk that is tolerable to them *if* they are given straightforward facts and answers to their questions and credible professional opinion. When answers are unavailable, fuzzy, or conflicting, the anxiety levels escalate.

In summary, the options available in the handling of a biting dog or cat are limited. They are:

a. Do nothing—this is undesirable in the eyes of the *bitee*, but often is the position of those in charge of the *bitor*.
b. Confine the biting dog or cat for ten days from the date of the bite to observe for the appearance of diagnoseable illness (confinement is frequently accomplished with difficulty for a variety of reasons).
c. Kill it immediately to examine the brain.

How Can Bites Be Better Handled Using New Technology?

Situation A: A dog bites a person and promptly escapes, never to be seen again. What better can be done?

The dog is gone so that no sampling can be done. However, the widespread knowledge that new technology is available will stimulate more lay persons, veterinarians, and physicians to seek out expert assistance. Advisors to these situations can use the best knowledge in behavioral and risk assessment. In other words, functioning laboratories will provide a focus to upgrade the entire advisory effort, even when laboratory services are inappropriate or impossible.

Occasionally, the person bitten has previously received antirabies treatment or vaccine; the blood of the person can be tested for antibodies to determine if adequate protection is already afforded from the previous immunization. In some cases, it is desirable to take a blood sample to determine the antibody level after the series of injections is completed (this is not routinely the case), to assure that the person has in fact responded to the vaccine. The increased use of advisory services, and the analysis of blood of certain persons exposed for antibodies should decrease the need for the use of antirabies vaccine.

Situation B: A dog bites a person, is clearly sick or acting abnormally, and is confined and available for examination.

The animal should be evaluated by a veterinarian immediately who should make a tentative diagnosis of the illness, securing appropriate samples for analysis. If there is a discreet, diagnosable illness involved or at least one that is clearly distinguishable from rabies, the probability of concurrent infection with rabies virus is remote, but not impossible. However, a positive response to treatment of that illness is incompatible with and lessens the likelihood of the animal being ill with the virus. If the animal has a blood antibody titer against rabies virus (the higher the titer the more reliable), the chance of it being infected by a previous exposure to rabies is remote (Koprowski et al. 1954; Dean et al. 1964; Cabasso 1965; Baer 1975; Fekadu and Shaddock 1984). A blood serum titer in response to rabies virus infection appears and rises during the clinical course of the illness (Hattwick and Gregg 1975; Anderson et al. 1984) and must be carefully interpreted along with the clinical condition of the animal. A reliable history of immunization would explain a high or very early titer and make rabies virus infection most unlikely. If the animal does not have a titer of significance, the decision of provocation or lack of provocation and further evaluation become important; if a negative titer converts to positive, or a low titer increases, rabies infection is established.

If evidence of unprovoked biting, and neurological or paralytic illness exists, immediate examination of brain tissue or skin biopsy specimens is strongly indicated, and the need can be balanced by the nature and severity of the bite exposure with the desirability of salvaging the animal.

If the illness is not strongly suggestive of being rabies, examination of skin biopsy specimens is indicated. In one study (Blenden et al. 1983), 133 animals (including many dogs and cats) with naturally occurring, undiagnosed illness, were tested for rabies virus using skin biopsy examination. Sixty-eight of seventy animals (97 percent) that were ultimately proven to have rabies had positive skin biopsy examinations. All of the sixty-three animals that were proven not to have rabies had negative skin biopsy results. These results are signficant because the animals did produce potential exposure of humans to rabies. This study thus suggests that such examination has high but not absolute sensitivity, and can of course be repeated should that be appropriate, as the passage of time (during the course of rabies) will make the next examination more likely to be positive (Blenden et al. 1983). As rabies in dogs and cats is unusual, the biopsy test results are most likely to be negative; the negative result must be considered within the context of the entire situation, and not taken as the last word. Following a negative biopsy, the animal is still alive, and the bite situation may dictate further evaluation.

In addition to skin and blood, cerebrospinal fluid can also be examined. Analysis of cerebrospinal fluid for antirabies antibodies will help demonstrate the immunization status of the dog, and whether this antibody is present as the result of vaccination. Thus, the dog that is sick and has an uncertain history of vaccination can be tested. If an antibody is present in the blood and absent in the cerebrospinal fluid, the dog can tentatively be assumed to not have rabies, and is still alive for appropriate observation. If the blood contains no antibody, it does not mean the illness is rabies, merely that the dog is more likely to be susceptible to rabies. If antibody is present in cerebrospinal fluid, and not in the blood, present or past infection with rabies virus is suggested (Bell 1975). Anderson et al. (1984) state that blood serum and cerebrospinal fluid antibody appear at about the same time in their sampling of human cases.

Situation C: A healthy-appearing dog bites a person, is captured, and is known to be a friendly type of dog.

The basic question in this situation is whether the bite reflects normal and expected behavior of the animal, or is an act of unexplained aggression, symptomatic of rabies. If the animal has a significant blood antibody titer (as from immunization) it is most unlikely that rabies infection is involved, although still not impossible. If the blood is negative, the possibility of rabies infection is not ruled out, but a second blood sample would likely show a titer if rabies was involved. As the skin biopsy test is relatively accurate in detecting rabies in a sick individual, a positive result is meaningful and high sensitivity is expected if rabies encephelitis has progressed to the point of producing biting behavior.

An animal in this category, healthy-appearing, having inflicted a bite under unprovoked conditions, and with a negative blood and skin biopsy, must be further assessed for the possibility of being a presymptomatic carrier. Therefore, further clinical observation, another skin biopsy (no less than three days after the first), and a repeat blood antibody level are indicated; all, however, on a living animal.

Situation D: A healthy-appearing dog bites a person, is captured, and is known to be an aggressive dog or habitual biter.

On the assumption that the bite was normal behavior for the dog, the remaining risk is to determine the likelihood that the dog is a presymptomatic carrier (i.e., incubating the disease, possibly shedding virus in the saliva, and destined to develop rabies within a ten-day observation period). The finding of blood antibody indicates that the dog has resistance to rabies virus and is most unlikely to be incubating the disease; its bite is therefore not considered a rabies exposure. Assuming the dog *was* actively incubating rabies (and the bite was thus dangerous), there is an estimated 25 percent chance that the skin examination would be positive. That chance increases every day that passes from that time on. Therefore, a negative biopsy should be followed by observation and perhaps another biopsy in three to five days, especially if the serum antibody test is negative. Serum antibody will appear if infection is present.

What Are The Strengths And Weaknesses of Application of These Methods?

The addition of specific technology of defined sensitivity to detect the presence of rabies virus infection can add significant confidence to existing methods of evaluation. It is quite feasible that observation periods can be reduced in many cases, although they cannot be eliminated. Conversely, it may on occasion be desirable to confine a few days longer than ten (perhaps fourteen), particularly dogs having had rabies exposure outside the United States (Fekadu et.al. 1982). The killing of dogs and cats to examine brain tissue can be reduced to only the most essential cases. The overall quality of risk assessments of bite cases should markedly improve, reducing the need for antirabies treatments in many cases; this will occur simply as medical professionals better realize that alternatives are available. As the technology is highly specialized, the services can be available in relatively few laboratories in the United States. The shipment of specimens unfortunately requires more time than the laboratory examinations. A distinct weakness of skin biopsy technology is that *early* clinical cases of rabies are detected at perhaps a 50 to 90 percent sensitivity level when 100 percent sensitivity is desirable; however, occasional cases are positive even before the onset of symptoms. Sensivity of the testing is adequate, however, to justify application as long as the results obtained are used in the proper context of the entire clinical situation. As is true with most laboratory tests for diagnosis of disease, complete reliance on a single technique is seldom justified. Some costs involved in confinement and antirabies treatments will be reduced, however, overall costs will not be reduced because of surgical and laboratory fees.

An important question in evaluating dog and cat bites relates to the immunization status of the animal. While rabies vaccine, when properly administered, is highly effective, it is not absolute in protective capability (as is true with any vaccine). Some animals inherently do not have the ability to respond adequately, and this fact cannot be known without highly specific testing. Also, improperly handled or administered vaccine loses immunogenicity. The properly immunized dog or cat has a minimal chance of contracting rabies if exposed. Exposure to a large dose of virus (as by the bite of a rabid skunk) can override the immunity, particularly if it is waning due to the passage of time. If the immunization history is inadequate or unreliable, it will not help the evaluation of rabies risk of a bite.

The presence of an anti-rabies antibody titer in the blood reveals much about the resistance of the animal to natural infection. Most properly immunized animals will respond with a blood titer, although a few may not. However, it is important to realize that those that do not respond with a titer probably have resistance to the infection anyway because of cellular forms of immunity not detectable by examination of blood serum. Conversely, an occasional animal with an antirabies titer can be infected with rabies virus (Dean et al. 1964) due to a large dose of virus in the exposure or inadequate cellular response within the animal. Very large challenge doses of virus probably are rather common in artificially induced rabies, and are not as likely to occur in nature.

An additional use of serological testing in evaluating the immune status of an animal is to administer one dose of rabies vaccine and secure a blood antibody titer two to three days afterwards. If the animal has been previously immunized, there should be a significant (and rapidly rising) antibody titer at that time. An animal that responds in a positive manner to this test, has minimal chance of being actively infected with rabies virus.

The Procedures Involved

Specimens acquired from the animal under test are relatively simple to obtain. Circulating antibody is measured in the blood; blood is easily obtained in small quantity for the purpose. To secure cerebrospinal fluid to measure antibody which is useful in determining whether antibody has been produced by infection or immunization, requires light surgical anesthesia, clipping and disinfecting a small area of skin at the base of the skull (back of the neck) and insertion of a needle into the spinal canal at that point. Only one to two milliliters of fluid are required. The comparison of antibody titers in the blood and cerebrospinal fluid are presented in Table 1. These antibody levels are guidelines only and must be interpreted by a veterinarian experienced in their use; "low" and "high" are relative terms needing supporting information.

Table 1. Neutralizing antibody levels in blood serum and cerebrospinal fluid as a result of clinical rabies or immunization against rabies virus: Guidelines for interpretation.

	Antibody Level		
Status	Blood	Cerebrospinal Fluid	Change
Immunization	Negative to high	Negative or low*	Stable
Infection	Negative early: then low to high	Negative early; then low to high	Increases

*The physiologic ratio of antibody between cerebrospinal fluid and blood is 6:100 (Adapted from Bell 1975; Hattwick and Gregg 1975).

The biopsy of skin tissue to examine under the microscope is a minor surgical procedure. From the dog, the ideal anatomical site is known as the lateral cheek papilla, a small raised area on the cheek (one or two on each side), having three to four tactile hairs or "whiskers" growing from each. The follicles of these tactile hairs, in the deeper layers of the skin, are surrounded by a complex of nerve fibers, and it is in these nerve fibers that the rabies virus is found in the infected animal. The dog is given a light surgical anesthesia, or local anesthetic is carefully infiltrated around (not into) the area, the skin clipped and disinfected, and a small (¼" diameter) plug of skin removed, making sure that the follicles of tactile hairs are included. A special biopsy punch is used for this purpose. The hole in skin is usually not sutured, merely kept clean with antispetics, and heals rapidly. Should any unusual type of infection develop, the wound requires further veterinary attention.

The tissue specimen is placed into a small specimen container, protecting it from drying, and refrigerated or frozen for delivery to the laboratory, the specimen must be packaged and shipped refrigerated or in dry ice in a molded styrofoam shipping container, sufficient to maintain the tissue cold or frozen until delivery to the laboratory; the best taken specimen is worthless if it partially decomposes en route. The day seems close when skin specimens can be sent in 10% formalin, not requiring refrigeration at all, but, as of today, there is no substitute for refrigeration; formalinized brain or other nerve tissue can be accurately processed now (figure 1, 2, 3).

The specimen is cut into ultrathin sections (10 nm), stained with special reagents (for immunofluorescence or immunoperoxidase staining) which react specifically for rabies virus, and are then examined under an ordinary or ultraviolet microscope, depending upon the procedure being used. In rabies, the virus gathers together in small clusters that are visible microscopically.

There are other tissues which can be utilized as well, in exceptional circumstances, in order to evaluate a specific case. For example, smear

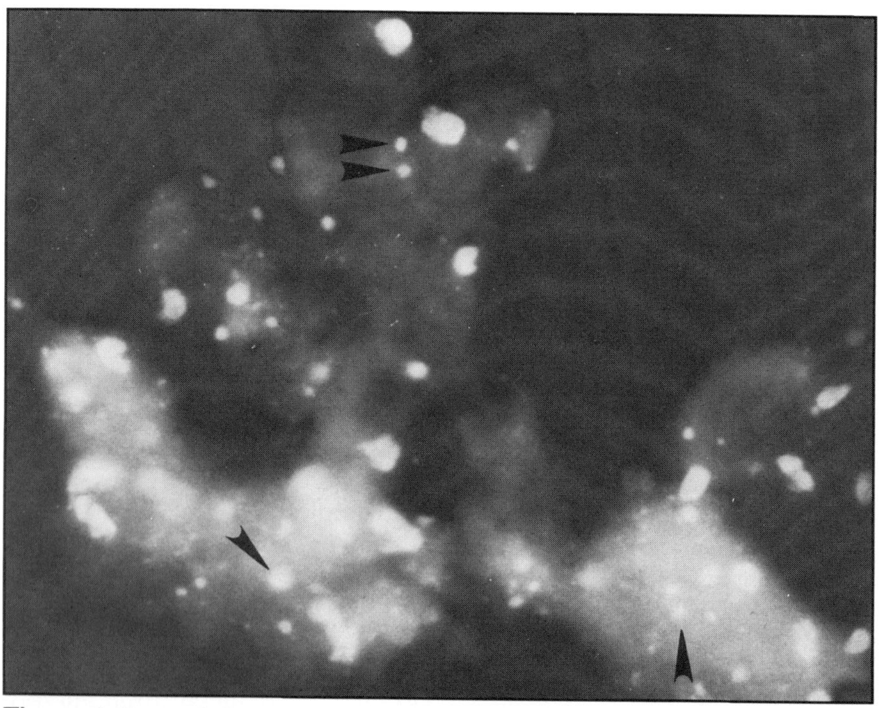

Figure 1: Fox cerebellum with natural rabies infection; immunofluorescent antirabies staining of tissue prepared by frozen sections. The tissue was stored in 10% formalin for three years and was not treated with trypsin. Magnification 1020X oil immersion, using ultraviolet illumination.

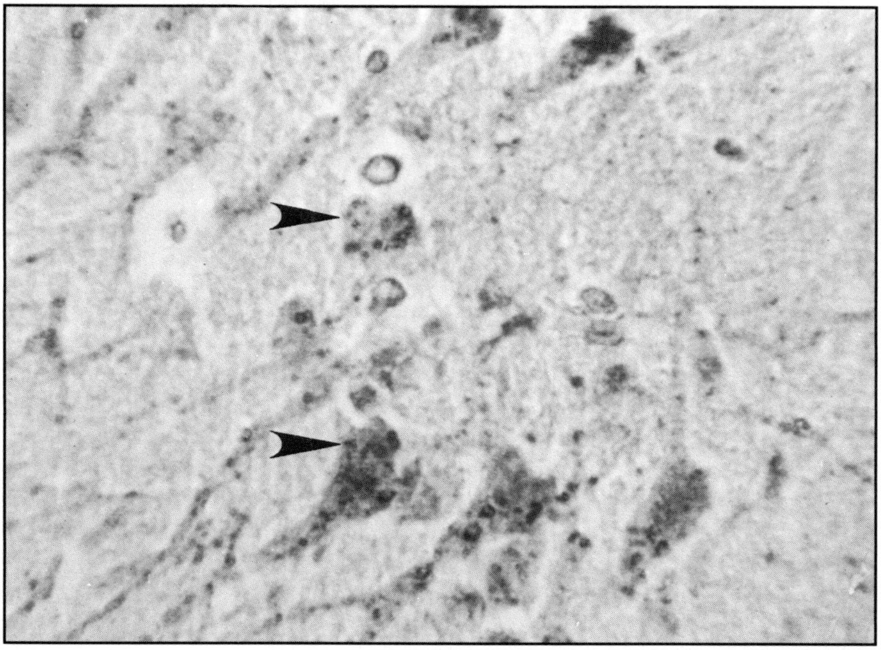

Figure 2. Fox cerebellum with natural rabies infection; immunoperoxidase antirabies staining of tissue preserved in 10% formalin for three years before paraffin embedding. The tissue was not treated with trypsin. Magnification 1020X oil immersion, using incandescent illumination.

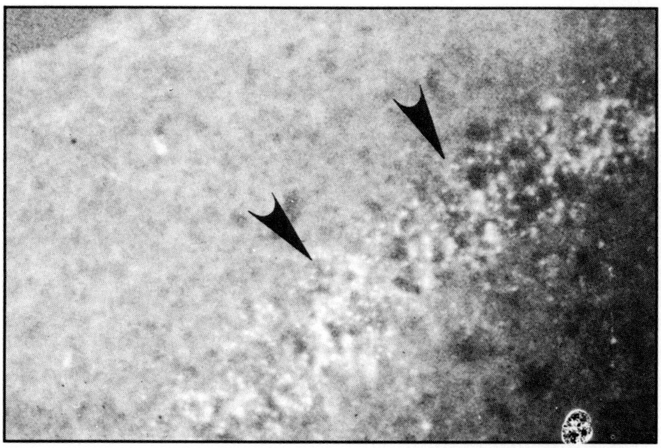

Figure 3. Mouse hippocampus infected with CVS-11; immunofluorescent antirabies staining of formalin-fixed paraffin embedded tissue. The tissue was acetone fixed and treated with 0.025% trypsin. Magnification 200X, using ultraviolet illumination.

preparations of the cornea can be carefully prepared and examined microscopically (Schneider 1975). This test seems comparable in sensitivity (when adequate numbers of cells are examined) to examining the nerves of the skin; it is quite specific when found to be positive. Acquiring the specimen correctly to have adequate cells to examine, and not damage the eye, is quite exacting. In exceptionally valuable animals it is also feasible to secure a biopsy specimen for microscopic examination from the brain itself by a neurosurgeon. Results obtained via this method also must be evaluated carefully, as the virus of rabies is not uniformly distributed throughout the brain tissue; the biopsy specimen secured may be just the area having little or no virus present (low or uncertain sensitivity; high specificity).

The rabies virus is widely distributed in other neural tissues close to the brain such as the cranial nerves (Umoh and Blenden 1982). These tissues can be examined when brain is unavailable, with high accuracy. Particularly suitable are the trigeminal nerve (gasserian ganglion), the optic nerve, and the ganglion cell layer of the eye, and the tongue (taste buds). Recent findings indicate these sensory nervous tissues are infected only centrifugally; thus the sampling of those sites for diagnosis increases the chances of success (Torres-Anjel et al. 1984a). Other cranial nerves also contain virus in the infected animal; it is wise to sample several of the cranial nerves as close to the brain as possible when brain is not available. The cervical and other portions of the spinal cord are also valuable tissues to examine, likely comparable to the brain (Fekadu and Shaddock 1984).

Especially useful is the ability to utilize tissues which have been fixed in formalin. This is accomplished by immunofluorescence using 0.25% trypsin digestion to decouple the polypeptide chains formed by the fixation and expose the virus antigen sites (Umoh and Blenden 1981). A trypsin and pepsin sequential digestion presumably works by the same mechanism (Reid et al. 1983). Improved results are obtained using only 0.025% trypsin (Torres-Anjel, M.J., unpublished data). We have had superior results without the use of enzymes using peroxidase-antiperoxidase staining on formalin fixed tissues which have been shipped internationally and stored for extended periods (Torres-Anjel et al. 1984a,b), (Figures 1, 2, 3).

The biopsy procedure is basically identical for the cat as the dog, except that the specimen must be taken from the muzzle, securing as many follicles of tactile hairs as possible. The wound resulting from the biopsy is slower to heal on the muzzle, as it easily becomes infected. Rapid healing of the wound requires scrupulous care with cleaning and antiseptics for a few days.

Sensitivity and Specificity of the Tests

One of the most difficult propositions to be faced in laboratory diagnosis of disease, is the theoretical reality that a relative few sick individuals have to be differentiated from within a much bigger pool of individuals. Those individuals with the disease and showing symptoms are more likely to be test positive, those with the disease and not showing symptoms are less likely to be test positive (more likely to be test negative) and that those without the disease are even less likely to be test positive (and even more likely to be test negative). Naturally, "disease" and "test" must be carefully defined.

As biological phenomena are rarely absolute, there is always the probability (and presence) of false positive and false negative results. Even individuals with the same disease within the population do not display identical signs. The distribution of both individuals and test

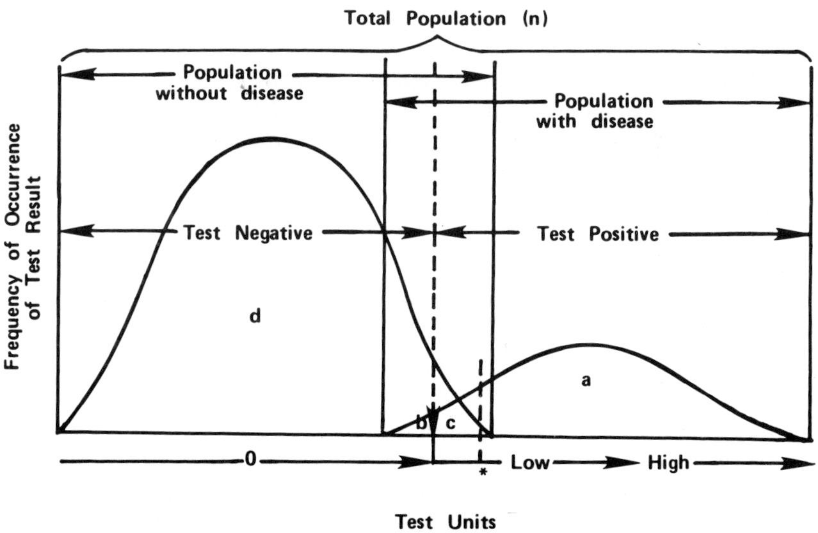

Test result threshhold of positive or negative is usually subjectively determined; depicted is estimated threshhold for skin biopsy testing for rabies (i.e., high specificity and lower sensitivity).

$$a+b+c+d=n$$

a = with disease and test positive (true positive)
b = with disease and test negative (false negative)
c = without disease and test positive (false positive)
d = without disease and test negative (true negative)

Figure 4. Determination of sensitivity and specificity of reference laboratory tests on a population of individuals.

results (in a population of adequate size) follows a typical sigmoid curve; problems producing confusion occur when the two sigmoid curves overlap. Referring to figure 4, curve "a" depicts those individuals that do have the disease (i.e., meet defined criteria); these are true positive test results. Curve "d" depicts those individuals that do not have the disease and are test negative (meeting defined criteria), representing the true negative test results. Subsegment "b" depicts those individuals that do have the disease and are test negative representing the false negative test results. Subsegment "c" depicts those individuals that do not have the disease and are test positive, comprising the false positive test results. In rabies testing, as the tests are highly specific, one expects to see a higher proportion of false negative than false positive tests.

Difficulties may be compounded when in reality we cannot even reach a theoretical truth with which to compare. This statistical approach assumes the calibration of a reference test against a true diagnosis. In practice, this model is much more complicated since one may be mostly calibrating a new (e.g., "field" or "screening", etc.) test against a reference test; the latter itself carries the statistical difficulties already mentioned and the new test will amplify the complications of sensitivity and specificity. There is not a perfect test, so that adequate management of imperfections is the clue to diagnostic decision-making. It is this ability on the part of the diagnostician that helps comprise the art of diagnostics.

This well-accepted concept of biomodal distribution has given rise to terminology and measurements of *sensitivity* and *specificity* as estimates of the accuracy and precision of a given test. Biologically, a test with a sensitivity and specificity of 1.0 (100 percent) does not exist; some examples may appear to do so, based on the particular sampling made available and observed from the universe of all true cases of the disease, including those cases not recognized. It is for the scientific, medical, and involved segments of our society to decide what degree of reliability (sensitivity and specificity) can be tolerated (table 2).

For example, in the laboratory diagnosis of rabies, the brain examination by fluorescent antibody microscopy is the recognized reference test, although not 100 percent sensitive and specific; extremely high to be sure, but not absolute. A problem immediately emerges as the tests for rabies have profound implications, so that anything less than 100 percent confidence and accuracy in interpretation escalates anxiety levels. Rabies diagnostic laboratories, when confronted with a test result that is not clear-cut, often report it as positive, as the results of the test will govern whether a person receives antirabies treatment or not. If error is involved, safety for the exposed individual must determine the result reported. The unwritten goal of routine diagnostic testing for rabies is to determine the need and appropriateness of treatment, rather

Table 2. Calculation of sensitivity and specificity of laboratory tests on populations of individuals.

		Diseased*	Not Diseased	Total
Test*				
Results	Positive	a	c	a + c
	Negative	b	d	b + d
		a + b	c + d	a + b + c + d = n

$$\text{**sensitivity of the test} = \frac{a}{a + b}$$

$$\text{***specificity of the test} = \frac{d}{c + d}$$

* "Test" and "diseased" must be specifically defined
** Ability to detect as positive those that have the disease (1.0 = 100 percent)
*** Ability to detect as negative those that do not have the disease (1.0 = 100 percent)

than to search for an absolute and accurate description of the presence or absence of infection by rabies virus.

An occasional case of rabies is not typical and requires additional effort and testing procedures to supplement the routine; additional time, high costs, and delay in treatment are involved, making this an unrealistic protocol for the routine diagnostic laboratory. Thus, the underlying goal of the testing (i.e., whether to treat or not) tempered by the realisms of time, money, and high specimen numbers in laboratories really determine the tolerable levels of specificity and sensitivity. Testing for diagnostic purposes has certain goals and limitations; testing for research purposes has a different set of goals and limitations. The search for 100 percent sensitivity and specificity even involves rather complicated statistics to assure significance (Buck and Gart 1966; Gart and Buck 1966).

Table 3 displays the calculated sensitivity and specificity of the examination of skin taken from various species and time-oriented situations. The commonly occuring figure of 1.0 in this table should not be construed to mean that the tests are perfect, which has been explained as unrealistic to expect; 1.0 should rather be considered as "close to 100 percent" as larger sample numbers would disclose an occasional discrepancy. Note also that specimens secured antemortem have lesser levels of sensitivity than those secured in terminal cases or postmortem;

Table 3. Sensitivity and specificity of skin examination for detection of rabies virus antigen in nerve fibers of skin secured antemortem and postmortem

Species	Total Observations	Sensitivity	Specificity
	Antemortem Experience		
Dogs, natural infection, all antemortem stages	47	.93	1.0*
Dogs, experimental infection, all antemortem stages	46	.68 or 0.0**	1.0
Dogs, experimental infection, first day of onset	46	.55	1.0
Human, all antemortem stages	20	.60	1.0
Mixed animal species with naturally occuring illness, all antemortem stages	136***	.98	1.0
	Postmortem Experience		
Mixed species, natural and experimental infections	251	.99	1.0
Dogs, two separate experimentally infected groups only	13	0.0	0.0
Goats, experimental infections	38	0.1	1.0

* All values of 1.0 should be interpreted as "close to 1.0."

** Two separate experimental groups of dogs, inoculated with two viruses produced totally negative and unexplained results; these (13) are not included in the total observations. The extensive collaboration of Dr. J.F. Bell is acknowledged.

*** One young skunk, naturally infected, had positive skin two days before symptoms developed.

the sensitivity on the day of onset of a series of experimentally infected dogs was .55 (55 percent), increasing through the course of the disease until it reaches 1.0 (100 percent) at the time of death (table 3). This increase through time (the course of illness) has been observed previously in experimentally infected mice (Blenden 1983) and in human cases of rabies (Blenden 1978). It is natural that the most critical need in the *in vivo* assessment of the biting dog or cat is as a predictor of the onset of rabies, or early in the clinical course of the illness as those with advanced illness are usually obvious. These types of data are virtually impossible to secure from naturally occurring cases, especially the dog and cat. There is reason to feel, however, that the onset of cases of dogs and cats may be predicted with a low degree of sensitivity (estimated .25 or below). Such predictive value has been observed in experimentally infected mice (Blenden et al. 1983) and in a naturally occurring case in a skunk kitten (Blenden 1981). Anderson et al. (1984) have observed that about 50 percent of human cases (which occurred between 1960-1979) were detected early in their clinical course by neck skin biopsy (three of four cases) or corneal impressions (four of twelve cases), a figure that agrees with our own experience (skin biopsy) on a larger number of cases (Blenden et al., unpublished data).

Some results relating to the sensitivity biopsy testing are quite baffling. For example, experimentally infected goats have a very low sensitivity of skin biopsy in detecting rabies infection antemortem. The same has been observed in some experimentally infected dogs, usually when the incubation period is short (abnormally short when compared to naturally occurring disease) (Umoh and Blenden 1982; Fekadu and Shaddock 1984). There is also likely a difference in the patterns of invasion of different strains of virus, and their dissemination into nerves of the skin. Virus strains used experimentally are uniform and used in groups of animals; only limited numbers of virus strains (even though they are "street virus") can be used. Naturally occurring infections on the other hand, are produced by a large and heterogeneous selection of virus strains, each differing slightly from another in their ability to infect and disseminate. Fortunately, skin biopsy seems more reliable in naturally occurring infections than in those which are artificially induced. Unfortunately, it is virtually impossible to secure a number of naturally occurring cases very early in their clinical course (when the information is most valuable), and so these data must be secured by experimental means.

An algorithm is presented (figure 5) to graphically depict the criteria and decision points which have been discussed and which may be considered in evaluating the rabies risk of dog and cat bites inflicted on humans. The early part of the algorithm, covering the common happening wherein the biting animal is not available for examination, has been previously published by other authors (Corey and Hattwick 1975).

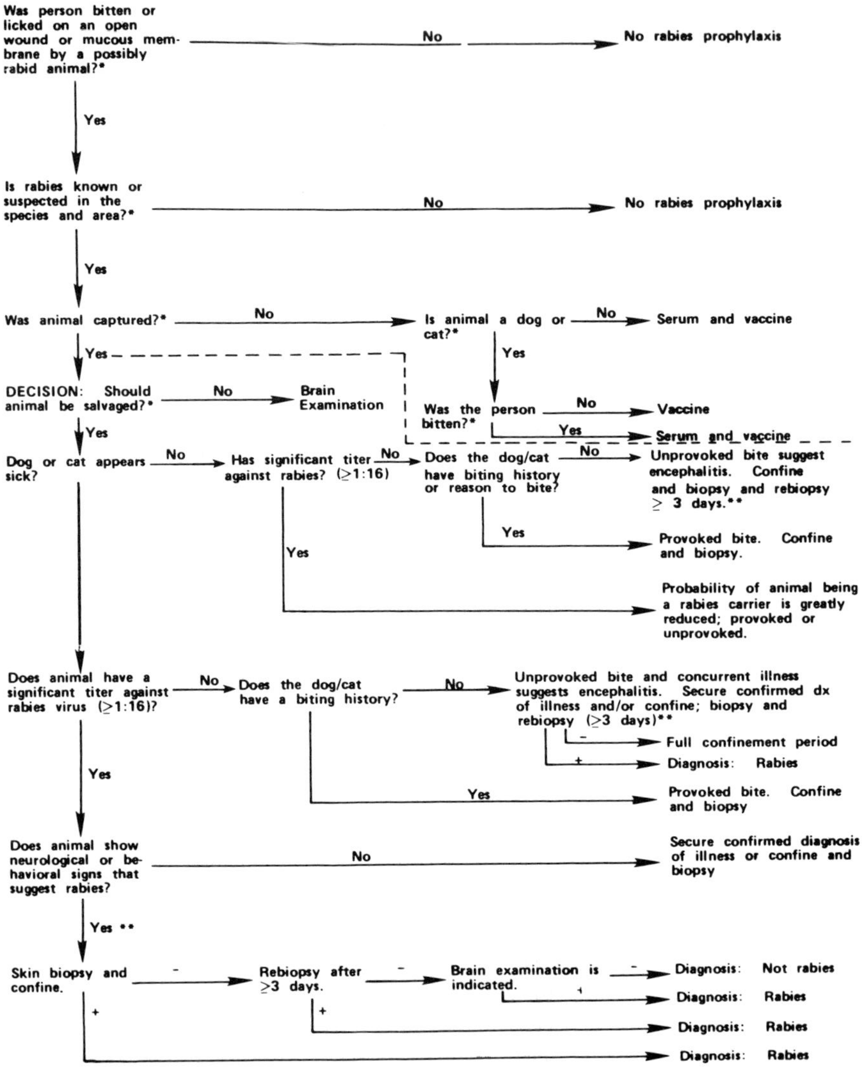

*Corey, Lawrence and Michael Hattwick. 1975. Treatment of Persons Exposed to Rabies. Journal of the American Medical Association. 232: 273.

**Initiation of anti-rabies treatment should be considered pending observations.

Figure 5. Steps to consider in the evaluation of rabies risk from dog or cat bites inflicted on humans (algorithm).

The remainder of the algorithm has been developed by blending traditional practices with new alternatives (in the form of laboratory examinations) into a decision tree. The decision pathways of the algorithm are constructed so that traditional means can be immediately resorted to if an unexpected event seems to warrant; it is likely that usage will suggest minor modification or refinement.

Summary and Conclusions

Dog and cat bites are increasing in importance to our society; dog bites especially are alarming in frequency and severity. Both species maintain a significant risk of rabies. Each bite represents a potential rabies risk requiring evaluation; some are slight or negligible in risk, other are high in risk. Concurrently, with the increase in dog bites, the relative risk of rabies exposure has decreased tremendously. In the 1950's, we officially recognized thousands of cases of dog rabies per year in the United States; due to immunization and stray control, the figure is now a few hundred per year. The technology of current evaluation for rabies risk of dog and cat bites was developed prior to and in the early 1960's, consisting of confinement and observation and immunofluorescence examination of brain tissue. Antirabies treatments administered to people are documented to be excessive (in retrospect), suggesting that easier availability and more active use of advisory services can reduce markedly the number of antirabies treatments. The evaluation processes of confinement and observation or examination of brain tissue can be reduced by the application of supplementary resources: i.e., better use of advisory services and the use of certain laboratory procedures to supplement information to make bite evaluations more objective.

A valid objective to consider is that positive and objective attitudes can be applied to these bite evaluations in order to accommodate for new technology and additional parameters. Considering the greatly reduced risk of dog bites and carefully separating the low risk majority from the high risk minority, the killing of dogs or cats solely to examine brain tissue is seldom justified. Periods of post-biting confinement and observation can be shortened or perhaps eliminated in selected cases; extended periods may be appropriate in select situations.* One must be careful not to compromise the sensitivity of the evaluation process, as even with greatly reduced risk, the exceptional cases will occur somewhere, and the "impossible" sometimes happens. At any rate, the

*Four of nine dogs artificially infected with an Ethiopian origin virus had virus in saliva thirteen days before onset (Fekadu 1984).

addition of new technology to the resources available can greatly reduce the killings for examination of brain tissue.

Laboratory technology which can complement existing methods centers around the detection of antirabies antibody both in the blood and cerebrospinal fluid (in order to differentiate antibody originating from infection versus immunization, and to establish the level of resistance of the animal) and the detection of virus antigen by examination of tissue available from the living animal (e.g. corneal impression smears and skin obtained by biopsy). The availability of alternative procedures will also focus on the easier availability of bite exposure counseling services to eliminate defensive and excessive antirabies treatments. The tremendous emotional distress which so often accompanies bite events can be greatly alleviated simply by developing more objective and accurate information about the degree of risk involved, and by having available laboratory technology to apply to the living animal, so that the common fear of brain examination can often be dispelled.

The sensitivity and specificity of laboratory tests, specifically as they apply to rabies are discussed. No test is perfect (even those in use today) so that reliance on a single laboratory test is seldom totally and absolutely justified. An algorithm is presented placing situations and actions regarding dog and cat bites into a decision tree.

Perhaps the biggest and most effective factor in the alleviation of this problem lies in the diligence used by owners with respect to their dogs and cats. It is well recognized that there is correlation between the level of responsibility assumed by dog and cat owners, and the bites that these animals inflict. If dogs and cats were properly and responsibly maintained, many less bites would occur, more dogs and cats would be immunized against rabies thus reducing the rabies risk of bites and the number of stray and unwanted dogs and cats would be reduced, resulting in less bites and a reduced reservoir of rabies.

Acknowledgements

The authors wish to gratefully thank B.N. Hamory, M.D. , J.F. Bell, M.D., Ph.D., R. Currier, D.V.M. and J. Martin, D.V.M. for review of portions of this manuscript and a continuum of advice and collaboration.

References

Anderson, L.J., Nicholson, K.G., Tauxe, R.V. and Winkler, W.G. 1984. Human rabies in the United States, 1960 to 1979: Epidemiology, diagnosis and prevention. *Ann. Int. Med.* 100(5):728-35.

Beck, A.M. 1981. The epidemiology of animal bite. *Compendium on Continuing Ed. for Pract. Vet.* 3(3):254-8.

Bell, J.F. 1975. Latency and abortive rabies. In: Baer, G. ed. *The Natural History of Rabies, Vol. 1.* New York: Academic Press.

Blenden, D.C. 1978. Identification of rabies virus antigen in the skin by immunofluorescent staining. *Zoonoses (PAHO)* I(1-2):7-11.

Blenden, D.C. 1981. Rabies in a litter of skunks predicted and diagnosed by skin biopsy. *J.A.V.M.A.* 179(8):789-91.

Blenden, D.C., Bell, J.F., Tsao, A.T. and Umoh, J.U. 1983. Immunofluorescent examination of the skin of rabies infected animals as a means of early detection of rabies virus antigen. *J. Clin. Micro.* 18(3):631-6.

Buck, A.A. and Gart, J.J. 1966. Comparison of a screening test and a reference test in epidemiologic studies. II. A probabilistic model for the comparison of diagnostic tests. *Am. J. Epidem.* 83:593-602.

Cabasso, V.J., Stebbins, M.R., Douglas, B.A. and Sharpless, G.R. 1965. Tissue culture rabies vaccine (Flury LEP) in dogs. *Am. J. Vet. Res.* 26:24-32.

Callaham, M. 1980. Dog bite wounds. *J. Am. Med. Assoc.* 244:2227-8.

Corey, L. and Hattwick, M.A.W. 1975. Treatment of persons exposed to rabies. *J. Am. Med. Assoc.* 232(3):272-6.

Dean, D.J., Evans, W.M. and Thompson, W.R. 1964. Studies on the Low Egg Passage Flury strain of modified live rabies virus produced in embryonating chicken eggs and tissue culture. *Am. J. Vet. Res.* 25:756-63.

Fekadu, M., Shaddock, J.H. and Baer, G. 1982. Excretion of rabies in the saliva of dogs. *J. Inf. Dis.* 145(5):715-9.

Fekadu, M. and Shaddock, J.H. 1984. Peripheral distribution of virus in dogs inoculated with two strains of rabies virus. *Am. J. Vet. Res.* 45(4):724-9.

Gart, J.J. and Buck, A.A. 1966. Comparison of a screening test and a reference test in epidemiologic studies. I. Indices of agreement and their relation to prevalence. *Am. J. Epidem.* 83:586-92.

Hattwick, M.A.W. and Gregg, M.B. 1975. The disease in man. In: Baer, G. ed. *The Natural History of Rabies, Vol. II.* New York: Academic Press.

Koprowski, H. and Black, J. 1954. Studies on chick embryo adapted rabies virus. V. Protection of animals with antiserum and living attenuated virus after exposure to street strain of rabies virus. *J. Immunol.* 72:85-93.

Marr, J.S. and Beck, A.M. 1976. Rabies in New York City, with new guidelines for prophylaxis. *Bull. N.Y. Acad. Med.* 52(5):605-16.

Reid, F.L., Hall, N.H., Smith, J.S. and Baer, G.M. 1983. Increased immunofluorescent staining of rabies infected formalin-fixed brain tissue after pepsin and trypsin digestion. *J. Clin. Micro.* 18:968-71.

Schneider, L.G. 1975. Spread of virus from the central nervous system. In: Baer, G. ed. *The Natural History of Rabies, Vol I.* New York: Academic Press.

Schnurrenberger, P.R., Martin, R.J., Merrdink, G.L. and Rose, N.J. 1969. Epidemiology of human exposure to rabid animals in Illinois. *Pub. Hlth. Rpts.* 84(12):1078-84.

Thomas, J.B. 1975. The serum neutralization, indirect flourescent antibody and rapid fluorescent focus inhibition tests. In: Baer, G. ed. *The Natural History of Rabies, Vol. I.* New York: Academic Press.

Torres-Anjel, M.J., Montano-Hirose, J., Cazabon, E.P.I., Oakman, J.K. and Wiktor, T.J. 1984a. A new approach to the pathobiology of rabies virus as aided by immunoperoxidase staining. *Amer. Assoc. Vet. Diag., 27th Annual Proceedings*. pp. 1-26.

Torres-Anjel, M.J., Blenden, D.C., Oakman, J.K., Frost, J.W. and Satalowich, F.T. 1984b. *International Symp. Med. Virology (Pan Am. Group on Rapid Viral Diagnosis)*. Dept. Pathology, Medical Center, Univ. of California, Irvine (In press).

Umoh, J.U. and Blenden, D.C. 1981. Immunofluorescent staining of rabies virus antigen in formalin-fixed tissue after treatment with trypsin. *Bull. W.H.O.* 59(5):737-44.

Umoh, J.U. and Blenden, D.C. 1982. The dissemination of rabies virus into cranial nerves and other tissues of experimentally infected goats and dogs and naturally infected skunks. *Int. J. Zoonoses*. 9:1-11.

U.S. Department of Health and Humane Services. 1983. Centers for Disease Control. Annual Summary 1980-82. *Rabies Surveillance.*

Vaughn, J.B., Gerhardt, P. and Paterson, J.L.S. 1963. Excretion of street rabies virus in saliva of cats. *J.A.M.A.* 184:705-8.

Vaughn, J.B., Gerhardt, P. and Newell, K.W. 1965. Excretion of street rabies in the saliva of dogs. *J.A.M.A.* 193:363-8.

Part III
Veterinary Ethics

TO WRITE A THERIATRIC OATH*

Gretchen Lockwood

Colorado State University
Veterinary Teaching Hospital
Fort Collins, Colorado 80523

The Veterinarian's Oath was a disappointment to me. When I first read it as a freshman, I suppose I was expecting something along the lines of the Hippocratic Oath; instead I was struck by the contrast to it—by the lack of eloquence, of poetry, of ancient power. As impressionable as I was then, a whole year and a half ago, it left me unmoved. Now, having had my eyes opened to its more troubling ethical difficulties, I feel the desire to create something better, something that is at least more meaningful to me. As an individual, particularly without extensive dialogue with my peers, I can't even pretend to create an oath suitable for all veterinary graduates for all time to come. This is, at best, my endeavor to write an oath which in the very writing can help clarify and define for me my moral stand, which will challenge me to be true to that stand, and to which I can honestly and earnestly hold myself responsible.

So here are two oaths sworn by those who make medicine their livelihood. I find the Veterinarian's Oath deficient and unsatisfactory on all counts. The Hippocratic, while admirable, is obviously not suited for a veterinarian's needs. Therefore I submit for my reader and myself a new oath.

The title is mostly a whim. What little significance it has is in its root, *ther*, meaning "wild beast." This is in contrast to the root of "veterinarian" which pertains to beasts of burden. It is to remind me that the animals I will deal with were all ancestrally wild, independent of humanity for their life and livelihood. In defense of the fact that this

*Reprinted with permission from *Intervet*, October 1984.

oath is even longer than the Hippocratic, let me say two things. First of all, life hasn't gotten any simpler since the latter was written. And second, I bow to Hippocrates' superior writing skill.

I begin with "I swear" as a statement of active commitment. I invoke the beings I do with reason. Apollon the healer is also Apollon the destroyer. As one who will have to destroy life as well as seek to aid it, I appeal to the god who was known to bring swift, painless death. Asklepios, son of Apollon and god of healing, is clearly a significant being to call upon and his close association with snakes ties him yet closer to veterinary medicine. Hygieia, the lady of health, should be strongly invoked by all in medicine as our emphasis should ever be more on nurturing health. Of all these gods, Cheiron is most powerfully and singularly important to veterinary medicine. The wise centaur was greatly skilled in medicine and was said to be the teacher of Asklepios himself. As both beast and man, he shows as none other the continuity of the natural and human world; he weaves the wisdom of both into a harmonious whole as no other centaur and very few humans have been able. There is importance in the fact that Cheiron, immortal and suffering from an incurable poison, chose as his final blessing the relinquishment of his immortality. Therein lies a message all healers should be mindful of. As to "the one God" to whom this oath is made—this is not the occasion to explain my religious beliefs. I will only emphasize that an oath must be made to a significant entity, preferably the most significant of all entities, whatever the swearer conceives that to be.

I have purposefully made a broad statement of goal: "to use all my skills," etc. I made an effort to include all abilities, not merely scientific, in the pursuit of the goals as I feel this is vital to halt the dehumanization of doctor, patient, and client in both human and veterinary medicine. It could be argued that considering acid rain, nuclear fallout, etc., the phrase "animals. . .touched by human activity" includes *all* animals on the face of the globe. Overwhelming as it is, I support that interpretation because as human beings we all have such responsibilities. As a veterinarian, I would narrow the interpretation to those animals within my sphere of influence, a condition sufficiently overwhelming.

I have quoted directly from the Veterinarian's Oath in "protection of animal health" because it was the most direct and appropriate wording. I fully realize that animal well-being, human health, and medical wisdom may come into conflict, and I've tried to deal with this below. Here I have made two stipulations: I support the growth of medical wisdom *when* it is to the benefit of human or animal health—and that it is *wisdom* I support. Knowing how long an animal will survive being blinded with hot needles may in some obscene sense increase medical knowledge but this has *nothing* to do with wisdom. I realize that I've said nothing directly about pure, unapplied research which is a troubling proposition. I fully believe that the need to discover is a deep part of human nature and, therefore, a right—but not an absolute one. This, like a number of other things, has to be toiled through case by case, weighing benefit against harm.

The portion concerning referral of patients is the only very specific point I make. Perhaps it is not vital to the oath. I leave it in partly in emulation of Hippocrates and partly because of two important statements contained therein—doing one's best on a daily basis and refusing to harm an animal for vanity's sake. The latter can and should be interpreted as a refusal to do harm for the client's vanity as well (e.g. ear-cropping).

In the last sentence of the first paragraph and all of the succeeding paragraphs, I try to address the conflicts of benefit and harm, human and animal welfare, and my responsibility to humans and animals. If I'm accused of being ambiguous, of resolving nothing, I have to plead guilty. These are some of the most difficult issues I know of. I have tried to acknowledge my inescapable responsibility to both humans and animals. There will be times when I have to wrong one to do good for the other, and I can't possibly resolve all those conflicts in advance. I can only hope my courage doesn't fail during those times. My last statement of the paragraph is not an abdication of responsibility; it is an assertion of my belief that all beings, humans included, have a right to ultimate loyalty to their own species.

Beyond these responsibilities as a veterinarian and a human being, I will have certain professional obligations to people, socially and individually. In the third paragraph I have tried to define and clarify these as well as emphasize my human, individual, and professional commitment to animal welfare. Passing this belief on in word and deed is the teaching to which veterinarians are obligated.

Life, as has been said, is not simple. I am convinced that there will always be situations where we all must act in ignorance of whether our acts are wrong or right. I also believe we have to accept the guilt in those situations, regardless. However, I hold with Aristotle that we are *not* guilty of those things we do unknowing and unwilling, and that no one need accept unnecessary guilt. I do not have Hippocrates' courage to call down a curse on myself for having failed, feeling that is all too likely to happen. I do hope and believe that trying counts.

Looking over this oath, I'm left with a number of impressions. It's idealistic; it's rough; I've probably set some impossible goals for myself. But I am willing to swear to it, as long as it can grow with me. If as I mature I see things unworthy of swearing to, then let them be changed. Otherwise, may I indeed be granted the courage, fortitude, and wisdom to carry out this oath. I'll need plenty.

A Theriatric Oath

I swear by Appollon the Healer, by Asklepios, by Cheiron, by Hygieia and to the one God whose children we all are, that to the best of my human power I shall keep this oath: to use all my skills, faculties, and sensitivities for the benefit of animals whose lives and deaths are touched by human activity. To this end, I shall work for the protection of animal health and the relief of animal suffering; for this purpose, and for the benefit of human health, I shall support the growth of medical wisdom. In my daily work, I shall use my abilities to their best extent, but where they are inadequate and I know of others who excel, I shall refer my patients to their skill; I shall not endanger an animal's health for vanity's sake. Knowing that benefit and injury are deeply interwoven in all things, especially medicine, I shall strive always to do more good than harm.

In all my actions I must recognize the possible benefit and harm to human well-being, especially to those people whose welfare depends upon animals. Knowing that animal and human good are closely tied, I will strive for the advancement of both whenever possible. When these interests conflict, I shall not lightly transgress the rights to life and nature of one for the benefit of the other. But I must realize that I am by choice and calling a veterinarian, by fate a human being; my final lot is cast with humanity.

My society has placed me in a position of respect and authority. I shall try to accept this position honorably and without arrogance. Knowing that people shall turn to me for knowledge and even wisdom, I will do my best to pass on such as I have, and especially by word and action to assert the inherent rights of animals to life according to their natures. Knowing that people may entrust to me their confidences as they would not to others because of my station, I will not lightly betray that trust. But neither will I allow insufferable wrongs to continue because of my silence. Knowing better than most that my colleagues are striving yet fallible human beings, I give them my respect and will be slow to judge their failings. But I shall not conceal wrong-doing under the aegis of Asklepios.

Knowing that I shall be called upon to weigh the many against the one, suffering against well-being, life against death; knowing that much of my life, even in these most important matters, I shall act in irremediable ignorance, I accept any guilt for whatever I do consciously and willingly. I ask the forbearance of others when I act in good faith to the best of my powers. I gladly embrace the commitment to grow in knowledge, skill, and wisdom the rest of my days.

As long as I strive to keep this oath, may I be granted courage, fortitude, and wisdom to do so. Where in good faith I fail, may I be corrected. Where I succeed, may I be granted to enjoy the fulfillment of life and my profession.

The Veterinarian's Oath

"Being admitted to the profession of veterinary medicine, I solemnly swear to use my scientific knowledge and skills for the benefit of society through the protection of animal health, the relief of animal suffering, the conservation of livestock resources, the promotion of public health, and the advancement of medical knowledge.

"I will practice my profession conscientiously, with dignity, and in keeping with the principles of veterinary medical ethics.

"I accept as a lifelong obligation the continual improvement of my professional knowledge and competence."

JAVMA. Vol. 17: 1970, p. 878.

The Hippocratic Oath

"I swear by Apollo the physician, by Aesculapius, by Hygeia, Panacea, and all the gods and goddesses, that according to my best ability and judgement, I will keep this oath and stipulation; to reckon him who taught me this art equally dear to me as my parents; to share my substance with him and relieve his necessities if required; to regard his offspring as on the same footing as my own brothers, and to teach them this art if they shall wish to learn it, without fee or stipulation, and that by precept, oral teaching and every other mode of instruction, I will impart a knowledge of the art to my own sons and to those of my teachers, and to disciples bound by a stipulation and oath, according to the law of medicine, but to no others.

"I will follow that method of treatment, which, according to my ability and judgement, I consider for the benefit of my patients, and abstain from whatever is deleterious and mischievous. I will give no deadly medicine to anyone if asked, nor suggest any such counsel; furthermore, I will not give to a woman an instrument to produce abortion.

"With purity and holiness I will pass my life and practice my art. I will not cut a person who is suffering with a stone, but will leave this to be done by practitioners of this work. Into whatever houses I enter I will go into them for the benefit of the sick and will abstain from every voluntary act of mischief and corruption, and, further, from the seduction of females or males, bound or free.

"Whatever in connection with my professional practice, or not in connection with it, I may see or hear in the lives of men which ought not be spoken abroad, I will not divulge, as reckoning that all such should be kept secret.

"While I continue to keep this oath inviolate, may it be granted to me to enjoy life and the practice of my art, respected always by all men, but should I trespass this oath, may the reverse be my lot."

VETERINARY CONDUCT AND ANIMAL WELFARE*

H. Rozemond

Chief Inspectorate
Veterinary Public Health
Section Animal Experimentation
P.O. Box 439
2260 AK Leidschendam,
The Netherlands

Introduction

In 1969 I had the honor to deliver a lecture to the 116th Annual Congress of the Royal Netherlands Veterinary Medical Association concerning the activities of veterinarians involved in herd health (Rozemond 1970). My lecture aimed to challege the veterinary aspects of a system of animal husbandry at that time new to Dutch circumstances; the system characterized by enlargement of scale and by species specialization. The thesis of this rather technical lecture read: "We have to build a new barn with a good climate." At that time, books such as *Animal Machines* by Ruth Harrison (1964), in which intensive rearing of farm animals was criticized, had barely attracted attention. That seemed unnecessary indeed: A Dutch agricultural journal had established Harrison as an adherent of an old-fashioned, useless and folkloristic belief. Much has changed since that time. The technical way of dealing with animals, not only in intensive rearing but also in other areas, is now facing increased criticism.

This paper is a lecture presented to the same Association but fifteen years later: the 131st Annual Congress in 1984. This second presentation contemplates two points: First, it tries to indicate how this criticism has gradually emerged and a historical outline is put forth of the development of veterinary medicine, a differentiation being made between a

---

*Translated from *Tijdschrift voor Diergeneeskunde* 1985, 110:21-30.

mythical, a technical, and a critical approach. Second, a discussion of how veterinarians have to associate themselves with this criticism in their professional conduct is presented. This discussion is necessary for two reasons. Veterinarians have increasingly become aware that they bear a professional responsibility not only for animal health but also for animal welfare; and, veterinarians are expected to give their views in concrete situations.

The Mythical Attitude

In a number of publications, the German veterinary historian Hausmann (1982a, b, 1984) has sketched the outlines of the centaur Cheiron, father of European medical and veterinary practice, a being from old mythical days: son of a god (Kronos) and a woman (Philyra); half man, half horse. These and other allurements of the Cheiron legend must not tempt us to doubt his historicity. The excavation of Troy was crowned with success because Schliemann took acknowledgement of the poems of Homer. Hausmann did the same to Cheiron. He made it plausible that Cheiron lived around 1270 B.C. in Mileai in the Greek Pelion mountains. Hausmann also asserts he can indicate the cave where Cheiron lived and worked.

During Cheiron's time, the cave was visited by people with various ailments: wounds, genetic disorders, diseases caused by summer heat or winter cold. Cheiron exorcized his patients with tranquilizing incantations, treated their wounds with herbs or with the scalpel. His care not only concerned man but also animals. This is evident from the history of the dogs of the Greek hero Aktaion. These animals, after the death of Aktaion, inconsolably searched for their master and eventually turned up at the cave of Cheiron, who allayed their grief by modeling a statue of their killed master.

The knowledge of Cheiron, we must assume, was experience-based. Man was linked with nature, partook with it, put to use the tools at hand or which were in sight, or performed what the gods instigated. Cheiron did not keep his knowledge to himself. He founded a school, passed knowledge to others, who were honored afterwards as gods and heroes in old Hellas: to Asklepios, to whom he taught medicine; to Hygieia, the goddess of health; to Panakeia (panacea); to Orpheus, to whom he also gave musical instruction; to Achilles, who learned from Cheiron the skills of hunting and foraging. In this way, Cheiron emerges from history as a man with universal knowledge and as one with his surroundings. In mythical times, the performance and technical skill of man were determined by his knowledge of, and his experience with, nature.

We may characterize this mythical attitude with some catchwords. Man participates in his environment; he uses the forces of nature and strives for a certain well-being. In summary, he lives with the notion "that" culture exists.

There is no reason to look down upon this mythical culture with self-conceit; but natural knowledge and natural experience can harden to magic and witchcraft. It has been pointed out that veterinary knowledge also was available in the middle ages, but at that time this knowledge was more often than not made up of a gathering of prescriptions, which were for centuries long transcribed, appended, and mutilated. Theriacum and asafoetida were the highest wisdom, and also elixirs, with up to sixty not too palatable ingredients, talismans, spells, uroscopy, cupping, leeches, holy water, relics, and saints. Till far into our century, the German rhyme was accepted: "Weisz man nicht mehr wie, was und warum, dann nimmt man Jod-jodkalium."* Dutch seventeenth century paintings conspicuously give an impression of the mistrust to prevailing (veterinary) medicine. The quack was a favorite subject for such painters as Jan Steen (1626-1679) and contemporaries (figure 1).

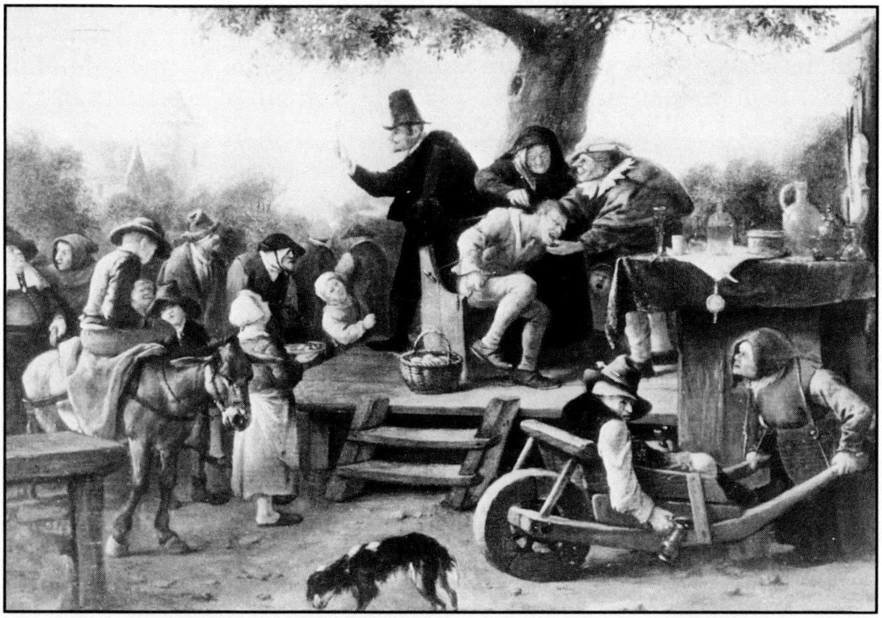

Figure 1. Jan Steen (1626-1679): *The Quack*. Rijksmuseum, Amsterdam.

*"When not is known who, what or why
potassium iodide you may try." (Author's translation)

The Technical Attitude

In the same period, however, other Dutch painters, e.g. Rembrandt van Rijn (1606-1669) were commissioned, mostly by City Guilds, to depict an "Anatomical Lesson." Such paintings portray a group of persons gathered around a prosector demonstrating the muscles and internal organs of a corpse. These paintings illustrate the changes that took place. Man not only makes use of the superficial but searches within the body. He has dissociated himself from his environment; he turns away from the familiarity of the mythical and focuses on observation. Experimentation has appeared; data are arranged, analytical, quantifying, systematical, controllable, causal. Science crops up and begins to flourish. A new age has emerged. The anatomists take the lead. They give descriptions of the substratum. Mondino de'Luzzi (fourteenth century) is the first in the Renaissance to perform dissections, not only of dogs and pigs but also of men. Leonardo da Vinci (1452-1519) and Albrecht Dürer (1471-1528) make their famous sketches. Andreas Vesalius publishes in 1543 the first standard work on human anatomy: *De Humani Corporis Fabrica*. Veterinary medicine barely lags behind: Carlo Ruini's *Anatomia del Cavallo* appears fifty-five years later. The foundations of a new science are laid. The painting of Cornelis de Man (1681) depicting an anatomical lesson to a group of scientists in the

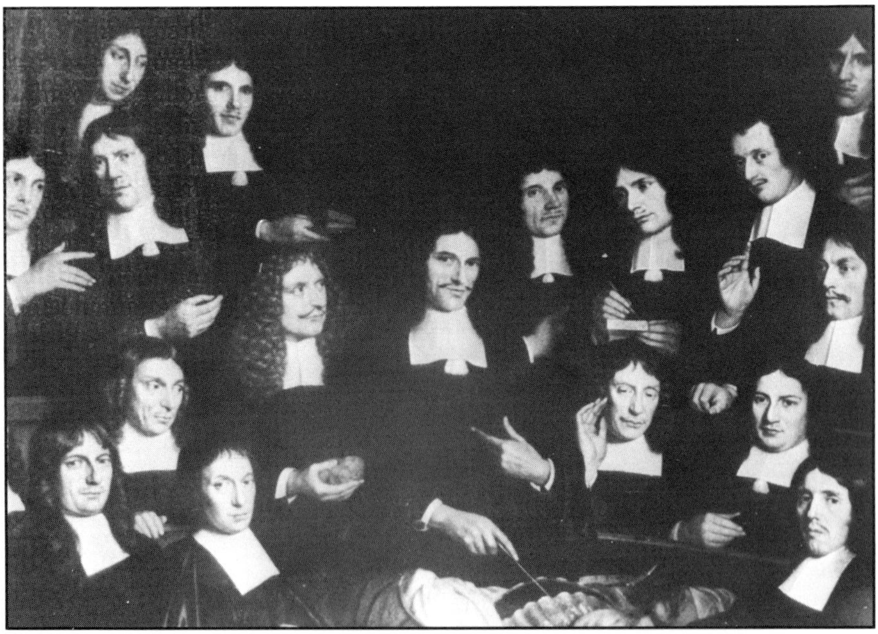

Figure 2. Cornelis de Man: *Anatomical Lesson of Isaac 's Gravensande.* Prinsenhof Museum, Delft.

small Dutch city of Delft (figure 2) characterizes the progress and dissemination of modern science albeit at Delftian level. However, this level must not be underestimated. In the painting, standing next to prosector Cornelis 's Gravesande, is a man wearing a peruke, Antoni van Leeuwenhoek, the father of microbiology and correspondent to the Royal Society of London for Improving Natural Knowledge. Reinier de Graaf, a contemporary Delftian physician, just missed appearing in the setting, as he died eight years before completion of the painting. De Graaf was the first to understand the significance of appearances on the ovaries which are now known as the graafian follicles. He was also able to perform fistulae to the pancreatic gland of dogs (without analgesics!) and to keep those animals alive (without antibiotics!). Unprecedented possiblities emerged. A wave of knowledge, not naive but scientific, spread throughout Europe. Ingenuity, medical and non-medical, yielded results and new technical possibilities. True, it needed time and immense energy. For example, to reach today's level of open heart surgery, it has been calculated that more than four thousand essential investigations had to be performed (Comroe and Dripps 1976). But the energy was available and also the money. Veterinary medicine again had not lagged behind. This may be deduced from the fact that the 1984 volume of the *Veterinary Bulletin* mentions more than eight thousand publications.

This representation—maybe it is better to speak of an accelerated film—gives an impression of a second cultural attitude, i.e., that of investigation and technique. Man no longer participates in his setting nor only uses what is at hand, but he takes distance; he devises principles and possibilities to interfere in nature. Technical ingenuity is placed into motion; production becomes the slogan; prosperity the aim. Man is no longer satisfied by ascertaining "that" he participates in culture; he seeks to answer the question, "what" can be done to develop culture. When we look about, the results seem to be nothing short of staggering indeed: a new barn, a good climate.

The Critical Attitude

It may be good to stop the film for just a moment. As a schoolboy, I learned that farming was a means of subsistence; today we speak of "agri-business." That sounds quite different and we observe that some animals in this business show severe and enduring behavioral aberrations. When referring to animal experimentation we speak of "animal models." In the Netherlands, 1.3 million of such models are used annually. We, as veterinarians, are able to geld, to spay, to amputate, to devocalize, to extirpate, to canulize, to declaw, to debeak, and to pinion.

Little by little we are able to do anything with animals, thanks to our ingenuity, and we do it when asked. Apart from the veterinary scene are also examples of technical possibilities and of their adversities. Acid rain, water pollution, nuclear weapons, and euthanasia, formerly far-off or unknown words are nowadays familiar eye-openers. They are catchwords for the crushing of our "what" culture, resulting from the unbridled self-reliance of the technical attitude.

Thus, technicians are summoned to solve these problems and when this seems to fail we clamor for legislation, in the way of: "Vivisection? A law! Continued vivisection? Higher fines!" But it becomes ever clearer, that it is not the technicians nor the legislators who can unravel our modern problems. What we need, is a new approach to culture, a third attitude. The principle question is no longer what we may conceive or perform: that is almost infinite. More important has become the question of how our judgement is on the technical potentialities we have and how we should handle our cultural inheritance. We can produce very well, but we must learn to benefit from it in a meaningful way. For the issue is not prosperity, but welfare. Obviously, we must learn to yield from distance (which causes disruption) and to concern us more with the equilibrium of involvement and companionship. The critical element which was kept out of my 1969 lecture was: "for what" functions our culture, "for what" functions veterinary medicine, "for what" function veterinarians.

It can be concluded that there is a distinction between the various attitudes towards culture. They are shown in the following diagram.

myth/nature	research/technique	judgment/criticism
participation	distance	relation
use	production	utilization
well-being	prosperity	welfare
"that"	"what"	"for what"

In addition, it can be reasoned that transition from one attitude to another usually occurs when culture is stumbling. In the above treatise this is marked by the prevailment of magic and by the surplus of technical influence respectively. However, transition does not emerge unless its need is recognized. A blind spot can prevent us from focusing on jammed circumstances. Eye-openers can be useful at this time.

Animal Welfare

One of the subjects for which we have a better appreciation is the welfare of animals. Since Cheiron, the veterinary profession has developed to an art of healing, alleviation, and prevention. We become increasingly aware that it also has to be attentive to the harmonious existence of animals both ethologically and physiologically. Veterinarians often work with animals in suboptimal circumstances, such as bare pens, plastic boxes, and apartment buildings. There, animals become resources, tools, and victims. Veterinarians should also care for the welfare of these animals to the extent possible.

Empathy to animals increases when they are less looked upon as tools or "whats." Other viewpoints have arisen, e.g. Schweitzer's idea of reverence for life (Schweitzer 1984) or Singer's principle of conditional equivalence (Singer 1975). The veterinary profession and each individual veterinarian has to reflect on such concepts in order not only to find the right attitude but also to meet the responses of society (Fox 1984). Veterinarians are expected to have a knowledge of these matters.

Professional Duties

Among the branches of the Royal Netherlands Veterinary Medical Association an inquiry was held concerning welfare bottlenecks in everyday practice. The responses can be placed into three categories.

First, there are difficulties with regard to careless or imperfect veterinary-technical performance. Veterinarians appear to experience difficulties with such interventions as castration, herniotomy, plastic surgery on teats, teeth-corrections, removal of warts, treatment of prolapsus ani et recti, use of coercive means, stunning for slaughter, choice of euthanasia methods.

The second group entails problems which result from nonmedical desires of individual owners with regard to an animal. To this category belong declawing, devocalization, partial tongue resection, penis deviation, tail docking, ear cropping, neurectomy, (sophisticated operations), euthanasia and its reverse, needless suffering, e.g., of disabled animals.

A third category is formed by the problems resulting from decisions made on a level beyond the direct relation of veterinarian/owner. At times tasks have to be performed at the instigation of employers or governmental agencies. Such problems relate to intensive animal farming, breeding of animals with genetic abnormalities, ritual slaughter, animal experimentation, or the like.

With regard to the first category, it has to be admitted that pain release or sedation are not always attended to in an optimal way in practice. Partly, these problems can be prevented by better application of available know-how. Veterinarians must possess this know-how and put it into practice. Neither economy nor convenience are motives to trifle with this principle. However, when technical knowledge is not available, specific research should be initiated.

Veterinary handbooks are not the place to find solutions for the second and third category of problems, for those problems are caused by technological successes, rather than by casual failures. It was the successes which brought us in a situation in which we can perform "everything." The tragedy is that this omnipotence results in disturbed relations. So, it is doubtful whether additional technology is the suitable means to do away with this disturbance. The most meritorious thing to do is to explore disturbed relations, to map them and to subsequently seek solutions in a creative and inventive way.

The endeavor to explore these relations is expressed by Boon (1983) in his definition of animal mistreatment as "the harming of an animal's welfare to a greater extent than is necessary to reach a meaningful (social) aim." This definition can be made operational by (1) a description of the use or intended use of the animal, (2) a description of the (direct and/or indirect) aim of the use, (3) a calculation or assessment of its social significance, (4) an assessment of its implications for the animal's welfare, (5) an assessment of alternatives, if any. In the end after a process of evaluation of this data and assessments (6) a judgement can (or cannot!) be made. Such a judgement can hold an accession, a conditional accession, a disclaimer or a suspended disclaimer.

In conclusion, our interrelationship with animals has to be incorporated in our society and culture. This means: not always for the benefit of economics, science or fashion, nor—granted—always in the interest of animals. Under discussion consequently comes the "for what" question. That question not only involves veterinary, medical, biological, or agricultural aspects, it also has religous, philosophical, ethical, juridicial, aesthetical, economical, sociological, historical, and political implications; in short, it is a human problem.

The Balance

The modern Dutch animal protection movement has understood that the "for what" question is a human problem. This movement is increasingly prepared to search for poised considerations. Here are some examples:

— membership of the Public Council of Veterinary Affairs, together with the Ministries of Agriculture and of Public Health, the Veterinary Association and organizations of farmers and industry;
— membership of the Committee on Health and Well-being of pet animals, together with the Veterinary Association;
— financial support of research into alternatives to animal experiments, at joint expense with government and industry;
— platform discussions with religious minority groups about ritual slaughter.

These examples have two characteristics in common: (1) the readiness to seek for logical solutions and (2) the willingness to do so with those who are faced with the same problem, but in a different viewpoint.

This should also hold true for the veterinary profession. The veterinary profession cannot pretend to be able to solve all animal welfare problems independently. It must listen to other disciplines as well.

The discussions about the "for what" question in relation to the position of animals is rather recent. As mentioned earlier, the "what" culture, reckoning from the Mondino dissections up to modern heart surgery took more than six centuries. The "for what" question occupies our minds but a fraction of that period. So it is not surprising that we now are in the state of only seeking after the right attitude. In fact, we are now just living in the Mondino phase of substrata description: how is the relation man-animal; what is pain and distress; when does it come to infringement of animal welfare; how can it be measured; do animals have an intrinsic value, do they have rights; what about intercultural differences, i.e., religious or urban-versus-rural traditions, and animal welfare. Such reflections ultimately must lead to better understanding and to new values and standards in society and in the veterinary profession. The broader the basis on which these problems are discussed and the greater the aptitude brought in, the more valuable results may be obtained.

Conscience

This brings us back to the question whether a veterinarian, minding all circumstances, should concern himself with particular interventions when he is asked by animal owners or decision-makers to perform: declawing, practice in intensive farming, animal experimentation. Such a question may lead to tension between a conscience that speaks out and the interests of others. Veterinarians are paid to dedicate themselves to the interests of their commissioners. However, they must also pay attention to animal interests, an entity with peculiar objective and subjective aspects. Welfare of man and animal are sometimes conflicting. Be that as it may, to perform in an ethically correct manner requires conscious reasoning, every time a decision has to be made.

Freedom of action is determined by values and standards. In concrete situations they allow us to make selections from alternatives. How such selections are made, does not concern us here. The point here is that our actions can at times barely be reconciled with our values and standards. So we must ask ourselves inventive and creative questions, not only the "what" questions, but also the "for what" ones. In sorting the answers we may come to an agreement with ourselves: I should, or I should not, declaw. The question may be put, whether it is the responsibility of the veterinarian to decide in such questions. Is not the owner the first to be addressed? The answer is that both are involved. The veterinarian as well as the owner has to account for his own decisions and the consequences. If necessary, veterinarians should make that clear to owners.

Quite different is the situation when the veterinarian functions in a peculiar task or role. This applies when his or her tasks are part of a framework, e.g., in an employment or a legal setting. In such situations the interests and the decisions of the organization are conclusive and the logic of it is determined at that "higher" level. Here two options are open for the veterinarian. He or she can do his or her job under protest and use the utmost endeavors to bring change in the rules. In this way, participation is not necessarily a matter of disgrace although it may be a painful embarrassment. The other option is that participation is felt to be unacceptable. This can result in the decision to not participate and the acceptance of the painful consequences of that decision. It can be reproached that in this manner the treatise gets stuck in a micro-ethical exploration, in a scanning of the individual responsibility of a veterinarian and that the burden of pain is charged on his or her conscience alone. Isn't there something like professional ethics as a whole? It can be replied that it is very difficult to avoid individual pain, because pain is a subjective feeling and a signal, here in particular a signal of disturbed relations which everyone experiences in his or her own manner. In addition, this author is insufficiently authoritative to decide for his whole profession which values and standards should prevail in future veterinary conduct. However, we do have some statements and acknowledgements. It is good to remember the recommendations and decisions on animal welfare of the Federation of Veterinarians in Europe (FVE) (van Riessen 1982) and of the draft International Guiding Principles for biomedical research involving animals of the Council for International Organizations of Medical Science (CIOMS 1983). However, such declarations are not yet fully accepted in society nor in the profession. So when we want to come to a meaningful attitude—and I believe this to be necessary—then critical discussions have to proceed and be amplified. Professional associations of veterinarians can be an important platform for it.

The Dutch poet Willem Elsschot wrote the verse:

. . . want tussen droom en daad
staan wetten in de weg en praktische bezwaren.
(From dream to deed you meet restraining laws and practical objections.)

If this be true, we have to critically assess such obstacles, for the aim still should be: a new barn with a better climate.

Acknowledgements

Translation of the original article was made possible by courtesy of the Editor of *Tijdschrift voor Diergeneeskunde*. The English version of this paper was improved tremendously by intelligent comments of Mr. R.P. Selman.

References

Boon, D. 1983. *Nederlands dierenrecht*. Arnhem, The Netherlands. Gouda Quint. B.V.

CIOMS 1984. *Biomedical Research Involving Animals*. Bankowski, Z. and Howard-Jones, N. eds. Council for International Organizations of Medical Sciences, Geneva.

Comroe, Jr., J.H. and Dripps, R.D. 1976. Scientific basis for the support of biomedical science. *Science*. 192:105-11.

Fox, M.W. 1984. Towards a philosophy of veterinary medicine. *The Veterinary Record*. 115:12-13.

Harrison, R. 1964. *Animal Machines*. London: Vincent Stuart Ltd.

Hausmann, W. 1982a. Ars Chironica, Antike Autoren über Cheiron. *Dtsch. Tierärztl. Wschr.* 89:407-11.

Hausmann, W. 1982b. Die medizinischen Höhlenschule des Cheirons. *Berl. Münsch. tierarztl. Wsch.* 95:94-5.

Hausmann, W. 1984. Cheiron. Eine weitere Sammlung und Auslegung von Zeugnissen. *Dtsch. tierärztl. Wschr.* 91: 24-6.

Riessen, H.A. van. 1982. Role of the Federation of Veterinarians in the EEC (FVE) in Animal Welfare. *Anim. Regul. Stud.* 3:145-52.

Rozemond, H. 1970. De veterinaire begeleiding van grote bedrijven *Tijdschr. Diergeneeskd.* 95:117-22.

Schweitzer, A. 1984. *Die Ehrfurcht vor dem Leben:* Grundtexte aus 5 Jahrzehnten. Beck, Munchen.

Singer, P. 1975. *Animal Liberation*. New York: Avon Books.

Part IV
Attitudes Towards Animals

THE GREEN MOVEMENT: IMPLICATIONS FOR ANIMALS

Ronnie Z. Hawkins

P.O. Box 13253
Gainesville, Florida 32604

Introduction

The Green movement, a newly emerging political movement that is both global in scope and firmly anchored to each local region at the grassroots level, is destined to be of great import to those concerned with the status of nonhuman animals in our society. Closely allied with deep ecology and bioregionalism, Green thinking embodies an alteration in our perception of the human organism: no longer seen as separate from and superior to all the other components of the ecosystem, our species is placed in context as one among many interdependent forms of life, with the attainment of a *sustainable balance* among all life forms being the desired goal in designing our human activities. Translation of this viewpoint into political action is the challenge of Green organizations on several continents today.

Green political organizations are springing up in one form or another all around the globe, including here in North America, but the West German *die Grünen*, the Greens, are perhaps the best known and have generated a detailed platform that will provide a helpful model for an examination of Green politics and its ramifications with regard to animal issues. Briefly, the policies of die Grünen are based on four fundamental principles: ecology, social responsibility, grassroots democracy, and nonviolence. The principle of ecology entails holistic thinking as well as ecological science, and deep ecology (to be discussed in greater detail shortly) as opposed to a shallow environmentalism which seeks ecosystem protection solely out of human-centered concern. Social responsibility has been defined as "social justice and an assurance that the poor and the working class will not get hurt by programs to restructure the economy and our consumer society ecologically," (Capra and Spretnak 1984b) and the *Federal Programme* of die Grünen contains a comprehensive set of guidelines for protecting and extending the rights and freedoms of human individuals. The political power of the West German Greens is deeply rooted in grassroots democracy, with many of the Greens' constituents coming from the various citizens' movements, including peace, antinuclear, ecology, feminist, and consumer groups. Priority is given wherever possible to participatory democracy, with most decision-making occurring at the level of decentralized, semiautonomous local units. The fourth principle, nonviolence, refers to a cessation of both personal and institutional violence; it is reflected in the Greens' active resistance to the nuclear arms race and other forms of militarism and in their call for an end to the oppression of women, children, and minority groups, an end to the economic exploitation of Third World peoples, and an end to the exploitation of nature and nonhuman animals as well. Three other principles are sometimes added to the first four: decentralization of all social structures into smaller, more manageable units that will have greater inherent flexibility and capacity for self-direction; post-patriarchal politics, empowering women at all levels of governance and incorporating feminist analysis in policy-making; and spirituality, appreciating and expressing an awareness of the unity of all life on a spiritual level. All seven principles, as a holistic understanding would have it, necessarily intermesh, but for purposes of discussion they have been separated and examined.

"Deep ecology" is the line of thinking that forms the philosophical backbone of the Green movement; it is currently being elaborated by philosophers such as Arne Naess, George Sessions, and Bill Devall. Its roots are traceable to the works of Spinoza, Heidegger, Saint Francis, American Indian religion, and some Eastern traditions. The writings of earlier ecological thinkers such as Thoreau, John Muir and Aldo Leopold, and poets Walt Whitman, Robinson Jeffers, and Gary Snyder have also played a significant role in the development of this philosophy. Deep ecology seeks to understand humans within the context of the entire biosphere, and this "total field" model allows us to envision the relationships among seemingly separate entities as interwoven within a single living system. In keeping with recent advances in physics and biology, natural phenomena are seen as vital, cyclical, interconnected, and diverse in qualitative ways, in addition to being describable under certain conditions as mechanical, separate, and reducible to quantifiable but nonliving parts and pieces. Beyond this integrative viewpoint, deep ecology grants what has been called *biospherical egalitarianism* (Naess 1973), that is, *"the equal right to live and blossom"*, to all forms of life. In a recent ecology journal, Naess and Sessions (1984) outlined a tentative formulation of eight principles of deep ecology:

1) The well-being and flourishing of human and nonhuman Life on Earth have value in themselves (synonyms: intrinsic value, inherent value). These values are independent of the usefulness of the nonhuman world for human purposes.

2) Richness and diversity of life forms contribute to the realization of these values and are also values in themselves.

3) Humans have no right to reduce this richness and diversity except to satisfy *vital** needs.

4) The flourishing of human life and cultures is compatible with a substantial decrease of the human population. The flourishing of nonhuman life requires such a decrease.

5) Present human interference with the nonhuman world is excessive, and the situation is rapidly worsening.

6) Policies must therefore be changed. These policies affect basic economic, technological, and ideological structures. The resulting state of affairs will be deeply different from the present.

7) The ideological change is mainly that of appreciating *life quality* (dwelling in situations of inherent value) rather than adhering to an increasingly higher standard of living. There will be a profound awareness of the difference between big and great.

8) Those who subscribe to the foregoing points have an obligation directly or indirectly to try to implement the necessary changes.

The perspective of the deep ecologist, therefore, has been shifted from the human-centered limitations of what is presently the dominant paradigm, expanding into the complexity and compassion of Leopold's (1949) "thinking like a mountain." Deep ecology embodies what is sometimes called *biocentrism* as opposed to anthropocentrism: it is a matter of putting *life* at the center of our concern—not just human life, but all life, life in balance.

A full grasp of deep ecology goes beyond scientific knowledge and ethical consideration to a sense of spiritual oneness with the cosmos; its implication for our status as humans, far from an anthropocentrically feared diminution, is profoundly elevating and transformative. In the words of Australian activist John Seed (1983):

> Alienation subsides. The human is no longer an outsider, apart. Your humanness is recognized as being merely the most recent stage of your existence, and as you stop identifying exclusively with this chapter, you start to get in touch with yourself as mammal, as vertebrate, as a species only recently emerged from the rainforest.

*The term "vital need" is left deliberately vague to allow for considerable latitude in judgement (Naess and Sessions 1984).

An integral part of deep ecology is the awareness of the need to take action to rechannel the present destructive course of human activity. Seed continues:

> As the fog of amnesia disperses, there is a transformation in your relationship to other species, and in your commitment to them..."I am protecting the rainforest" develops to "I am part of the rainforest protecting myself. I am that part of the rainforest recently emerged into thinking."

In their recently published *Deep Ecology*, Devall and Sessions (1985) discuss at some length the obligation to engage in nonviolent witnessing of and direct action to halt the injuries being inflicted upon the planetary systems, action which can range from public speaking, filing lawsuits, and educating politicians to sitting down in front of bulldozers. They describe *ecological resistance* as acting on the principles of deep ecology, likening it to befriending another species, or a mountain or river, and taking steps to preserve the peace of the greater neighborhood when the need arises. In his foreword to *Ecodefense* (Foreman 1985), Edward Abbey extends this analogy by comparing the latest assault upon American wilderness* to a stranger breaking down the door of one's house, threatening one's family with deadly weapons, and ransacking the place, a crime that one must defend oneself against by whatever means are necessary. Detailing the techniques of "monkeywrenching," Foreman goes beyond civil disobedience to include the incapacitation of the machinery of destruction in this defense, being careful to exclude violence to human or nonhuman life in such measures. He asserts:

> Monkeywrenchers—although nonviolent—are warriors. They are exposing themselves to possible arrest or injury. It is not a casual or flippant affair. They keep a pure heart and mind about it. They remember that they are engaged in the most moral of all actions: protecting life, defending the Earth.

Foreman states that a widespread and serious ecodefense could protect millions of acres of wilderness and hundreds of threatened life forms more effectively than a Congressional act or an army of game wardens. He concludes:

> John Muir said that if it ever came to a war between the races, he would side with the bears. That day has arrived.

---

*The Development Activities in Roadless Nonselected plan of the U.S. Forest Service, now getting under way, aims to cut over 75,000 miles of new roads into presently roadless areas and in many cases log from the center outward, thus destroying most of the last remaining large areas of natural diversity in the continental United States. Of 140 million acres of undeveloped public lands, only about 24 million are likely to be protected as wilderness; the rest will face ecological devastation within half a decade.

Deep ecology thus provides the Green-oriented individual with both spiritual affirmation and an impetus toward action that can entail a very high degree of personal commitment.

If deep ecology forms the philosophical foundation of the Green movement, the translation of its concepts into appropriate human activity unique to each particular place on the planet occurs through bioregionalism. An awakening that has been taking shape predominantly in North America, bioregionalism has to do with reintroducing a sense of *place* into our disconnected and homogenized Western culture, rediscovering how the web of life interplays in any given natural region, be it a watershed, a mountain range, a coastal plain, or whatever, binding together the topography, climate, floral, faunal, and human communities found therein. Emphasizing that the human has a rightful place within each bioregion (or, at least, within many of them), Peter Berg has introduced the term *reinhabitation*, signifying the active process of learning to *live in place* once again. In *Reinhabiting a Separate Country*, Berg (1978) notes:

> The boundaries of a bioregion are best described by people who have lived within it, through human recognition of the realities of living in place. All life on the planet is interconnected in a few obvious ways and in many more that remain barely explored. But there is a distinct resonance among living things and the factors which influence them that occurs specifically within each separate place on the planet. Discovering and describing that resonance is a way to describe a bioregion.

The American Indian tradition has always had a strong sense of living in place, and indeed the lack of a sense of place combined with an overemphasis on historical *time* has been an American Indian criticism of European culture (Deloria 1973); even European societies, however, were by necessity adapted to the conditions of their particular geographical areas until the coming of industrialism, which offered the illusion of having freed us from that seeming obligation while hastening our loss of regional character and widening the gap of our separation from the rest of the natural world. Bioregionalism is the obvious answer to the question "Decentralize into what?"—so logical a unit is it for human activity and organization that one may well wonder why our society has for so long overlooked the natural unit in deference to what is an often unwieldy, abstract demarcation arising predominantly out of historical contingency. But perhaps the most critical quality of a bioregion is found in this definition by Thomas Berry (1984): "A bioregion is simply an identifiable geographic area whose life systems are self-contained, self-sustaining and self-renewing." The concept of *sustainability*, once raised, forces us to confront the fact that most of our present activities are neither self-contained in space nor self-sustaining over time, from the metropolis that can exist only by spatially exploiting other bioregions to obtain its food and energy and relieve itself of wastes, to mistakenly self-congratulatory "growth" regions like the American Sunbelt that are seemingly unaware of the temporal limitations to the prosperity accompanying the first phase of that exponential curve. Applying the criterion of sustainability necessitates recognizing an optimal, and certainly a maximal, limit determined by the human carrying capacity for each bioregional unit, and once we achieve this realization we can begin a conscious leveling off into a steady state of appropriate design.

Decentralization into the bioregional unit can be a powerful concept to embrace if we are to free ourselves from several serious dilemmas caused by the bigness and bureaucracy to which our society currently clings. As Ozark organizer David Haenke (1984) discusses in his pamphlet *Ecological Politics and Bioregionalism*, recognition of natural or ecological law, as it operates specifically within each place, shows us what will work best for us too—the deceptive abstractions of economics notwithstanding, it is most efficient to operate *with* rather than *against* nature, and in decentralized units we can exercise the utmost flexibility in doing so. The present deadlock of forcing a choice between the problems of nuclear power and acid rain thereby breaks down into utilizing windpower here, capturing solar energy there, and generating some biomass for fuel across the way, depending on what is most available and practical. The myth that we must accept topsoil-depleting, pesticide-soaked monocultures of machine-harvested crops shuttled thousands of miles to market, or run the risk of starvation, dissolves into embracing permaculture, integrated pest management, regional and seasonal crop variety, and community gardens tended with local pride for satisfying local appetites. Decentralization into the bioregional unit also points us in a direction leading away from the nuclear weapons impass, since recognizing the natural law that sets a maximum size limit to fully self-governing groups of human beings and rediscovering responsible, participatory democracy enables us to let the nation-state, upon which planetary nuclear war is predicated, recede into the background and fade away.

The ways in which Green thinking and Green policies will affect nonhuman animals, directly and indirectly, are numerous. Most importantly, the old anthropocentric bias that gave humans automatic priority in every situation has been swept away; while all Green-oriented individuals may not agree on just what the animals' rights are, recognition has been granted to nonhuman animals as fellow beings whose concerns we must consider. On one level, the problems of animals cannot be separated from those of the ecosystem at large, just as those of humans as a group cannot, and hence all policies dealing with ecological considerations are of relevance to animal species. But appreciation of animals as our spiritual relations entails protection of individual creatures as well as members of population groups, and the platform of the West German Greens reflects this position also.

The preamble to the Federal Programme of die Grünen (1983) contains the statement "We consider ourselves part of the Green movement throughout the world," and among the most urgent of the issues they address are global ones. If our goal is sustainability of the planetary ecosystem, each diminution or disappearance of a species represents another failure in moving toward that goal, a further weakening of the web of life that supports us all. Actions must be taken at once to halt and reverse those processes leading to species extinction, from a cessation of whaling to an end to rain forest destruction, and indeed the Federal Programme calls for both. Trade in endangered species and their products is to be totally prohibited; West Germany is instructed to campaign actively for international species protection, and immediate measures are to include a ban on importation of products such as sealskins and a license requirement for certain other items. Appreciation of the gravity of the human overpopulation problem is present along with the desire for partnership with Third World peoples, and the Programme specifies that assistance for birth control must be supplied to overpopulated countries upon request. Likewise,the destructiveness of the Western development model, which is particularly severe when abruptly applied to "underdeveloped" areas, and which results in known mistakes that need not be duplicated, is recognized in the provision: "Vocational training of the less developed peoples must be promoted not so as to impart to them the failed ideas of the industrialized countries but rather to allow them to solve their problems within their means and in a way appropriate to their environment." And with the awareness that nuclear holocaust is an even quicker means of planetary destruction than the ongoing ecological degradation, the Greens demand an immediate beginning to worldwide disarmament and a global ban on the production and storage of nuclear weapons. Understanding that present economic policies underlie and encourage all these undesirable activities, die Grünen reject the major assumption made by both ends of the old political spectrum. Proclaiming "we are neither left nor right, we are in front," (Capra and Spretnak 1984a) the Greens seek to correct the mistaken belief that infinite expansion of industrial production is possible or desirable in a finite system, an error that both capitalist and communist forms of government have incorporated. While it may take many decades, indeed centuries, to restore the planet to a truly harmonious balance among populations of its different life forms, implementation of the global objectives of the Greens will assure that at least the overall trend of our society will be heading in that direction rather than in the reverse—we would sleep at night secure in the knowledge that our children's children will inherit a planet at least as stable, diverse, and sustainable as the one we have now, something that, sadly, cannot be said at present.

With regard to their own country, the Greens' Federal Programme contains extensive and detailed provisions aimed at protection of the ecosystem. The Greens take the position that "Protection of native animals and plants in their natural surroundings must be given priority over economic development plans." Large areas are to be maintained or restored as nature preserves, and native species which have been exterminated in areas are to be reintroduced. Attention is paid to protection of shorelines, saltmarshes, and wetlands, and further drainage measures are to be prohibited. In addition to preserves, protection of species and natural areas is to be extended into the places where people live and work. "Open planning" is demanded in regard to all new building, with environmental protection organizations to be included in all planning procedures and granted the right to bring citizen lawsuits. Wooded areas, thickets, and hedges removed by building are to be completely replaced. Road building is to be restricted to the completion and maintenance of the existing road system (in effect delimiting an optimal size for the society as well as ensuring protection of natural areas), with the people formerly employed in road building to be retrained, perhaps in landscape preservation or energy conservation activities. A ministry of the environment is to be established to correct present conditions of habitat degradation and species extirpation, deforestation, soil erosion, and contamination of soil, water, and air by toxic chemicals and radioactivity. Immediate measures are to be taken to reduce the emission of pollutants by industry, power plants, and motor vehicles, with an absolute ban on known carcinogenic pollutants; emphasis is to be put upon recycling, as well as minimizing and detoxifying the waste that is produced. The Greens oppose the construction and operation of nuclear power plants.

Agriculture is to be closely scrutinized as to its effects on the ecosystem: "As far as damage to the environment goes, agriculture can now compete with industry." The Federal Programme states that "The supreme aim of agricultural policy must be the healthy nutrition of the population," which presupposes healthful foodstuffs produced on healthy soil through an ecologically oriented mode of production. Economic policies which have heretofore favored large, centralized, industrialized and chemically dependent methods of agriculture and adversely affected organic or ecological agriculture and small- to medium-sized farms must be reversed. Monocultures and intensive livestock production are to be replaced by mixed farming, with on-site interchange of fertilizer, feeds, and energy sources where possible. Chemical pesticides and herbicides will eventually be completely supplanted by appropriate cropping, biological controls and other ecologically sound, soil health-enhancing measures; and during the readjustment period, stricter legal limits are to be imposed on pesticides, and residues closely monitored.

Fishing and forestry are also to be readjusted to ecological soundness. The Federal Programme makes the (for some) radical statement that "The main task of forestry is to sustain the ecological stability of the forest. Timber production for profit must be subordinate to this aim." There is to be a shift away from the species-poor stretches of even-age monoculture to more natural, mixed foliage of native types and differing age composition which are much more favorable to a diversity of wildlife. Individual selective felling is to replace clear-cutting, accompanied by a restriction of large machinery and the eventual banning of chemical controls. Corrective measures with respect to fisheries include immediate reduction of catch quotas on certain depleted species to allow stocks to recover, protected zones, closer controls over fishing grounds, mesh sizes, and closed seasons, a prohibition on catching young fish as fish meal, steps to reduce waste of fish products, and support for techniques that favor small- and medium-sized fishing companies.

Going beyond protection of the species within the ecosystem, the Federal Programme of die Grünen includes a number of provisions for protecting the rights of individual nonhuman animals. "Animals must no longer be legally considered as 'objects,' but should be granted a special legal status." Torture of animals is prohibited and to be "severely punished," and strict regulations on the keeping and transport of domestic and captive wild animals are proposed. In agriculture, animals are to be kept in ways that are "fair to their species and nature," and "Cruel battery farming must finally be abolished." As an immediate measure, obligatory labeling of animal products as to their origin (e.g., battery vs. free-range eggs) is demanded. Animal breeding must also be "fair to the species," and genetic manipulation of animals as well as humans is rejected. Industrial animal production, in addition to its cruelty to the animals in question, is to be curtailed also in the interests of supporting small farms and protecting human jobs.

The issue of laboratory experimentation upon animals is also raised specifically: "In the name of science, thousands of animals daily undergo fatal experiments, e.g., for the testing of chemicals, weapons, medicines and cosmetics. . . .Experiments on animals should be replaced by suitable proven alternative methods (e.g., tissue culture or computer simulation in the medical sphere). A comparison must be made by legal experts between the expected benefit from the experiment and the right to life of the animals concerned." Repetition of experiments is to be avoided by establishment of a central data bank for all permitted animal experiments and the obligation to publish data already obtained. The value of psychological experiments on animals is noted to be "highly questionable." Responsibility for enforcement of animal protection guidelines in both agriculture and research is to be transferred from the ministry of agriculture to a ministry of the environment, to be created.

While this platform may not go quite far enough to satisfy the most committed animal rights activists, it clearly provides a framework within which many improvements in the status and condition of animals can be made. All of those who care about animals should agree on the necessity for vigorous pursuit of ecosystem stabilization and rehabilitation of endangered and threatened wild species. In regard to domestic animals, certain changes—decentralization and scale reduction, with the aim of eventual elimination of industrialized agriculture, for instance—will go far to correct the worst institutional abuses. But much more work needs to be done on this front, and, since the Green program, taken as a whole, represents an attempt to define an optimal scheme for all our human activities, what constitutes an ideal position for domestic animals must be reexamined critically in the years to come if we are to move away from all forms of exploitation. There are those who would advocate the eventual elimination of all human-animal dependence, including the phasing out of all farm and companion animals over a period of time, allowing them to revert over generations back to autonomous wild beings. Others consider the small farm situation in which the animals are accorded respect and a pleasant livelihood in exchange for certain "products," which might or might not include flesh, to be an appropriate, minimally exploitative and overall mutually beneficial state.

Certainly the application of an ecological analysis to our companion animals is overdue: we must assume responsibility for correcting an overabundance of domesticated carnivores, the excess of which is not supportable by the ecosystem and individuals of which, having weakened survival skills and disrupted social patterns, are doomed to prolonged suffering and starvation when not in the care of a human. An accounting must also be made of the meat presently being used to maintain them, which may ultimately be contributing to a toll taken on marine mammals and other diminishing species as well as domestic cattle and poultry. Trade in wild-captured tropical birds, coral reef fish and exotic reptiles for the "pet" trade should be curtailed on ecological grounds, and a total ban on removal of any wild species, endangered or not, from its native habitat, except perhaps for the most pressing scientific purposes in the interests of that species, is not unthinkable. The raison d'être of the fur trade likewise needs reevaluation, and a new definition of our relationship to so-called "pest" species is clearly called for, with peaceful coexistence as a goal. In regard to laboratory experimentation on nonhuman animals, the shift to emphasis upon a holistic understanding of health should hasten the cutting back on invasive exploitation, as we recognize the inherent limitations of the mechanistic "animal model": neither the importance of the total field of interaction in health and illness, nor the importance of inner motivation in the active pursuit of health, can be addressed adequately by studying caged and coerced animals. Under the new model, much scientific progress can be anticipated in the area of interspecies communication, through noninvasive exploration, in the appropriate context, of the language structure and social organization of the species in question—meeting wherever possible on the animal's terms rather than solely on human ones.

The West German Greens make no mention of vegetarianism in their Programme, although one would expect a considerable number of adherents among them by personal choice, out of concern for ecological, health, and spiritual considerations; there is also no specific attention to the issue of hunting, though presumably if such activity is to occur it will be only under strict ecological guidelines. As we fashion an optimal level of human-animal interaction, we humans are faced with the choice of just how predatory we shall allow ourselves to be. Our biological capacity provides us with a high degree of flexibility, and arguments can be made both for the predatory role being as much our right as that of many other members of the ecosystem, as well as for the minimalization of our carnivorous practices so as to be more in keeping with the dietary habits of the great apes, and hence with our own physiological adaptations. Another facet to the hunting question concerns the traditions of native peoples throughout the world. While appreciation of the cultural diversity of human beings is perhaps as much a Green value as preservation of biological diversity, it must be admitted that in many areas irreversible changes have occurred, and where the introduction of technological advantages to traditional hunting is working to the detriment of the hunted species, such practices will have to be curtailed. It is to be hoped that, where new cultural norms will inevitably arise from cultural mingling, respect for the lives of nonhuman animals will prevail and the conscious choice for a reduction in exploitation will be made.

In working out their ambitious program, the West German Greens have not been free of conflict, which has arisen as much out of the diversity of their constituency and the struggle to maintain noncompetitive ideals within the established structure of government as out of the difficulty of introducing new ideas, some of which require considerably more development, into the political arena. Perhaps the remarkable thing is that the party has functioned as well as it has to date. Temporary allies on different pieces of legislation may come from either camp of old-paradigm politics, as illustrated by the Freiburg proposal to ban the salting of streets in winter because of its detrimental effect on trees; the right-leaning Christian Democrats voted with the Greens, while the traditionally left-wing Social Democrats put the protection of human jobs, in this case those of the street-salters, above the ecological considerations. The split is indicative of the kinds of conflict and compromise that will arise in making the transition to an ecologically sound society, and demonstrates the need for the kind of conversion programs and job retraining called for by the "social responsibility" principle of the platform. Obviously, since the vote that sent a Green contingent into the West German *Bundestag* in March of 1983 was barely over the mandatory 5 percent necessary for inclusion under their system of proportional representation, there is a long way to go before many of the more visionary proposals set forth begin to see implementation. What is perhaps most significant at this time is that the goals, in particular the overriding goal of attaining a sustainable human society on the planet, have been drawn up for all to see, and the presence of a Green voice, however small, in government will assure that they are kept before our eyes.

There are now Green political organizations within Great Britain, most European nations, Australia, New Zealand, Canada, and Japan, and a Green organization is currently taking shape at the national level in the United States. The Cumberland Greens, the Los Angeles Greens, and other Green groups have already formed at the local and regional level, and they join a number of bioregions that have already developed a high degree of ecopolitical awareness, such as Shasta, in northern California, and Ozarkia, straddling Arkansas and Missouri. In the "Green Alternative—It *Can* Happen Here," the concluding chapter of *Green Politics*, by Fritjof Capra and Charlene Spretnak (1984b), several possible forms are outlined for the Green movement in the United States, including a network linking decentralized Green groups, a national membership organization that might include a political action committee but would not sponsor candidates, Green caucuses that could work within both the Republican and Democratic parties, and an actual Green party that would run candidates in elections. Since the United States, unlike West Germany and some other countries, does not have a system of proportional representation, and since a third party traditionally fares poorly in American politics, the success of an actual Green party appears somewhat dubious in America at present. However, while electoral politics at the national level may present disadvantages for the budding Green movement, other American traditions are in its favor, from a historical beginning arising out of grassroots democracy to considerable recent experience with activism through the peace movement, the feminist movement, and different environmental and animal protection organizations, to name a few, and many of these latter groups are beginning to appreciate the way in which their various agendas begin to merge past a certain point. Spretnak suggests five layers for Green organization: local, bioregional, state, macroregional, and national; the major thrust of most Green political activity will most likely take place at the local and bioregional level, with the preexisting bioregional consciousness in some areas providing a ready-made framework for initiating an ecological politics. One such group is the

Ozark Area Community Congress, which has convened five successive participatory congresses and maintains standing committees dealing with almost every aspect of living in the Ozarks: agriculture and forestry, water, energy, health, education and communications, economics, communities, spiritual and cultural concerns, feminism, and peace; committee members educate themselves, make resolutions to translate ecological law into appropriate human activity in each category, and as much as possible put these activities into practice.

One of the first steps in awakening people to Green awareness is introducing them to their bioregion's characteristic plants and animals and their habits, and a number of efforts in that direction are currently ongoing in the United States. The Ozark Area Community Congress, for example, puts out a "bundle," a sampler packet containing materials representative of life in the Ozarks, among which is information on Ozark flora and fauna and their seasonal changes within the Ozark year. Other groups working to focus attention on the nonhuman life in their area include Peter Berg's Planet Drum Foundation, putting on programs in and around San Francisco and generating publications including a tri-annual bioregional newspaper entitled *Raise the Stakes*, and Nancy Morita's "Wild in the City" project (sponsored by Planet Drum), which is seeking to reintroduce and strengthen the populations of some of San Francisco's native wild species, such as peregrine falcons, brown pelicans and California sea lions. To make San Franciscans aware of the wild creatures that once inhabited the area as well as of present indigenous species, her "Wild in the City" poster/map compares the city of today with the native bioregion of 250 years ago, and she and others have been known to paint "ghost" hoof prints and paw prints of the vanished tule elk and grizzly bear down city sidewalks where, before the sidewalks came, these wild ones used to roam. All Species Day celebrations, initiated in 1978 in San Francisco by Ponderosa Pine and continued through the efforts of Chris Wells and others, have now been held in over a dozen different cities; children are encouraged to choose a species they feel close to, learn about its habits and needs and personify it in some way through costume and theatre, coming away with a new understanding of the animals' lives as well as their own.

More than two hundred participants gathered for the First North American Bioregional Congress in May of 1984, just outside Kansas City, Missouri; at that time a Green politics committee took shape to address the interest in formation of a Green political organization within the United States. The following August, a meeting of sixty activists, predominantly representatives of ecological, community, and peace groups, was held in the Minneapolis-St. Paul, Minnesota, area, out of which has emerged the Interregional Committee of Correspondence to facilitate the growth of the Green movement in America. A formal founding convention for a Green organization on the national scale is being planned for the near future. Those who manifest a concern for nonhuman animals and who are interested in what the coming Green movement will portend in their regard are strongly urged to become involved at some level.

For more information on the Wild in the City Project, readers may contact Nancy Morita, director, at 6 Cypress, San Anselmo, CA, 94960. Information on Planet Drum publications, activities, and newspaper subscriptions may be obtained from: Planet Drum Foundation, Box 31251, San Francisco, CA, 94131. Information on sponsoring an All Species Day celebration may be obtained from Chris Wells, 538 Aqua Fria, Sante Fe, NM, 87501. The Interregional Committee of Correspondence may be reached at PO Box 40040, St. Paul, MN, 55104.

References

Berg, P. 1978. *Reinhabiting a Separate Country.* San Francisco: Planet Drum Foundation.
Berg, P. 1981. Devolving beyond global monoculture. *CoEvolution Quarterly.* 32:24.
Berry, T. 1984. Bioregionalism: A better way to understand where you live. (Interview). *The Tarrytown Letter.* 41:3-5.
Capra, F. and Spretnak, C. 1984a. Who are the Greens? *New Age Journal.* April: 34.
Capra, F. and Spretnak, C. 1984b. *Green Politics: The Global Promise.* New York: E.P. Dutton, Inc.
Deloria, V., Jr. 1973. *God is Red.* New York: Grosset and Dunlap, Inc.
Devall, B. and Sessions, G. 1985. *Deep Ecology.* Layton, Utah: Peregrine Smith Books.
die Grünen. 1983. *Programme of the German Green Party.* Fernbach, H., trans. London: Heretic Books.
Foreman, D. 1985. *Ecodefense: A Field Guide to Monkeywrenching.* Tucson, AZ: Earth First! Books.
Haenke, D. 1984. *Ecological Politics and Bioregionalism.* Drury, MO: New Life Farm.
Leopold, A. 1949. *A Sand County Almanac.* Oxford University Press, Inc.
Naess, A. 1973. The shallow and the deep, long-range ecology movement. A Summary. *Inquiry.* 16: 95-100.
Naess, A. and Sessions, G. 1984. The basic principles of deep ecology. *Earth First!* 4(6): 19.
Seed, J. 1983. Anthropocentrism. *Earth First!* 3(6): 15.

HUMAN PERCEPTIONS OF ANIMALS AND ANIMAL AWARENESS: THE CULTURAL DIMENSION*

Elizabeth A. Lawrence

Tufts University
School of Veterinary Medicine
Boston, MA. 02111

Introductory Overview

Culture is generally a powerful determinant of human perceptions of animals and the treatment animals receive in a given society. For example, Plains Indians' views of the status of animals—their capacities, their awareness, and their place in the world relative to mankind—differ radically from those characteristic of Western thought. Many of the contemporary Crow Indians, a group of native Americans among which I have recently carried out anthropological field research, continue to look upon their horses according to traditional tribal belief. Their particular attitude toward horses conflicts with that of the dominant white society with which the Indians and their horses must interact. Mutual hostility results from a lack of understanding between members of the two cultures who, though living in proximity, remain worlds apart in ethos. Two other examples from ethnographic literature involving the habitual treatment of mules in a community of farmers and of sled dogs by a group of Eskimos also highlight the importance of cultural attitudes in affecting interactions with animals in those societies. It is vital to strive to understand the many complex factors which determine views toward animals, including their capacities for awareness, in alien cultures whose value-systems may be foreign to our

*Paper presented at the Institute for the Study of Animal Problems Symposium on Animal Awareness and Human Perceptions: Implications for Animal Welfare, November 3, 1982.

own. Since human actions toward animals are rooted in perceptual concepts concerning the intrinsic nature of those animals, it is only through empathy resulting from understanding such concepts that a beginning can be made in solving the many problems involved in human relationships with animals.

Plains Indian Worldview

See, Brothers; Spring is here.
The earth has taken the embrace
of the Sun, and soon we shall see
The children of all that love.
All seeds are awake, and all animals.
From this great power we too have our lives.
And therefore we concede
to our fellow creatures
even our animal fellows,
The same rights as ourselves
To live on this earth.

(Fuchs and Havighurst 1972, p. xv)

Speaking these words in 1877, the great Sioux leader, Sitting Bull, was expressing the viewpoint of his Plains Indian culture and society toward animals. Embodying a holistic concept of all creation, this outlook is at opposite poles from that of the white Anglo-American ethos which was aggressive and exploitative toward nature—the attitude characteristic of the dominant society which had all but defeated and subjugated the Plains tribes, even as Sitting Bull spoke. For in the minds of the whites, nothing could stand in the way of westward expansion and the progress of "civilization": Indians and nature were both considered as part of the wild which must be cleared away.

Plains tribes generally embrace a mode of thought in which all forms of life on earth exist on a dynamic circular plane. One form of life is not considered to be above another, in a linear hierarchy with man at the top, as in the Judaeo-Christian scheme. As one articulate native American expresses it, "All of life is living—that is, dynamic and aware, partaking, as it does, in the life of the All-Spirit, and contributing, as it does, to the ongoing life of that same Great Mystery" (Allen 1975). There is essential harmony in the world, and primary assumptions are that all of nature, both animals and people, "are seen to be brothers or relatives, all are offspring of the Great Mystery, children of our mother, and necessary parts of an ordered, balanced, and living whole." Such an ideology makes no separation between nature and mankind and no dualistic division between material and spiritual: all are expressions of the same reality (Allen 1975).

No people have been more closely attuned to the earth and to nature than have the nomadic tribes of the Great Plains, and their beliefs developed out of keen observations of their living environment. It was clear to them that other animals besides man possessed many capacities. People could see that animals had certain powers and believed that it was reasonable that they could think and communicate. Sitting Bull related how as a boy he was saved from the attack of a grizzly bear by the warnings of a meadowlark. The alert songbird had been aware of the boy's danger and communicated it. Thereafter, this bird, along with others of its kind, became Sitting Bull's special protector, whose speech he could henceforth understand (Vestal 1932). Such occurrences were by no means uncommon, and even today some individuals who still follow old traditions continue to experience them.

Native American creation tales, differing radically from Genesis, reveal insights about the status of animals as perceived by Indians. Unlike the Judaeo-Christian God, who made everything and then gave commandments as to the way it all was to function, the Cheyenne All-Spirit, for example, consulted the animals concerning the process of creation, once it had begun (Allen 1975). In virtually every native explanation for the beginning of the earth or the origin of the first human beings, feelings of close kinship with animals and great respect for other creatures and their powers are evident. In some versions, water birds were asked to dive down and bring up mud to form the earth (Burland 1970). Often the human race is believed to have come into existence with the aid of animals or through transformation from an animal (Emerson 1965). Certain tribes assert that mankind resulted from the union of two different species of animals, such as the snail and the beaver who were parents to the first Osage people (Marriott and Rachlin 1975).

Crow Indians and Horses

Today, although acculturation to the dominant society has brought many changes for native Americans, there are still some groups which have managed to retain much of their own culture. One of these is the Crow tribe of southeastern Montana, a Plains people among whom I have carried out field work (1975-80) focusing on attitudes toward nature and animals. A large majority of the Crows still speak their native language, and many tribespeople have retained traditional beliefs, customs, and ceremonies. One aspect of the Crow attitude toward animals—that of their relationship with their horses—illustrates the relevance of the cultural dimension in affecting perceptions of animals and their treatment. Crow interaction with horses, I found, exemplifies the sharp contrasts which exist between the Crow ethos and the views of the members of the dominant white society who live on or near the reservation and with whom the Indians and their livestock must interact.

Horses are very important to contemporary Crows, and are abundant today on the reservation. The vital significance of horses in the lives of these people results from a combination of factors from the past and from the present. For Plains tribes such as the Crows, acquisition of horses early in the eighteenth century vastly improved the quality of their lives in virtually every way. Horses revolutionized transportation, hunting, and war, and the many benefits they conferred upon their riders soon made the animals the tribe's most treasured possessions. So great was their worth that they became the measure of all value, synonymous with prestige and wealth. Yet this did not mean, as it might have in another context, that the relationship with horses was purely utilitarian. As admired partners, horses became part of the human spiritual and aesthetic spheres as well as the pragmatic. Horses imparted special knowledge and power to people who established rapport with them, and could provide help in time of trouble. A strong sense of reciprocity supported the belief, still widely held, that considerate treatment of horses brings good fortune to a person and that mistreatment of the animals will be punished. Traditional taboos, originating out of gratitude, continue to dictate against killing horses and eating their flesh. Plains riders became as one with their mounts, and communication based on mutual understanding was a natural occurrence. As the great Crow chief, Plenty Coups, expressed it:

> My horse fights with me and fasts with me, because if he is to carry me in battle he must know my heart and I must know his or we shall never become brothers. I have been told that the white man, who is almost a god, and yet a great fool, does not believe that the horse has a spirit (soul). This cannot be true. I have many times seen my horse's soul in his eyes. And on this day on that knoll I knew my horse understood. I saw his soul in his eyes. (Linderman 1930, p. 100)

One of the most tragic aspects of the Plains natives' experience after they were confined to reservations was the cessation of active participation in the horse-related activities which had made life meaningful as mounted nomads. For the Crows, adverse reaction to this loss was a significant factor contributing to the difficult adjustment to a sedentary existence. It is the period of their tribal history between the introduction of the horse and the end of nomadic life by which Plains Indians are still characterized, even by the natives themselves. Today the Crows continue to look back to the Horse Era of their history with nostalgia and enduring pride. Partnership with horses had given their people new freedom and dignity, and their dynamic interactions with these animals charged the tempo of life with the force of expanded dimensions of experience and awareness.

In recent times, the Crows were fortunate in being able to bring about a return of horses to their reservation. Renewed interest in them has meant that horses have been adapted to recreational activities compatible with modern reservation life. For many Crows, association with their horses is essential to the maintenance of their identity as Indians. Horses, though, do not have to be ridden or handled individually to be important. Repeatedly, the Crow people made clear their deep satisfaction in simply having abundant horses grazing around them. This is perceived as the way life should be for Crows, who told me "horses are part of our nature, and love of horses is instilled into the spiritual makeup of all Crows from the time they are little." They reveal that the satisfaction derived from the prevalence of horses on tribal lands is a source of encouragement in facing the difficult problems of daily existence which natives feel are imposed upon them by the dominant white society.

Despite the vital importance of interaction with horses in contemporary Crow society, however, the role of the animals is not understood by local non-Indians and officials who deal with the Indians and their horses. Such people, lacking empathy, generally view animal relationships only by standards set by their own culture and the values it espouses. Whites claim, for example, that the Crows are negligent in allowing their horses to overgraze the land, that they should fence in their livestock, and control their animals at all times. But the Crows, with their enculturation from a nomadic background, do not have the same sense of "management" of animals and the manipulation of nature that are ingrained in the Western ethos. Thus differing points of view cause frequent conflicts. Neighboring whites often criticize the Crows for what non-Indians perceive as cruelty to their horses. The traditional practice of leaving horses to "winter out" in the northern Montana Plains without providing shelter or supplementary feed brings accusations of inhumanity and neglect. But the Crows' perceptions of animals and their capacities are different. Crows know that a horse will paw through the snow to eat the grass below, just as in the old nomadic days, and that this ability shows intelligence and adaptiveness. Tribesmen recall that throughout Crow history cottonwood bark served as winter feed for horses on the Northern Plains. The efficacy of this practice in keeping horses well-nourished all winter has been documented (Boller 1972).

Crow horsemen insist that horses left out to fend for themselves are usually in far better condition in the spring than those which have been sheltered and provided with artificial feed. The intense pride these people take in their horses' toughness reveals the Crows' sense of identification with their animals and their concept that animals are not creatures of another order, but close kin. Crows today feel that even though their fellow tribesmen may be losing their former physical strength and endurance by succumbing to a "soft" life on the reservation, at least their horses—their "other selves," as it were—are perpetuating the hardiness which was formerly necessary to sustain life on the Plains. Indeed, the Crows' own historic ability to survive, surrounded as they once were by powerful enemies, and later to endure white domination while retaining much of their culture, has come to be symbolized by the hardihood of their horses.

This idea about wintering of horses is expressed in the story told to me by a Crow who in his boyhood had observed the government-organized killing of so-called "worthless range horses" on tribal land. He made special reference, again and again, to the fact that *all* the horses had been shot indiscriminately, not just the weakest or the "locoed" ones (poisoned by eating loco weed), as the official horse-killers had claimed. Equine victims of the slaughter included, he stressed, "the horses that could winter by themselves and survive alone." His words echoed disbelief as he reiterated his feelings about what was to him a preposterous aspect of the horse slaughter. "Many that were killed were hardy, and needed no care in a hard winter. Those horses knew what to do. They could make it themselves, on their own. But even the horses who were used to the hard winter were killed off with the rest!"

Winter care of equine animals is directly related to religion in the minds of many with whom I spoke. Crow elders explained that one of the reasons such great supernatural powers are ascribed to animals in their traditional belief system is that "they can get along alone, unaided, without clothing, shelter, and without fire." This remarkable ability distinguishes nonhuman creatures from mankind, who requires these artificial elements for survival, and helps to explain the animals' roles as intermediaries with the Great One. "There is power vested in animals," Crow traditionalists say, "because they can survive with no contribution from man." Thus, what constitutes "cruel treatment" in the minds of whites is for the Crows a sign of deep admiration for their horses' physical endurance and special mental and spiritual endowments. In this important matter concerning animal abilities, human perceptions resulting from cultural differences act to preserve social distance between two peoples who live in proximity and yet are worlds apart.

It must be emphasized that along with considering the particular ethos by which a society views its animals, it is essential that peoples' standards for treatment of animals be considered in the light of the standards they set for themselves. Without considering this comparative dimension, a distorted picture emerges. Life in the Great Plains, the context in which Crow culture developed, for example, was demanding. Strength and endurance, above all, were required and merited society's approval—no less for animals than for people.

Mules as Victims

Turning now to a different society for a brief comparison, a study of tenant farmers in the Deep South as described by James Agee in his classic work, *Let Us Now Praise Famous Men* (1978), provides an intimate portrait of a culturally distinct group of people living in extreme poverty. Probably lost upon the average reader within the vast welter of information the writer gives about every observable detail of life for these downtrodden people, are a few remarkably revealing passages about the treatment of the mules who work with the sharecroppers. "Even in harnessing him his head is knocked around some, and in all his motions relevant to his users he is used with the gratuitous sort of toughness an American policeman uses against anyone (except the right people) who happen to fall into his power" (Agee 1978). "The farmer," Agee goes on to say, "is liable to be an expert within the whole range of bullying, battering, and torturing this particular animal, and to have peculiarly urgent egoistic and sexual needs to exert full violence and domination over something living, preferably something at least as large and strong as himself" (1978).

With insight, Agee explains that "the mule stands readier victim than any other animal because he is used in the main and most hopeless work, because he is an immediate symbol of this work, and because by transference *he is the farmer himself* (italics mine), and in the long tandem harness wherein members and forces of a whole world beat and use and drive and force each other, if they are to live at all, is the one creature in front of this farmer" (1978). The writer confesses his own lack of ability to fully explain the observed sadism, the "casualness, apathy, self-interest, unconscious, offhand, and deliberated cruelty, in relation toward extra-human life" which is "terrible enough to freeze your blood or to break your heart or to propel you toward murder." Sadly, he concludes that it is "unlikely that enough of the causes can ever be altered, or pressures withdrawn, to make much difference" (1978).

Unfortunately for purposes of analysis, the sharecroppers Agee observed so closely never told him of their perceptions of animals or of animal awareness. It *is* clear, however, that in their life stories there is revealed no sense of reciprocity or kinship with their fellow creatures, no belief in a harmonious world. The explanation that the almost unbearable hardship of their own lives bears directly upon the sharecroppers' treatment of animals is inescapable. The sense of identity with his mules which Agee noted on the part of the farmer must be a powerful determinant. Related to this is the awful and unspoken truth that if awareness were not somehow attributed to the mules, such abuse as they received would yield no satisfaction to the drivers. This is one of the dilemmas in attempting to understand the roots of cruelty: do the perpetrators lack empathy, or do they indeed have it in excess, torturing in fact because they *do* have sharpened cognizance of the pain they inflict? Undoubtedly, many causative factors are involved in the dynamic relationship between sharecropper and mule which habitually results in the beast as victim of human brutality. A vitally important element here, as in the next example of sled dogs, is that such relationships are deeply ingrained, having the full force and endorsement of societal and cultural sanction. One carries out actions toward animals not just as an individual who is so disposed, but is motivated, at least in part, by a strong sense of belonging to a group which shares and upholds this particular mode of behavior.

Treatment of Sled Dogs

Sled dogs among arctic peoples are invariably described by observers as, according to our standards, inhumanely handled and often cruelly abused. In my experience the comment routinely following any discussion of this matter is that such treatment is inevitable, since it is not feasible to make "pets" out of working animals. Yet the whole question of the necessity for such harshness actually remains unanswered. Once again, there is a lack of data on native belief concerning their dogs' awareness. What is known is that in interaction with sled dogs, reciprocal kindliness and devotion between man and animal, whatever their untested effects may be, generally do not have the sanction of Eskimo societies that have so far been studied. Whether this attitude toward dogs has its origin, as some would say, in pure utility, or whether it results from a more complex combination of deep-level psychological and sociological characteristics of the Eskimo ethos has yet to be explained.

Resulting from her intensive long-term field research in the Canadian arctic, Jean Briggs' remarkably detailed ethnography, probes virtually every aspect of the Eskimo group with whom she lived. Expressively titled *Never in Anger* (1972), the study lays bare the central characteristic which ensures social cohesion in a difficult environment: individuals must never express or show outward signs of anger toward other people. Repressed hostility may be one cause, then, of the sadistic treatment of animals. Briggs describes the children's delight in killing the unwanted newborn puppies, "dashing them with squeals of excited laughter against boulders or throwing them off the high knoll edge into the rapids below" (1972). It is clear that this behavior is not just an individual affair; the practice has social approval, cultural acceptance. "Killing puppies was a child's job." One youngster, "her eyes gleaming with pleasure, beat two small puppies with a stick until they cried piteously." Her mother paid no attention (Briggs 1972). Another child "squeezed a longspur (small bird) until its heart burst through its skin" (1972). Significantly, one particular Eskimo woman, the object of derision and virtual social ostracism because of her many atypical and unconforming behavior patterns, was the only person observed by the anthropologist who "rolled on the ground playfully with the puppies" (Briggs 1972).

Discussion

Answers to the dilemmas posed by the above examples and many more which could be cited are, unfortunately, difficult to find. Scholars must search, and probe ever more deeply, in an attempt to shed light on the complexities involved in human interactions with animals. Although there is no one solution, it is essential to realize that culture, as a vital force in people's lives, must be recognized as a powerful determinant of patterns in the treatment of animals, as in other dimensions of human experience. "It's that kind of world here" is an expression Crows frequently use in describing their lives and beliefs. They are speaking not only of the outer world of interactions, but of the inner world of attitudes as well. Where cultural perceptions determine that animals and people share many important qualities and can cooperate and communicate, it follows that the treatment of animals generally is based on respect. In human-animal interactions, the degree of awareness attributed to the beasts works in dynamic equilibrium: the more an animal is downgraded as an object whose worth is measured only by usefulness to mankind, the less it is possible for that animal to have meaningful input into a relationship with people. Whatever potential it has, like that of an abused child reared in a closet, can never be realized.

One feature in a society's ethos which I have found to play a particularly significant role in determine relationships to animals is the aesthetic element. In communicating with informants of different cultures about their perceptions and treatment of animals, I have found that if appreciation for the beauty and uniqueness of the animal is lacking, treatment is less humane. Possession of beauty in its deepest dimension implies individual worth beyond what is central to human concerns. Like all of us who have thought long and hard about such questions, James Agee, in the book referred to earlier, wonders about the human "sense of beauty," asking "is this an 'instinct' or a product of 'training'" (1978). Portraying the poverty-stricken sharecroppers of his study with compassion, and finding them beautiful to him, he nonetheless admits that the people themselves are totally without a sense of beauty. Questioning whether this lack is due to the necessity of overwork leading to the exclusion of all that is not pragmatic, their poverty, their living only among "man-built things," or their low social status, Agee is unable to give a satisfactory answer. He goes on, however, to provide a remarkable observation about animals: "It is very possible, I would believe probable, that many animals are sensitive to beauty in terms of exhilaration or fear or courting or lust; many are, for that matter, accomplished and obvious narcists [*sic*]: in this sense I would also guess that the animals are better equipped than the human beings" (1978). More than through any other mechanism it appears that by means of culturally-defined perceptions of animals as intrinsically beautiful and valuable, and as possessing significant shared capacities including awareness, that we come to grant to animals, as the Plains Indians did, "the same right as ourselves to live on this earth."

References

Agee, J. and Evans, W. 1978. (1st ed. 1939) *Let Us Now Praise Famous Men*. New York: Ballantine Books. pp. 193, 194, 285, 286.

Allen, P.G. 1975. The Sacred Hoop: A Contemporary Indian Perspective on American Indian Literature. In: Chapman, A. ed. *Literature of the American Indians: Views and Interpretations*. New York: New American Library. pp.111-35.

Boller, H.A. 1972 (1st ed. 1867) *Among the Indians: Four Years in the Upper Missouri, 1858-1862*. Lincoln, Nebraska: University of Nebraska Press. pp. 204-5.

Briggs, J.L. 1972. (1st ed. 1970) *Never in Anger*. Cambridge, Massachusetts: Harvard University Press. p. 174.

Burland, C. 1970. (1st ed. 1965) *North American Indian Mythology*. New York: Hamlyn House. p. 69.

Emerson, E.R. 1965. (1st ed. 1884) *Indian Myths*. Minneapolis, Minnesota: Ross and Haines, Inc. p. 127.

Fuchs, E. and Havighurst, R.J. 1972. *To Live on This Earth*. Garden City, N.Y.: Doubleday and Co.

Linderman, F.B. 1970. (1st ed. 1930) *Plenty-Coups: Chief of the Crows*. New York: John Day Co.

Marriott, A. and Rachlin, C.K. 1975. *Plains Indian Mythology*. New York: Thomas Y. Crowell Co. p. 24.

Vestal, S. 1932. *Sitting Bull: Champion of the Sioux*. Boston: Houghton Mifflin Co. p. 21-22.

IS MAN'S INFLICTION OF SUFFERING ON ANIMALS IMMORAL?

Robert Welborn

P.O. Box 208
Franktown, Colorado 80116

Must not the first step in the consideration of this question be definition: what is moral? *Webster's Dictionary* says it is that which is "conforming to generally accepted ideas of what is right and just in human conduct" but let us propose another definition: that conduct which is compassionate, rational, and vital in relation to the preservation and enhancement of life itself.

If it is believed that man is properly in dominion over the earth and that he may do with it and all things on it as he will, then the first definition is sufficient. If generally accepted ideas in man's community are to the effect that man's infliction of suffering on animals is right, then such is not immoral.

If it is believed, however, that life, all life, as it has evolved in its beauty and complexity is the consideration upon which conduct should be judged, then the second definition must apply. Man being the dominant species that consciously and by plan produces suffering or harmony, beauty or ugliness, can do or fail to do what is right in relation to all life. Of course the first definition does not rule out ideas for human conduct that are determined in relation to life but it does not require such ideas.

If a person should put a dog in a cage and then abandon it to die slowly for want of food and water, it would be said that such conduct is immoral under both the first and second definitions. If, however, a person in a white coat for experimental purposes injects lye into the esophagus of a dog and the dog experiences pain and loneliness for days or weeks before death, it would be said by many that this is moral under the first definition because it is generally accepted that animals should be used in laboratories for the benefit of mankind. (This usage of dogs and many other horrendously cruel usages of animals are reported in authentic detail by Dallas Pratt M.D. in his books: *Alternatives to Pain in Experiments on Animals* and *Painful Experiments on Animals*. Anyone wanting to know what life is really like on this globe under man's dominion should read these books.) But this type of laboratory use is immoral without question under the second definition. It is the infliction of prolonged unnatural suffering on a sentient creature, an abuse of life.

The world and life on it, including man's life, will be secure from extinction and life will be profoundly satisfying only when the first and second definitions mean the same thing, when man fulfills his dominant and self-conscious part in the life process with compassion, reason, and vitality. Those who are concerned with animal welfare must strive toward the merging of the definitions so that the second is really a part of the first, must be imbued not just with the horror of man's cruelty to other living things but with the reverence for all life, its evolution and its beauty.

One approach to this merging of the definitions is to teach, and hopefully bring people to the realization, that humanity's welfare is intertwined with the welfare of all life on this earth. This certainly is an approach that should be followed but it suggests an acceptance of the first definition alone with man's welfare still being the sole consideration and with man, although broadening his purview, still determining what life serves his purpose and what does not. This selective evaluation would seemingly permit whatever action man conceived to be in his own self-interest with other life being subservient to it. The goal is the unity of human self-interest and the interest of all life. When this goal is achieved, and thus people revere all life as they revere their own part, there will be a merging of the definitions. (See Mary Midgley—*Animals and Why They Matter*, 1984, University of Georgia Press, for further fine discussion.)

The other approach to the merging is to seek moral propriety outside of man. It seems fundamental that if there is no value determinant outside of man, if there is no God, then morals are a matter of the dominant expediency. (Thomas Jefferson invoked the Laws of Nature and Nature's God to establish the values, life, liberty and the pursuit of happiness, as against the temporal expediency that was dominant.) We can urge that it is expedient for people to realize that their welfare and the welfare of all life are interdependent. But expediency is a vagrant thing. It varies according to the situation; it is not the same from one society to the other, from one generation to the next. It simply teaches that that which seems to work in a particular society will be the determinant of the morals of that society. Assault and battery will be punished because it is inimical to the peace and comfort of the society. The torment of animals in laboratories, in entertainment spectacles, and in food production procedures will not be punished because it is felt that these uses of animals contribute to the pleasure and comfort of the society, such being a proper test of propriety and morals. There are no universal, permanent values, only values for a particular time and place.

It is, therefore, only with a consideration outside of man that universal values are found, the second definition made universally applicable and the merger of the two definitions made secure. This consideration is God and God is manifest in the life that has evolved on this earth. God is not supernatural or mystical but the essence of the natural, the truth of the universe and the truth of the meadowlark and the blade of grass. This is not the god of any particular religion or cult. No confined doctrine or teaching of any sect can lay claim to God—only life itself and man as a part of that life.

The truth that is God is all encompassing. There is no separation of fact and value; there is no distinction between science and compassion and no isolation of science from the moral sphere. Each element of reality, each element of life, the seen and the unseen, the known and the felt, the proved and the believed, is involved in and is a part of those values which are consummate in beauty. This is the purpose, the harmony and the balance, and includes the minutest part of life and each particle that makes up the sunset and the sea.

Man's anthropocentrism is nowhere more evident than in the gods he chooses and thus those gods are basically called upon to have as their primary concern the salvation of man. Man mostly conceives that he alone of the species has a soul worthy of consideration by a divine being. There is no realization that man's function is fulfilled and happiness achieved by serving God and that this can only be done by serving life and beauty which are the manifestation of God. This service calls for the second definition.

People shy away when one talks about God as the universal being not defined by a particular doctrine. They cannot stand the broad responsibility and seeming uncertainty of service to God through the preservation and enhancement of life, through the inspired and rational creative process of love for that life. They want their book to tell them what to do. They seek refuge from the discomfort either in the dogma of some organized religion which teaches the propriety of man's dominion or in the dominion itself which they assume justifies all, without God.

Acceptance of the second definition is the real hope for the cause of animal welfare, for the reduction and elimination of the suffering which man inflicts on other living things. Although there may seem to be more people aware of this suffering, the massive obstacle of indifference enlarges and the number of animals used and abused each year increases. Without a new and true morality people will continue with their approval of the torture of rabbits, monkeys and calves for the benefit of cosmetics, science, good food and entertainment.*

The truth that people fail to grasp is that only by respecting and serving all life for its own sake will they achieve for themselves meaningful and satisfying lives. The callous and irrational preoccupation with the use of all other things on this earth, animate and inanimate, for present and often perverted physical comfort and gratification portends certain deterioration. Man fails even to protect his own progeny by conservation and the reasonable use of natural resources, and fails to realize the happiness that would come from a compassionate and rational relationship with other forms of life.

Several years ago Mortimer Adler of the Great Books program discussed the arguments of the humanists as against those he called animalists. The humanists, he said, take the position that animals do not have inherent dignity or inherent rights but that people might do moral damage to themselves by being cruel to animals, (The *Great Ideas Today—1975,* Encyclopaedia Britannica, Inc.). There is no felt or understood awareness of the sanctity of all life, of the capacity of the dog or bird for pain or love or joy. Man, the tormentor and destroyer, is the only important thing. These humanists never saw or found the dignity of the cow with her calf, the hen with her chicks, the mother gorilla with her baby. Under their theory the covert torment of animals in laboratories would be acceptable because no one but the attendants and experimenters sees the animals, society is not exposed to the atrocities and thus the human race does not suffer moral damage. The attendants and experimenters are indifferent to the suffering of the animals and therefore the cruelty has no affect on them.

A contrast to this failure to understand and be inspired by the significance of all life is the thought and feeling of Loren Eiseley who had the completeness of perception to believe and know that all life is sacred, from the vagrant seed drifting in the air to the violet and the tree frog. He spoke from the expertise of his profession, anthropology, and with the sensitivity of an Emily Dickinson. From personal experience he told of the capacity of the hawk and the fox for pain and love and joy. For him there was companionship and familial oneness with this hawk and this fox and with the bittern in whose life there was a fundamental element like an element in his own. (See Loren Eiseley's

*This is a reference to the United States government-sanctioned Draize test in which the substance to be tested is placed in the eye of a live conscious rabbit to see how long it takes to cause irreparable damage to the eye; to the misery of primates restrained in vice-like chairs for endless days of psychological or surgical experiments; to the confinement of veal calves in boxes; and to the brutal torment of calves and steers in roping contests at rodeos or practice arenas.

The Star Thrower, a collection of essays and *Another Kind of Autumn,* a collection of poems.)

The insensitive rationalization that only man has dignity or rights underlies the first definition and that definition is predominant. How then do we effectively invoke morality in our presentations to those people who could do something for animal welfare—by legislation, by teaching, or by direct action? We unequivocally assert the second definition. We sustain it affirmatively by the perception of people of science such as Loren Eiseley. We sustain it negatively by the teaching of authorities such as Jonathan Schell and Paul and Anne Ehrlich. (Jonathan Schell's *Reflections on The Fate of the Earth* received wide recognition when they first appeared in *The New Yorker* in 1982. The Ehrlichs' book entitled *Extinction* deals with just that.) This is the perception and this is the teaching that man may well be in the process of ending life on this earth, either abruptly or gradually.

Some may question the relevance of this reference to the extinction of life in a paper dealing with the subject of animal welfare. It may be said that man can determine what life forms continue and what do not and that whether or not living things suffer at the hands of man is irrelevant to the question of survival. But this is precisely the danger—man's assumption that he can be the determinant of life. Man has failed completely in this regard and this establishes that only a respect for all life will unify humanity and carry it through the destructive forces it has created. This respect is the basis for the second definition, a moral standard existing outside of man. One cannot respect life and permit its torment. This is fundamental. The infliction of suffering is by definition immoral.

Let us not hesitate to urge this morality on all persons to whom supplication is made for animal welfare. There will be deaf ears and bored expressions but this is our only hope for man's proper relationship with animals and for the balance and development of life itself. Unless the humane treatment of animals is made a part of the most basic and affirmative moral considerations, it will continue to be treated by the lawmakers and the teachers and by society in general as a minor matter in relation to what man conceives to be his major concerns and desires.

Through the process of evolution and refinement man has come to have the capacity for compassion and reason, the two attributes that must be constantly combined, and to have the power of domination. This capacity and this power make possible the responsible custodianship of the earth and all life on it. If the capacity is unused, the power becomes the devolutionary force it is today and all life suffers.

What are the responsibilities of this custodianship? They are to conserve and nurture the earth's natural resources, the minerals, the vegetation, the soils, the contours, the air and the water so that they are an ever-present source of life and beauty; and they are to protect and care for those animals that are under or affected by man's dominion so that they will have lives no less vital than in natural conditions with suffering minimized as much as humanly possible.

Suffering is a fact of life. Man cannot eliminate it for himself or for other creatures. But the suffering imposed by man on other living things is different in kind from the suffering of animals in nature. With man animals are in an alien world; with nature they are in their own environment. Man need not and should not interfere with the natural environment, even in an attempt to alleviate natural suffering. His function is to deal with the suffering he creates. This he can control and prevent.

The moral charge to man is to have the same fervor and diligence for the preclusion of animal suffering that he has for the preclusion of his own. The implementation of this charge must be accomplished by laws and standards as detailed as those man has conceived for his own governance, realizing that different laws and standards would be appropriate in many respects for different species or different conditions of particular animals. For example, these laws or standards would require that laboratory animals live in comfortable, non-stressful conditions and be protected from pain by anesthetics, analgesics or other appropriate care, with the elimination of the use of animals in laboratories as the ultimate requirement; they would deal with the care and humane raising, handling, transportation, and slaughter of animals used for food; and they would preclude the use of animals for or in connection with entertainment if such use would cause stress or pain.

Surely all of this responsibility involves something very affirmative, not the passive approach of those who feel only that cruelty to animals might be bad for human morals nor the approach that relies on sensitizing people and making them feel uncomfortable about cruelty, however commendable such an approach might be. This affirmative responsibility involves man leading himself into the inspired, rational, and vital state of being in which there is respect, and indeed reverence, for all life with man's life being relevant as a part of the whole. Only this completely positive way will preclude extinction and bring balance, harmony, and constructive relationships among all living things. This then is the morality, some may call it religion, for animal welfare because it is the morality for all life, including man's.

Perhaps those professors of human and divine morality who speak from temple and mosque, from synagogue and church could be persuaded that all life is involved in the constitution of morality and in morality's purview and protection. Perhaps those people who are moved to tears by Bach's great Saint Matthew Passion as it profoundly sings of the suffering of a great human being can be moved to tears by the suffering of the dog and the calf as they are tormented by human cruelty. Because this is the hope: the uniting and the unity of those passions which make up the religious, the music and the humanitarian experience in compassion for life itself.

Instructions to Authors

All manuscripts submitted and solicited are subject to prior review and approval by members of the Manuscript Review Committee. Authors may submit manuscripts to: Dr. Michael Fox, The Humane Society of the United States, 2100 L St., N.W., Washington, D.C. 20037. Manuscripts not adhering to the style outlined below will be returned to the author.

Manuscripts: Footnotes, references, tables, and figure legends are to be typewritten, double-spaced on 8½ × 11 inch bond paper leaving generous margins. Manuscripts must be in English using the preferred spelling in the *Webster's Third International Dictionary.* Submit original and two (2) copies.

Manuscript organization: Title page (p. 1) containing title of the manuscript, author(s) and author(s) affiliation, present address wherever proofs should be sent; Text (beginning p. 2), with introduction, methods, procedures, results, discussion, conclusion, acknowledgements, references, tables, and figure legends. Special instructions to the copy editor or printer should be affixed to the original copy.

Abbreviations and units: Standard dictionary abbreviations are generally accepted. Other abbreviations should be explained when first mentioned in the text. SI units are preferred.

References: The Author-Date system, not a numbering system, is to be used for the citation of references in the text, e.g., Jones (1977) or (Jones and Smith 1977) or (Jones et al. 1977) for more than two authors of one citation. When citing the authors of such papers in the reference list, *all* authors must be listed for citations using et al. in the text. Where more than one paper by the same author(s) has appeared in one year, the reference should be distinguished by "a," "b," "c," etc. (e.g., 1971a). The list of references should be arranged alphabetically by authors' last names, and chronologically per author.

Titles: Journals should be abbreviated in accordance with the *Chemical Abstract Service Source Index.* References to books/monographs should include editors, edition/volume number, city, state, publisher and relevant page numbers. A paper in press may be referenced if it has been accepted for publication. References to personal communications and unpublished works are permitted in the text only. *Proceedings* and talks given at meetings are to be treated as published material.

Sample references: (in accordance with the University of Chicago, *A Manual of Style.)*

Journal article:

Smith, J. 1970. The effect of heat stress on hogs. *J. Anim. Sci.* 5(1): 127-8.

Book:

Smith, J. and Jones, A. 1970. *Animals and Environment.* New York: Academic Press.

Chapter or paper in book:

Smith, J. 1970. The effects of farrowing system on piglet health. In: Jones, A. ed. *Animal Husbandry.* New York: Academic Press.

Tables: These should be concise and double-spaced throughout.

Figures: Submit three sets of glossy prints (no negatives) with identifying arrows and letters contrasting sharply with the background. Indicate on the back the author's name, figure number, and "top." *Do not* write this material on the back of the print with felt-tip or ball-point pen; a separate typewritten sheet attached to the back is preferable. Prints will not be returned to the author(s).

Figure legends: Captions should contain sufficient information allowing the figures to be clearly understood without reference to the text.